Lung Imaging and CADx

Lung Imaging and CADx

Edited by

Ayman El-Baz and Jasjit S. Suri

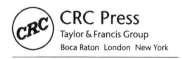

CRC Press is an imprint of the
Taylor & Francis Group, an **informa** business

CRC Press
Taylor & Francis Group
6000 Broken Sound Parkway NW, Suite 300
Boca Raton, FL 33487-2742

First issued in paperback 2023

© 2019 by Taylor & Francis Group, LLC
CRC Press is an imprint of Taylor & Francis Group, an Informa business

No claim to original U.S. Government works

ISBN-13: 978-1-138-05091-4 (hbk)
ISBN-13: 978-1-03-265256-6 (pbk)
ISBN-13: 978-0-429-05595-9 (ebk)

DOI: 10.1201/9780429055959

Library of Congress Cataloging-in-Publication Data

Names: El-Baz, Ayman S., editor. | Suri, Jasjit S., editor.
Title: Lung imaging and CADx / [edited by] Ayman El-Baz and Jasjit Suri.
Description: Boca Raton : Taylor & Francis, 2018.
Identifiers: LCCN 2018054774 | ISBN 9781138050914 (hardback : alk. paper)
Subjects: | MESH: Lung Neoplasms—diagnostic imaging | Image Interpretation, Computer-Assisted
Classification: LCC RC280.L8 | NLM WF 658 | DDC 616.99/424075—dc23
LC record available at https://lccn.loc.gov/2018054774

Visit the Taylor & Francis Web site at
http://www.taylorandfrancis.com

and the CRC Press Web site at
http://www.crcpress.com

With love and affection to my mother and father,
whose loving spirit sustains me still

Ayman El-Baz

To my late loving parents, my wife, and loving children

Jasjit S. Suri

Table of Contents

Acknowledgments

The completion of this book could not have been possible without the participation and assistance of so many people whose names may not all be enumerated. Their contributions are sincerely appreciated and gratefully acknowledged. However, the editors would like to express their deep appreciation and indebtedness particularly to Dr. Ali H. Mahmoud and Ahmed Shaffie for their endless support.

Ayman El-Baz

Jasjit S. Suri

Preface

This book covers the state-of-the-art approaches for automated noninvasive systems for early lung cancer diagnostics. Lung cancer is the second most common cancer after prostate cancer in men and after breast cancer in women. Moreover, it is considered the leading cause of cancer death among both genders in the United States and worldwide as the number of people who die each year of lung cancer is more than the people who die of breast and prostate cancers combined. According to the American Cancer Society, in 2017, 1,688,780 new lung cancer cases were diagnosed, and 600,920 lung cancer deaths are estimated to occur in the United States. This means that lung cancer claims more lives each year than all other forms of cancer.

Fortunately, early detection of lung cancer increases the chances of patients' survival. Current noninvasive lung imaging includes positron emission tomography (PET), computed tomography (CT), and magnetic resonance imaging (MRI). Today's computer-aided diagnostic (CAD) systems can analyze images from these different modalities for detecting lung cancer and determining its aggressiveness. Generally, the CAD systems analyze the images in three steps: (1) segmentation, (2) description or feature extraction, and (3) classification of the status. These steps are discussed in the book.

In summary, the book aims at advancing scientific research within the broad field of early detection of lung cancer. It focuses on major trends and challenges in this area, identifies new techniques, and presents their use in biomedical image analysis.

Ayman El-Baz

Jasjit S. Suri

Contributors

Mohammad Reza Ahmadzadeh
Department of Electrical and
    Computer Engineering
Isfahan University of Technology
Isfahan, Iran

Samr Ali
Department of Electrical and
    Computer Engineering
Abu Dhabi University
Abu Dhabi, United Arab Emirates

Mohanad AlKhodari
Department of Electrical and
    Computer Engineering
Abu Dhabi University
Abu Dhabi, United Arab Emirates

Estanislao Arana
Department of Radiology
Valencia Oncology Institute Foundation
Valencia, Spain

Ulas Bagci
Center for Research in Computer
    Vision (CRCV)
University of Central Florida
Orlando, Florida, USA

Deniz A. Bölükbas
Lung Bioengineering and Regeneration
Department of Experimental
    Medical Sciences
and
Wallenberg Center for Molecular
    Medicine and Stem Cell Centre
Lund University
Lund, Sweden

G. Buonanno
Department of Civil and
    Mechanical Engineering
University of Cassino and
    Southern Lazio
Cassino, Italy
and
Queensland University of Technology
Brisbane, Australia

Meghan Cahill
Department of Radiology
New York-Presbyterian Hospital/Weill
    Cornell Medical College
New York, New York, USA

Kimberly Del Mauro
Department of Radiology
New York-Presbyterian Hospital/Weill
    Cornell Medical College
New York, New York, USA

Neal Dunlap
Department of Radiation Oncology
University of Louisville
Louisville, Kentucky, USA

Ayman El-Baz
BioImaging Laboratory
Department of Bioengineering
University of Louisville
Louisville, Kentucky, USA

Amany F. Elbehairy
Department of Chest Diseases
Faculty of Medicine
Alexandria University
Alexandria, Egypt
and
National Heart and Lung Institute
Imperial College
London, United Kingdom

Adel Elmaghraby
Department of Computer Engineering
  and Computer Science
University of Louisville
Louisville, Kentucky, USA

Mohammed Ghazal
Department of Electrical and
  Computer Engineering
Abu Dhabi University
Abu Dhabi, United Arab Emirates
and
BioImaging Laboratory
Department of Bioengineering
University of Louisville
Louisville, Kentucky, USA

Georgy Gimel'farb
Department of Computer Engineering
  and Computer Science
University of Auckland
Auckland, New Zealand

Guruprasad Giridharan
BioImaging Laboratory
Department of Bioengineering
University of Louisville
Louisville, Kentucky, USA

Victor Gonzalez-Perez
Department of Medical Physics
Valencia Oncology Institute Foundation
Valencia, Spain

Hassan Hajjdiab
Department of Electrical and
  Computer Engineering
Abu Dhabi University
Abu Dhabi, United Arab Emirates

Sarfaraz Hussein
Center for Advanced Machine Learning
  (CAML) at Symantec Corporation
Atlanta, Georgia, USA

Rosminah M. Kassim
Department of Diagnostic Imaging
Kuala Lumpur Hospital
Kuala Lumpur, Malaysia

Robert Keynton
Department of Bioengineering
University of Louisville
Louisville, Kentucky, USA

Fahmi Khalifa
BioImaging Laboratory
Department of Bioengineering
University of Louisville
Louisville, Kentucky, USA

Ali Mahmoud
BioImaging Laboratory
Department of Bioengineering
University of Louisville
Louisville, Kentucky, USA

Hadi Moghadas-Dastjerdi
Department of Electrical and
    Computer Engineering
Isfahan University of Technology
Isfahan, Iran

David Moratal
Center for Biomaterials and
    Tissue Engineering
Universitat Politècnica de València
Valencia, Spain

Chuen R. Ng
UTM Razak School of Engineering and
    Advanced Technology
Universiti Teknologi Malaysia
Kuala Lumpur, Malaysia

Mizuho Nishio
Department of Diagnostic Imaging
    and Nuclear Medicine
Kyoto University Graduate School
    of Medicine
Kyoto, Kyoto, Japan
and
Preemptive Medicine and Lifestyle-
    related Disease Research Center
Kyoto University Hospital
Kyoto, Kyoto, Japan

Norliza M. Noor
Department of Engineering
UTM Razak School of Engineering
    and Advanced Technology
Universiti Teknologi Malaysia
Kuala Lumpur, Malaysia

Ikenna Okereke
Division of Cardiothoracic Surgery
University of Texas Medical Branch
Galveston, Texas, USA

Brooke Crawford O'Neill
Department of Radiology
New York-Presbyterian Hospital/Weill
    Cornell Medical College
New York, New York, USA

Sumathi Poobal
Department of Electronics and
    Communication Engineering
KCG College of Technology
Karapakkam, Chennai
Tamil Nadu, India

Michele Porcu
Azienda Ospedaliero Universitaria di
    Cagliari
Polo di Monserrato
Università di Cagliari
Cagliari, Italy

Bradley B. Pua
Department of Radiology
New York-Presbyterian Hospital/Weill
    Cornell Medical College
New York, New York, USA

K. Punithavathy
Department of Electronics and
    Communication Engineering
Hindustan Institute of Technology
    & Science
Padur, Chennai, Tamil Nadu, India

M. M. Ramya
Centre for Automation & Robotics
Hindustan Institute of Technology
    & Science
Padur, Chennai, Tamil Nadu, India

Omar M. Rijal
Institute of Mathematical Sciences
Faculty of Science
University of Malaya
Kuala Lumpur, Malaysia

Luca Saba
Azienda Ospedaliero Universitaria
    di Cagliari
Polo di Monserrato
Università di Cagliari
Cagliari, Italy

Ahmed Sadaka
Faculty of Medicine
Alexandria University
Alexandria, Egypt
and
Royal Brompton Hospital and Harefield
    NHS Foundation Trust
London, United Kingdom

Ahmed Shaffie
BioImaging Laboratory
Department of Bioengineering
    and Department of Computer
    Engineering and Computer Science
University of Louisville
Louisville, Kentucky, USA

Abbas Samani
Department of Electrical and
    Computer Engineering
Western University
London, Ontario, Canada
and
Department of Medical Biophysics
Western University
London, Ontario, Canada
and
Imaging Research Laboratories
Robarts Research Institute
Western University
London, Ontario, Canada

Ahmed Soliman
BioImaging Laboratory
Department of Bioengineering
University of Louisville
Louisville, Kentucky, USA

L. Stabile
Department of Civil and
    Mechanical Engineering
University of Cassino
    and Southern Lazio
Cassino, Italy

Harman S. Suri
Brown University
Providence, Rhode
Island, USA

Jasjit S. Suri
Global Biomedical Technologies Inc.
Roseville, California, USA
and
AtheroPoint LLC
Roseville, California, USA
and
Department of Electrical Engineering
Idaho State University
Pocatello, Idaho, USA

Joel C. M. Than
UTM Razak School of Engineering
    and Advanced Technology
Universiti Teknologi Malaysia
Kuala Lumpur, Malaysia

Darcy E. Wagner
Lung Bioengineering and Regeneration
Department of Experimental
    Medical Sciences
and
Wallenberg Center for Molecular
    Medicine and Stem Cell Centre
Lund University
Lund, Sweden

Brian Wang
Department of Radiation Oncology
University of Louisville
Louisville, Kentucky, USA

Alison Wenholz
Division of Cardiothoracic Surgery
University of Texas Medical Branch
Galveston, Texas, USA

Courtney Yeager
Department of Radiology
New York-Presbyterian Hospital/Weill
    Cornell Medical College
New York, New York, USA

Ashari Yunus
Institute of Respiratory Medicine
Kuala Lumpur, Malaysia

Editors

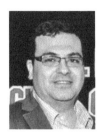 **Ayman El-Baz** is a professor, university scholar, and chair of the Bioengineering Department at the University of Louisville, Louisville, Kentucky. He earned his bachelor's and master's degrees in electrical engineering in 1997 and 2001, respectively. He earned his doctoral degree in electrical engineering from the University of Louisville in 2006. In 2009, he was named a Coulter Fellow for his contributions to the field of biomedical translational research. He has 17 years of hands-on experience in the fields of bio-imaging modeling and noninvasive computer-assisted diagnosis systems. He has authored or coauthored more than 500 technical articles (132 journals, 23 books, 57 book chapters, 211 refereed-conference papers, 137 abstracts, and 27 U.S. patents and disclosures).

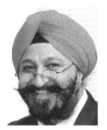 **Jasjit S. Suri** is an innovator, scientist, a visionary, an industrialist, and an internationally known world leader in biomedical engineering. He has spent over 25 years in the field of biomedical engineering/devices and its management. He received his doctorate from the University of Washington, Seattle, and his business management sciences degree from Weatherhead School of Management, Case Western Reserve University, Cleveland, Ohio. He was awarded the President's Gold Medal in 1980 and named a Fellow of the American Institute of Medical and Biological Engineering for his outstanding contributions in 2004. In 2018, he was awarded the Marquis Life Time Achievement Award for his outstanding contributions and dedication to medical imaging and its management.

1

Computer-Aided Diagnosis of Chronic Obstructive Pulmonary Disease Using Accurate Lung Air Volume Estimation in Computed Tomographic Imaging

Hadi Moghadas-Dastjerdi, Mohammad Reza Ahmadzadeh, and Abbas Samani

Contents

1.1 Introduction

According to World Health Organization reports, lung diseases are among the leading causes of death around the world. The death rate due to lung diseases is still on the rise, while other causes of death, such as cancer and stroke, are declining. Among all pulmonary disorders, chronic obstructive pulmonary disease (COPD) is one of the most prevalent and fatal diseases. About 7% of the global population is affected by this disease, leading to an economic burden estimated at $2.1 trillion in 2010 [1]. The main effect of COPD is the lung's air ventilation reduction, which may occur due to two different mechanisms. The first mechanism is the obstruction of small airways as a result of clogging by mucus or as a consequence of shape change. The second mechanism, emphysema, involves destruction of the alveoli's wall and a reduction of the elasticity of the alveoli sacs and consequently a reduction of the gas–blood exchange surface. In general, these two mechanisms lead to the limitation of airflow throughout respiration and immobility of old inhaled air in the lungs, referred to as air trapping. The trapped air has no beneficial function in the pulmonary system, as it includes a low amount of oxygen and a high amount of carbon dioxide.

Since COPD is associated with a reduction in the lung air volumes, the diagnosis, severity assessment, and treatment monitoring of COPD can be assessed through measurement of the lung air volume. There exist several lung volume measurement techniques, such as spirometry, body plethysmography, image processing, and so on. Among these techniques, image processing has the following important advantages:

1. Image processing techniques can be used for all patients, including those who are unable to undergo other clinical testing methods, such as children or elderly people who are unable to hold their breath during the test.
2. In comparison with other techniques, it is more convenient for patients, and the test time is shorter.
3. It is more accurate while being capable of providing local assessment in addition to global assessment, whereas other techniques are capable of providing only global assessment.

The image processing techniques used in lung air volume measurements are comprised mainly of registration or segmentation techniques. Image registration techniques are capable of measuring changes of lung air volumes, while segmentation techniques can measure the air absolute volumes as well as relative volume changes. Among available segmentation techniques (e.g., region growing, active contours, etc.), thresholding is more suitable for use in lung air volume measurement because of its ability to handle the complex geometry of the lung, efficiency with very large image data sets, high computation speed, and straightforward implementation. The main drawback of the thresholding method is its high dependence on the segmentation threshold values. As such, in recent years, researchers have invested substantial efforts in developing effective methods for finding optimal threshold values in lung air segmentation. In most studies, researchers utilized predetermined threshold values obtained empirically in this application. For example, threshold values of −1,000, −950, −650, and −350 HU were utilized as the air intensity, the upper and lower intensity threshold values of the lung's air, and the lung tissue intensity, respectively [2–5]. However, it has been demonstrated that such empirically determined values do not lead to accurate segmentation for the lung air segmentation application. This is due partly to the fact that the measured computed tomographic (CT) attenuation coefficient of the lung varies significantly with different scanners, reconstruction kernels, and CT protocol parameters, including tube voltage (kVp), tube current (mAs), and voxel size [6–8]. Moreover, lung lesions in COPD patients affect how the air flows and fills different regions of the lung, which consequently impacts how the image intensity of voxels varies throughout the lung CT images. In current clinical practice, airflow and distribution are usually assessed by pulmonary function tests (PFT), using, for example, spirometry or plethysmography. As stated earlier, this assessment may be made more effective by utilizing effective image processing techniques. In one of the early relevant studies, Hayhurst et al. [9] reported that emphysema could lead to an increase in the number of the voxels with intensities in the range of −1,000 to −900 HU. However, Müller et al. [6] used −910 HU as the upper threshold value for calculating the percentage of low-attenuation areas (LAA%). They showed that this parameter is highly associated with the degree of pathological grade of emphysema. During the following years, researchers used various threshold values to improve their results. Upper threshold values of −910, −950, −960, and −970 HU were used to calculate LAA% in end-inhalation lung CT images for quantifying the assessment of emphysema [2, 10–12], while upper threshold values of −850, −856, −900, and −910 HU were utilized to calculate LAA% in end-exhalation lung CT images for quantitative assessment of air trapping as a symptom of small airway disorders [13–16]. It should be emphasized that the threshold values are known to vary under different conditions (e.g., different equipment, settings, reconstruction techniques, etc.). As such, to assess the lung air volumes, their distributions throughout the lung volume and their variations over the respiration cycles without using predetermined threshold values is highly advantageous. To this end, a fully automatic framework will be introduced here that is capable of finding optimal segmentation threshold values from end-inhalation/end-exhalation CT images based on lung parenchyma biophysics, including tissue incompressibility in addition to the principle of air mass conservation. The method also offers an effective technique for partial volume effect compensation to improve the accuracy of lung air estimation. Furthermore, the technique was developed to be capable of assessing the air distribution within the lung over the respiration cycle. As such, the segmentation technique was exploited for COPD stage assessment. For this purpose, the segmentation technique was used to obtain lung air distribution. Using this distribution, several image-based features are extracted and used through a machine learning framework to automatically diagnose and determine COPD severity measured by its stage. Utilizing the proposed highly accurate air volume and distribution estimation technique, which is founded on adaptive computation of optimal thresholds, led to highly accurate results that paved the way for the successful development of an effective technique for COPD stage assessment.

1.2 Clinical Study Protocols

The gold standard for diagnosis of COPD consists of forced expiratory volume in 1 second (FEV_1) and forced vital capacity (FVC) measurements by spirometry. These measurements are exploited through a standard protocol called the Global Initiative for Chronic Obstructive Lung Disease (GOLD) staging system to assess COPD severity stages. Table 1.1 shows the criteria on the diagnosis and staging of COPD based on the FEV_1 and FVC measurements. Individuals are classified into normal or patient based on the value of FEV_1/FVC, while the severity of the disease measured by GOLD[1] stage for patients cohort is determined based on the value of FEV_1.

Lung lesions in COPD caused by tobacco or other irritants are permanent, and there is no reliable therapy available to cure this disease. Therefore, early detection

TABLE 1.1   COPD Diagnosis and Severity Determination Criteria Based on Spirometric Measurements and the GOLD Staging System

GOLD Stage	GOLD Severity	$\dfrac{FEV_1}{FVC}$	FEV_1
0	Normal	≥0.7	—
1	Mild	>0.7	≥80%
2	Moderate	>0.7	50%–79%
3	Severe	>0.7	30%–49%
4	Very severe	>0.7	>30%

that aims at controlling, slowing down progress, and minimizing the symptoms and side effects of COPD is of great importance [17]. It should be noted that the fast, progressive evolution of COPD may increase the probability of late diagnosis of the disease or even the failure of its diagnosis.

As stated earlier, utilizing PFT measurements involves some drawbacks. As such, in recent years, developing other methods based on various criteria other than PFT measurements (e.g., image processing and machine learning algorithms) for the diagnosis and determination of COPD severity stage has gained the attention of many researchers [18]. However, due to some issues, these methods have not been embraced by clinicians to be routinely used in clinical diagnosis; hence, the GOLD criterion is still known as the gold standard. To overcome these issues, we introduce a method based on image-based lung air volume measurements. The general framework of the method is depicted in Figure 1.1. The first step in this procedure is to acquire inspiratory/expiratory CT images from both normal individuals and COPD patients. The COPD patient cohort includes all possible severity stages (stages 1–4). In the next step, several features that are hypothesized to include significant information about the state of the disease are extracted from the CT images. Then correlation coefficients of the extracted features and spirometric measurements (FEV_1/FVC and FEV_1) are investigated to assess the relationship between PFT measurements and image features. In the next step, the discriminatory power of the features and their possible

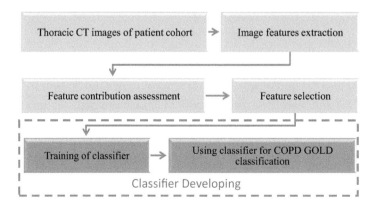

Figure 1.1   General framework of development of the classifier for automatic assessment of COPD severity based on the GOLD staging system.

TABLE 1.2   Combination and Distribution of the Subjects in the Data Set Based on Gender and Disease States

Individuals	Normal	GOLD 1	GOLD 2	GOLD 3	GOLD 4	All
Male	8	10	8	9	5	40
Female	5	7	7	5	5	29
All	13	17	15	14	10	69

combinations are analyzed to find the best combination of the feature that could lead to the best performance for training and classification procedures. The selected features are then exploited to train a classifier. After the training procedure, the classifier is ready for use as a computer-aided diagnostic (CAD) system to assess both the presence of disease and its severity stage. These steps will be described in details in the following sections.

1.2.1 Data Sets

The data set used in this part of the study consists of inspiratory/expiratory 3D CT images, PFT measurements, COPD diagnosis, and GOLD stage for 69 individuals who were distributed in five groups: normal and COPD GOLD stages 1–4. This data set was acquired from the COPDgene Study database. Table 1.2 shows the characteristics of the subjects, including their gender and disease state.

The inclusion criteria in this study were adult subjects, 45–80 years of age, with a diagnosis of COPD or at least a 10-pack-year smoking history. Each pack-year is equal to smoking one pack (or 20) of cigarettes per day for 1 year or, similarly, smoking two packs per day for 6 months. Moreover, subjects who were unable to undergo CT imaging (e.g., pregnant women and subjects who had a history of thoracic surgery or thorax radiotherapy) were excluded. Exclusion criteria also included subjects suffering from concurrent respiratory disorders in addition to COPD in their medical records. All the subjects were provided with a comprehensive explanation of the study and its objectives before their oral and written consents were obtained.

1.3 Lung Air Estimation

The lung air estimation from 3D CT images in end-inhalation and end-exhalation phases is the main core of image features extracting procedure. The general framework of the lung air estimation algorithm is demonstrated in Figure 1.2. In the first step, a pair of CT images in end-inhalation and end-exhalation phases are acquired from all the subjects. Next, these images are fed to two separate procedures: (1) computing optimal segmentation threshold values and (2) computing lung region mask.

In first procedure, the histograms of each pair of images are exploited to find the respective combined histogram. The optimal threshold values are calculated using an optimization framework [19, 20] where the cost function is developed based on the

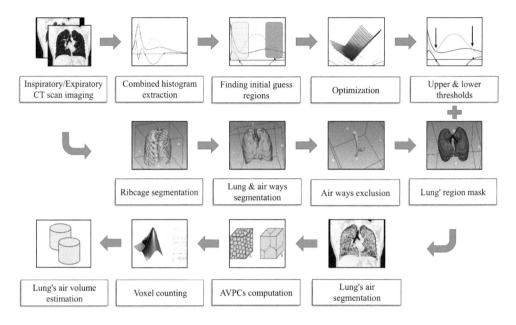

Figure 1.2 Block diagram of the lung air estimation algorithm.

imaging principles and on lung tissue incompressibility and air volume conservation principles. In this framework, the intersection of the first and second peaks and the intersection of the second and third peaks in the combined histogram are considered as the initial guesses for the optimal lower and upper segmentation threshold values, respectively. As such, two large enough neighboring regions around the initial guesses can be considered as the solution domain used to solve the optimization problem. The cost function of optimization problem, that is, $J\left(I_x,I_y\right)$, which is constructed based on tissue incompressibility and air mass conservation principles, is given below:

$$J\left(I_x,I_y\right)=\left|\sum_{I_{min}}^{I_x}\left|Hd[I]\right|-\sum_{I_x+1}^{I_y}\left|Hd[I]\right|\right|+\omega\sum_{I_y+1}^{I_{max}}\left|Hd[I]\right| \tag{1}$$

where $Hd[I]$ and ω are the difference of paired-image histograms and a weight coefficient, respectively. Moreover, I_{min}, I_{max}, I_x, and I_y are the minimum and maximum intensity values in CT images and lower and upper intensity segmentation thresholds, respectively. The optimal threshold values can be obtained by solving this optimization problem with respect to I_x and I_y considering the solution domain surrounding the computed initial guess value as follows:

$$\left\{I_\alpha,I_\beta\right\}=\arg\min_{I_x,I_y} J\left(I_x,I_y\right) \tag{2}$$

where I_α and I_β are the optimal lower and upper thresholds, respectively.

The main purpose of the second procedure is to find a mask corresponding to the lung region of paired CT images in which lower and upper threshold values should be exploited to segment the voxels corresponding to the lung's air. To this end, the first step is to find the lung surface by segmenting the rib cage, where the bones possess a clearly distinct intensity in thoracic CT images. Consequently, the lung, including airways, can be segmented by finding voxels that contain intensity values in the range of intensity of air within the rib cage region. The lung region then can be obtained by excluding the main airways from the segmented region in the previous step. To segment the main airways before their subtraction, a region-growing algorithm was utilized that starts from the uppermost slice along the SA axis. The highest slice along the SA axis intersects with the trachea, and consequently a round region with an intensity in the range of air intensity is found in the center of this slice. As such, the whole main airway segment can be obtained by starting the confidence connected region-growing algorithm from this disk. Finally, the lung region mask is achieved by excluding the main airway regions from the whole lung volume segmented earlier.

After finding the lung region mask and optimal segmentation threshold values, the lung air voxels can be segmented by finding all the voxels within the lung region that possess intensity values between the optimal lower and upper threshold values of I_α and I_β. Thus, the air voulme of lung will be computed as

$$AV = V_{vox} \sum_{i=I_\alpha}^{I_\beta} N_{vox}\left[i\right] \tag{3}$$

where V_{vox}, $N_{vox}\left[i\right]$, and AV are the volume of each voxel, the number of the voxels with intensity value of i, and lung air volume, respectively.

The limitation of X-ray dose received by a patient leads to a limitation of CT image resolution. As such, the sizes of voxels (typically about 1 mm³) are generally considerably larger than those of alvoli sacs, where their diameters vary from 150 to 500 µm over respiration periods and different individuals. As such, all voxels corresponding to the segmented lung air region contain a large amount of air and a small amount of alveloi tissue, leading to what is known as the partial volume effect. The air-to-tissue ratio in each voxel is not constant, and it varies over respiration time as illustrated in Figure 1.3. The alveoli expand through different mechanisms as illustrated in Figure 1.4. All of the mechanisms lead to a reduction in the amount of tissue within the voxels. However, isotropic expansion and shape change are the most prevalent mechanisms in a healthy lung. Therefore, to increase the accuracy of lung air volume estimation, it is necessary to compensate for the patial volume effect. Fortunately, the relationship between the attenuation coefficient and density is linear for the lung. Therefore, the air portion of each voxel can be determined based on its intensity.

We introduce a coefficient called the air volume portion coefficient, which is determined for each voxel, $AVPC_{vox}$. This coefficient is computed as follows:

$$AVPC_{vox} = \frac{I_{vox} - I_{air}}{I_{tis} - I_{air}} \tag{4}$$

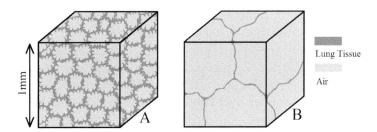

Figure 1.3　The variation of air-to-tissue ratio in a lung air voxel over respiration in end-exhalation phase (A) and end-inhalation phase (B). The amount of tissue is reduced in (B) due to expansion of the alveoli.

(Adapted from [19])

where

$$I_{air} = \frac{\sum_{I=I_{min}}^{I_\alpha-1} H[I]\,I}{\sum_{I=I_{min}}^{I_\alpha-1} H[I]}, \quad I_{tis} = \frac{\sum_{I=I_\beta+1}^{I_{max}} H[I]\,I}{\sum_{I=I_\beta+1}^{I_{max}} H[I]}. \quad (5)$$

In these equations, I_{vox} is the intensity of a given voxel, and H is the histogram of the CT image. Using this coefficient, which accounts for the partial volume effect, the following equation can be used to obtain a highly accurate estimate of the lung air volume:

$$AV = V_{vox} \sum_{i=I_\alpha}^{I_\beta} N_{vox}[i]\, AVPC_{vox}[i] \quad (6)$$

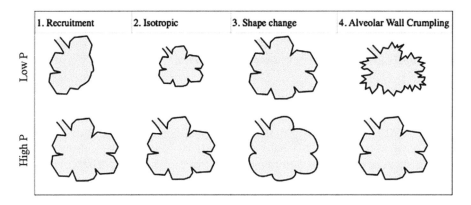

Figure 1.4　The four mechanisms by which alveoli expand: (1) recruitment, (2) isotropic expansion, (3) shape change, and (4) alveolar wall crumpling. All of these mechanisms reduce the amount of tissue within the lung's air voxels in the inhalation phase. Upper and lower rows correspond to low (exhalation) and high (inhalation) pressure statuses, respectively.

(Adapted from [21])

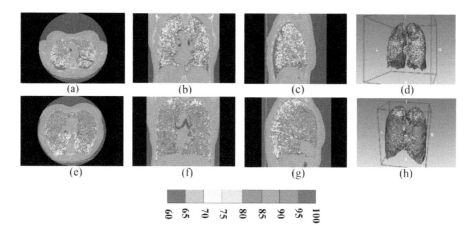

Figure 1.5 Air distribution within the lung in end-exhalation (upper row) and end-inhalation (lower row) phases. The color map is constructed based on the $AVPC_{vox}$ coefficients, and it demonstrates the variations of air concentration within the lung over respiration. (a, e), (b, f), and (c, g) illustrate end-exhalation, end-inhalation pairs of air distribution in axial, coronal, and sagittal views, respectively. (d, h) show an end-exhalation, end-inhalation pair of 3D-reconstructed volumetric distribution.

Figure 1.5 demonstrates the results of lung air segmentation displayed in axial, coronal, sagittal, and 3D constructed views. In this figure, the $AVPC_{vox}$ coefficients are utilized to construct a color map that can describe the air distribution within the lung in CT images. The regions with low, medium, and high concentrations of air are shown with red, light green, and blue, respectively.

1.4 Feature Extraction

In this study, four groups of features are extracted from CT images. It is hypothesized that these features contain both local and overall information about air ventilation ability and function of the lung. Each group of these features will be described in the following sections.

1.4.1 Group 1: Lung Air Volume Changes

The simplest feature that can be extracted corresponds to the amount of air ventilated through the lung over inspiration and expiration. In COPD, the capacity of the lung increases in response to efforts to compensate for the conditions imposed by air trapping, elasticity reduction of alveoli wall tissue, and expiratory airflow reduction [22, 23]. However, this occurs while the ventilation capability of the lung declines. In order to establish a fair comparison between different lung functions based on their respective image information, the lung air volume variations should be normalized. This can be achieved by normalization with respect to inspiratory or expiratory lung volumes. As such, the lung air volume changes of ΔV_{Inh} and ΔV_{Exh} normalized with respect to end-inhalation and end-exhalation volumes can be computed as follows:

$$\Delta V_{Inh} = \frac{AV_{Inh} - AV_{Exh}}{AV_{Inh}} \tag{7}$$

$$\Delta V_{Exh} = \frac{AV_{Inh} - AV_{Exh}}{AV_{Exh}} \tag{8}$$

where AV_{Inh} and AV_{Exh} are the estimated lung volumes in the end-inhalation and end-exhalation phases, respectively. These volumes are equal to TLC and FRC in PFT measurements, which are made consistent with respect to the supine position. ΔV_{Inh} and ΔV_{Exh} are considered as criteria of overall lung capability for air ventilation over the respiration cycle. In respiratory disorders, the amount of ventilated air during respiration usually declines as a result of lung tissue elasticity reduction and small airway obstruction. As such, any reduction in these two features can be considered as an indication of disease.

1.4.2 Group 2: Lung Air Distribution in the Inspiration Phase

The second group of features are computed as the percentage of voxels in the end-inhalation CT image, which contains equal or more than 95%, 90%, ..., and 65% of air. These features are denoted by V_{95Inh}, V_{90Inh}, ..., and V_{65Inh}, respectively. The extension of areas with medium to high concentrations of air within the lung in the inspiration phase is highly associated with the occurrence of emphysema, according to reported research [10–12]. The first step to compute these features is to find the intensity corresponding to a certain amount of air within the lung voxels, which can be computed using the following:

$$I_{n\%} = I_{tis} + \left(I_{air} - I_{tis}\right) AVPC_{n\%}$$

$$= I_{tis} + \frac{\left(I_{air} - I_{tis}\right)n}{100}, \quad n = 95, 90, ..., 65 \tag{9}$$

where $I_{n\%}$ is the intensity corresponding to $n\%$ of air within the lung voxels. Then the percentage of voxels containing an equal or more than a certain amount of air throughout the lung volume in end inhalation can be obtained as follows:

$$V_{nInh} = \frac{\sum_{i=I_{\alpha}}^{I_{n\%}} N_{vox}[i]}{\sum_{i=I_{\alpha}}^{I_{\beta}} N_{vox}[i]} \times 100 \tag{10}$$

where V_{nInh} can be any of the features of V_{95Inh}, V_{90Inh}, ..., and V_{65Inh}.

1.4.3 Group 3: The Lung's Air Distribution in the Expiration Phase

Analogous to the second group, the third group of features are computed as the percentage of voxels in the end-exhalation CT image, which contains an equal amount or more than 95%, 90%, …, and 65% of air. These features are called $V_{95\,Exh}$, $V_{90\,Exh}$, …, and $V_{65\,Exh}$, respectively. They describe the air distribution and concentration within the lung during the expiration phase. The equations utilized for computing these features are the same as the previous set of equations except that the end-exhalation image is used instead of the end-inhalation one. Research has demonstrated that the extension of areas with medium to high concentrations of air within the lung in the expiration phase is highly associated with the occurrence of air trapping [13–15].

1.4.4 Group 4: Overall Statistical Features

A feature combining the second and third features may include invaluable information. To investigate the influence of such features, a weighted summation of these features is considered where the correlation coefficient of each feature is used as the weight. To this end, the mean values of the correlation coefficients of the second and third groups of features and PFT measurements are computed before the vectors of features and correlation coefficients are calculated as follows:

$$F_{Exh} = \left\{ V_{95\,Exh},\ V_{90\,Exh},\ V_{85\,Exh},\ V_{80\,Exh},\ V_{75\,Exh},\ V_{70\,Exh},\ V_{65\,Exh} \right\} \tag{11}$$

$$F_{Inh} = \left\{ V_{95\,Inh},\ V_{90\,Inh},\ V_{85\,Inh},\ V_{80\,Inh},\ V_{75\,Inh},\ V_{70\,Inh},\ V_{65\,Inh} \right\} \tag{12}$$

$$R_{Exh} = \left\{ \frac{r\left(V_{95\,Exh},\ FEV_1\right) + r\left(V_{95\,Exh},\ \dfrac{FEV_1}{FVC}\right)}{2},\ \ldots,\ \frac{r\left(V_{65\,Exh},\ FEV_1\right) + r\left(V_{65\,Exh},\ \dfrac{FEV_1}{FVC}\right)}{2} \right\} \tag{13}$$

$$R_{Inh} = \left\{ \frac{r\left(V_{95\,Inh},\ FEV_1\right) + r\left(V_{95\,Inh},\ \dfrac{FEV_1}{FVC}\right)}{2},\ \ldots,\ \frac{r\left(V_{65\,Inh},\ FEV_1\right) + r\left(V_{65\,Inh},\ \dfrac{FEV_1}{FVC}\right)}{2} \right\} \tag{14}$$

where $r(.)$ indicates the correlation coefficient. Afterward, the normalized weight of every feature is computed by dividing the absolute value of the feature vector elements by the maximum absolute values of the correlation coefficients as follows:

$$W_{Exh} = \left| \frac{R_{Exh}}{max\left(|R_{Exh}|\right)} \right| \tag{15}$$

$$W_{Inh} = \left| \frac{R_{Inh}}{max\left(|R_{Inh}|\right)} \right|. \tag{16}$$

Finally, the weighted summation of features can be computed through

$$F_{Exh}^{w} = \frac{\sum_{i=1}^{7} W_{Exh}(i) \, F_{Exh}(i)}{7} \tag{17}$$

$$F_{Inh}^{w} = \frac{\sum_{i=1}^{7} W_{Inh}(i) \, F_{Inh}(i)}{7} \tag{18}$$

where F_{Inh}^{w} and F_{Exh}^{w} are the weighted summations of the second and third group of features, respectively.

While all features contribute to the computation of the weighted summation of F_{Inh}^{w} and F_{Exh}^{w}, features with low correlation coefficients may skew the results. To avoid this issue, one may use only the features with high correlation coefficients. To investigate this idea, two new features of V_{Inh}^{w} and V_{Exh}^{w} are introduced that are the weighted summation of the second and third groups of features that highly correlated with PFT measurements (i.e., correlation coefficient ≥ 0.7, respectively). The correlation coefficient computation results indicated that the first three features of the second group and the last six features of the third group of features have a correlation coefficient ≥ 0.7. As such, these features can be computed using the following equations:

$$V_{Exh}^{w} = \frac{\sum_{i=2}^{7} W_{Exh}(i) \, F_{Exh}(i)}{6} \tag{19}$$

$$V_{Inh}^{w} = \frac{\sum_{i=1}^{3} W_{Inh}(i) \, F_{Inh}(i)}{3}. \tag{20}$$

Moreover, the mean and standard deviation values of the second and third groups of features may include invaluable information about overall air distribution within the lung. Therefore, four features of M_{Inh}, S_{Inh}, M_{Exh}, and S_{Exh} are introduced that are the mean and standard deviation values of the second and third groups of features, respectively. These feature can be computed using the following equations:

$$M_x = \frac{V_{95x} + \cdots + V_{65x}}{7} \tag{21}$$

$$S_x = \sqrt{\frac{\left(V_{95x} - M_x\right)^2 + \cdots + \left(V_{65x} - M_x\right)^2}{7}} \tag{22}$$

where x indicates the *Inh* an *Exh* indices corresponding to the second group (inhalation phase) and third group (exhalation phase) of features, respectively.

1.4.5 Statistical Study of Features

In addition to the TLC and FRC volumes, spirometric data (e.g., FEV_1) of the subjects were acquired using an EasyOne spirometry device (ndd Medical Technologies). The data were recorded such that the time difference between recording the spirometric test data and CT imaging was less than half an hour. The spirometric data were analyzed by an expert in our group to ensure that reliable data were used in the study.

To assess the relationship between PFT measurements and extracted features, the Pearson correlation coefficients and linear regression coefficients were computed. The magnitude of each coefficient indicates how efficient the extracted feature is; hence, the most effective features can be identified and used for classification. Figures 1.6 to Figure 1.12 illustrate the results as scatter plots of V_{xxInh} and V_{xxExh} versus FEV_1 and $\frac{FEV_1}{FVC}$ along with computed correlation coefficients and linear regression coefficients, where xx indicates indices of 95, 90, or 65. Moreover, the correlation coefficients between the first group of features and FEV_1 and $\frac{FEV_1}{FVC}$ are summarized in Table 1.3. The results indicate that ΔAV_{Inh} has higher correlation values of $r = -0.77$ and $r = -0.69$ with both FEV_1 and $\frac{FEV_1}{FVC}$, respectively. The scatter plots indicate various degrees of separation for data corresponding to subjects with COPD GOLD 1, 2, 3, and 4 and normal subjects.

TABLE 1.3   Correlation Coefficients Between the Lung's Air Volume Variation Features and Corresponding PFT Measurements

Feature	Correlation Coefficient (r)	
	ΔV_{Inh}	ΔV_{Inh}
FEV_1	0.77	0.75
FEV_1/FVC	0.69	0.68

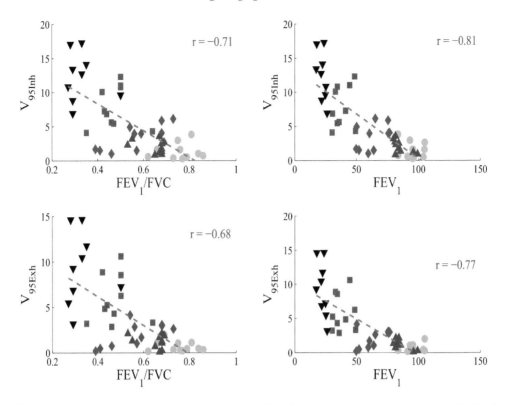

Figure 1.6 Scatter plots showing the relationships between V_{95Inh}, V_{95Exh}, FEV_1, and $FEV_1/$ FVC along with respective correlation coefficients. The black ▼, red ■, pink ◆, blue ▲, and green • symbols correspond to COPD GOLD 1, 2, 3, and 4 and normal subjects, respectively. The dashed line shows the best fit obtained by linear regression.

Table 1.4 shows the correlation coefficients between the second group of features and FEV_1 and $\dfrac{FEV_1}{FVC}$. Results indicate that V_{95Inh} has the highest correlation coefficient of $r = -0.81$ with FEV_1, while the highest correlation coefficient of $r = -0.74$ with $\dfrac{FEV_1}{FVC}$ belongs to V_{90Inh}. Furthermore, the correlation coefficients between the third group of features and FEV_1 and $\dfrac{FEV_1}{FVC}$ are summarized in Table 1.5. This table

TABLE 1.4   Correlation Coefficients Between the Lung's Air Distribution Features in Inhalation Images and Corresponding PFT Measurements

	Correlation Coefficient (r)						
Feature	V_{95Inh}	V_{90Inh}	V_{85Inh}	V_{80Inh}	V_{75Inh}	V_{70Inh}	V_{65Inh}
FEV_1	−0.81	−0.78	−0.77	−0.69	−0.58	−0.48	−0.23
FEV_1/FVC	−0.71	−0.74	−0.71	−0.62	−0.50	−0.41	−0.21

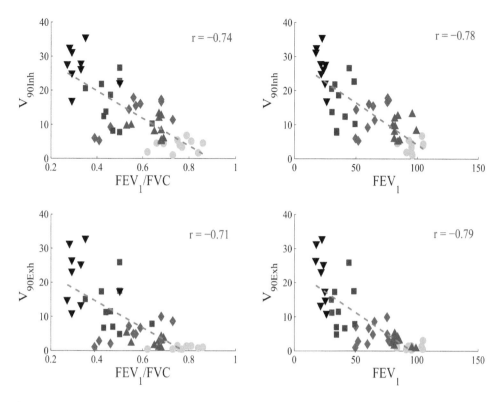

Figure 1.7 Scatter plots showing the relationships between V_{90Inh}, V_{90Exh}, FEV_1, and FEV_1/FVC along with respective correlation coefficients. The black ▼, red ■, pink ◆, blue ▲, and green • symbols correspond to COPD GOLD 1, 2, 3, and 4 and normal subjects, respectively. The dashed line shows the best fit obtained by linear regression.

indicates that V_{70Inh} has the highest correlation coefficient with both FEV_1 and $\dfrac{FEV_1}{FVC}$ at $r = -0.89$ and $r = -0.86$, respectively. Results in Table 1.4 and Table 1.5 indicate that the V_{70Inh}, V_{75Inh}, V_{90Inh}, V_{95Inh}, and AV_{Inh} features have the highest correlation with PFT measured data. The mean and standard deviation values of all features of the second and third groups are summarized in Table 1.6. Results in these tables show that almost all of the feature values increase with higher COPD GOLD (i.e., higher COPD severity). However, some of the features do not show meaningful trends.

TABLE 1.5   Correlation Coefficients Between the Overall Features in Exhalation Images and Corresponding PFT Measurements

	Correlation Coefficient (r)						
Feature	V_{95Exh}	V_{90Exh}	V_{85Exh}	V_{80Exh}	V_{75Exh}	V_{70Exh}	V_{65Exh}
FEV_1	−0.77	−0.79	−0.81	−0.79	−0.86	−0.89	−0.79
FEV_1/FVC	−0.68	−0.71	−0.72	−0.70	−0.79	−0.86	−0.78

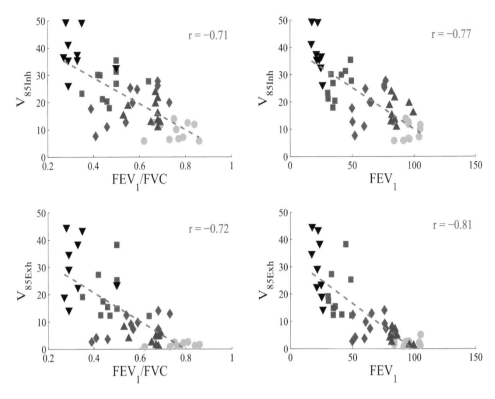

Figure 1.8 Scatter plots showing the relationships between V_{85Inh}, V_{85Exh}, FEV_1, and FEV_1/FVC along with respective correlation coefficients. The black ▼, red ■, pink ◆, blue ▲, and green • symbols correspond to COPD GOLD 1, 2, 3, and 4 and normal subjects, respectively. The dashed line shows the best fit obtained by linear regression.

TABLE 1.6   Mean and Standard Deviation (SD) Values of the Lung's Air Distribution Features in the Inhalation and Exhalation for All the 69 Subjects, Including Normal Subjects and Subjects with COPD GOLD Stages 1 to 4

	Mean ± SD (%)				
Feature	Normal	GOLD 1	GOLD 2	GOLD 3	GOLD 4
V_{95Inh}	1.48 ± 1.20	2.06 ± 0.97	3.47 ± 1.91	7.80 ± 3.01	12.32 ± 3.59
V_{90Inh}	3.85 ± 1.75	8.92 ± 2.97	12.97 ± 4.69	16.25 ± 6.65	27.27 ± 5.61
V_{85Inh}	9.53 ± 3.15	16.43 ± 4.25	19.32 ± 6.93	26.45 ± 5.55	38.35 ± 7.51
V_{80Inh}	19.84 ± 7.30	32.86 ± 9.28	36.33 ± 12.27	48.70 ± 12.77	59.87 ± 15.79
V_{75Inh}	39.11 ± 13.79	45.98 ± 9.10	47.07 ± 12.76	60.93 ± 10.45	66.85 ± 11.13
V_{70Inh}	55.98 ± 12.07	67.62 ± 7.46	66.23 ± 9.85	73.08 ± 11.43	75.82 ± 8.63
V_{65Inh}	84.36 ± 6.91	85.63 ± 7.47	84.03 ± 7.49	86.44 ± 7.64	88.34 ± 6.07
V_{95Exh}	0.69 ± 0.57	1.27 ± 0.74	1.99 ± 1.33	5.82 ± 2.69	9.28 ± 3.97
V_{90Exh}	1.11 ± 0.78	2.72 ± 1.39	5.12 ± 2.93	12.47 ± 6.51	21.76 ± 7.94
V_{85Exh}	2.04 ± 1.24	4.45 ± 2.29	8.41 ± 4.02	19.51 ± 8.44	30.07 ± 10.91
V_{80Exh}	3.72 ± 2.08	7.31 ± 3.35	13.10 ± 4.49	28.94 ± 15.16	43.89 ± 13.31
V_{75Exh}	6.61 ± 2.63	13.19 ± 4.72	19.59 ± 5.28	36.38 ± 12.30	52.49 ± 11.90
V_{70Exh}	15.60 ± 5.58	20.81 ± 5.68	32.78 ± 5.03	48.70 ± 7.23	60.91 ± 8.64
V_{65Exh}	30.13 ± 8.69	36.57 ± 11.10	45.87 ± 7.64	60.49 ± 12.56	69.98 ± 11.16

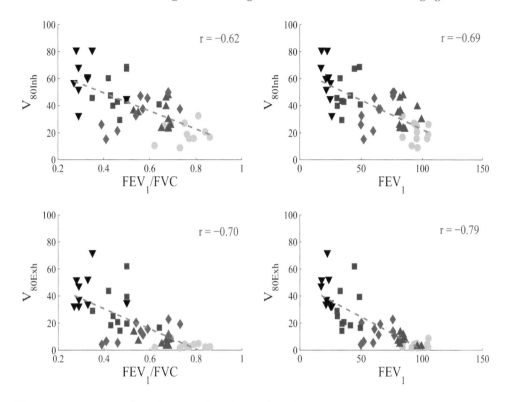

Figure 1.9   Scatter plots showing the relationships between V_{80Inh}, V_{80Exh}, FEV_1, and FEV_1/FVC along with respective correlation coefficients. The black ▼, red ■, pink ◆, blue ▲, and green • symbols correspond to COPD GOLD 1, 2, 3, and 4 and normal subjects, respectively. The dashed line shows the best fit obtained by linear regression.

1.5 Classification Algorithm

Recently, significant efforts have been made to develop CAD systems for COPD diagnosis and treatment planning and monitoring. The human eyes have limited capability in discriminating between various grayscale values, as they can detect only 30 to 40 distinct gray levels in CT images [25]. As such, subtle but significant differences may be ignored by human observers. In addition, the large number of patients where each has large image data sets to be interpreted by a radiologist can be time consuming and exhausting, increasing the probability of human error and misdiagnosis.

Many investigations have led to publications that report the correlation between image-extracted features and symptoms of pulmonary diseases. As such, some researchers have now focused on developing automatic diagnosis and staging determination tools by exploiting features extracted from clinical studies and image data [26]. However, limited discriminatory power and insufficient accuracy of features and classifiers involved in these methods indicate a gap, hence the necessity for developing more sophisticated tools aiming at developing highly effective CAD systems. The following section describes the development of an effective automatic CAD system for

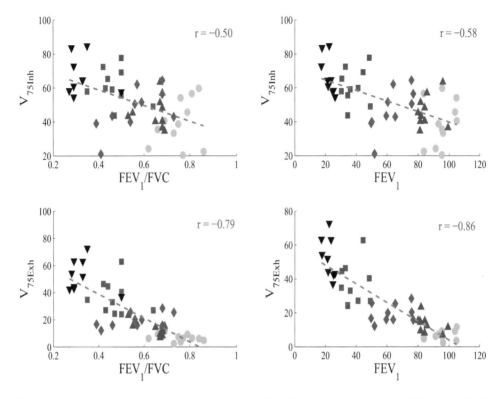

Figure 1.10 Scatter plots showing the relationships between V_{75Inh}, V_{75Exh}, FEV_1, and FEV_1/FVC along with respective correlation coefficients. The black ▼, red ■, pink ◆, blue ▲, and green • symbols correspond to COPD GOLD 1, 2, 3, and 4 and normal subjects, respectively. The dashed line shows the best fit obtained by linear regression.

diagnosis and staging severity of COPD based on inspiratory/expiratory CT images extracted features with high discriminatory power.

1.5.1 Feature Selection

Using a smaller number of features in a classifier is known to be advantageous. Such classifiers facilitate better interpretation as a result of simplification, improved model generalization resulting from reduced overfitting, and reduced training time [27]. One of the techniques that can be utilized to find the best combination of features is the sequential feature selection algorithm. This technique can be applied in both forward and backward directions. In the sequential forward selection (SFS) method, the procedure starts with a null vector, and in each iteration, the feature that could improve the performance of the classifier the most is added to the vector. In contrast, in the sequential backward selection (SBS) method, the procedure starts with a full vector that includes all the features, and in each iteration, the feature that improves the performance of the classifier the least is removed from the vector. Improvement

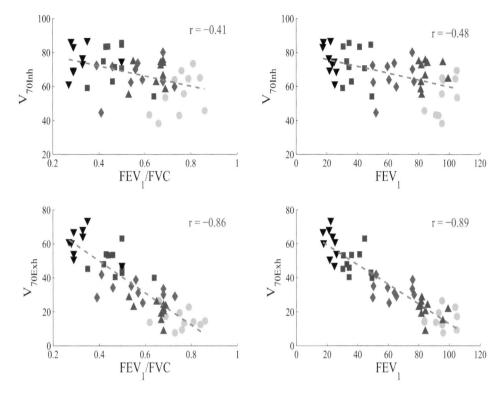

Figure 1.11 Scatter plots showing the relationships between V_{70Inh}, V_{70Exh}, FEV_1, and FEV_1/FVC along with respective correlation coefficients. The black ▼, red ■, pink ◆, blue ▲, and green • symbols correspond to COPD GOLD 1, 2, 3, and 4 and normal subjects, respectively. The dashed line shows the best fit obtained by linear regression.

(Adapted from [24])

of classifier performance is assessed by a certain criterion. In this study, the sum of misclassification rate (SMR) is used and can be computed as follows:

$$SMR = \sum_{i=1}^{n}\left(1 - D_{i,i}\big/100\right) \tag{23}$$

where $D_{i,i}$ denotes each of the diagonal elements of the confusion matrix. The less the SMR, the better the performance of the classifier. Table 1.7 summarizes the results obtained from applying the SFS and SBS methods. It indicates that the least SMR was achieved in the 11th and 12th iterations in the SFS and SBS methods, respectively. According to the third and fifth columns of Table 1.7, all the most effective features are the same in both directions except feature numbers 5, 6, and 19, that is, V_{70Inh}, V_{75Inh}, and V_{Exh}^{w}. As such, the performance of the classifier was investigated independently with or without each of these three features. Results demonstrated that the performance of the classifier improved when features 6 and 19 were added to the features vector. Consequently, features 1, 2, 3, 4, 6, 13, 16, 17, 18, 19, 20, and 21 were selected as the appropriate features, while the other features were removed from the vector. The selected features were used

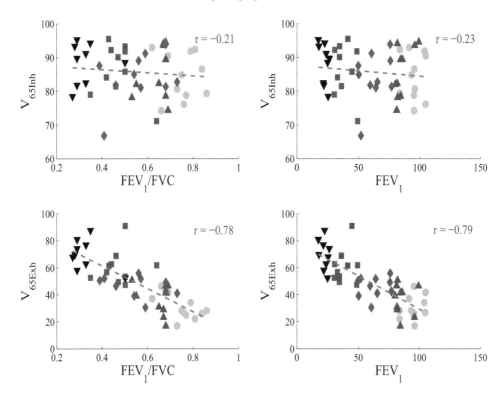

Figure 1.12   Scatter plots showing the relationships between V_{65Inh}, V_{65Exh}, FEV_1, and FEV_1/FVC along with respective correlation coefficients. The black ▼, red ■, pink ◆, blue ▲, and green • symbols correspond to COPD GOLD 1, 2, 3, and 4 and normal subjects, respectively. The dashed line shows the best fit obtained by linear regression.

for training and developing the classifiers. In the next sections, implementation of the Naive Bayes (NB) classifier, as a supervised learning method, and the k-nearest neighbors classifier, as an unsupervised learning method, is discussed.

1.5.2 k-Nearest Neighbors Classifier

The k-nearest neighbors (k-NN) classifier is one of the most frequently used classifiers. In this method, a cluster, which consists of k-nearest neighboring objects, is considered, and the corresponding class of a given object is assigned the most common class of the k-nearest neighbors. In this classifier, in order to find the nearest neighbors, it is necessary to evaluate the distance of the features. In this study, the standardized Euclidean distance was utilized to assess the distance between the features. Moreover, the performance of the classifier was investigated for various values of k from 1 to 10, where the best performance was achieved with $k = 3$. The performance of the classifier was evaluated using the leave-m-out (LMO) method because of the limited number of subjects in the study data set; m is chosen to be equal to 7, almost 10% of the size of the data set. In this method, the data corresponding to 62 subjects out of all of the

TABLE 1.7   Order of the Discriminatory Power of Features with Respect to Both of the FSF and SBS Schemes

	SFS Scheme		SBS Scheme	
Order	Feature Number, Feature Name	SMR	Feature Number, Feature Name	SMR
1	17, V_{70Exh}	1.294	All	0.829
2	4, V_{85Inh}	0.997	8, V_{65Inh}	0.830
3	1, ΔV_{Inh}	0.981	23, F_{Inh}^{w}	0.829
4	6, V_{75Inh}	0.917	7, V_{70Inh}	0.828
5	13, V_{90Exh}	0.886	10, M_{Inh}	0.826
6	16, V_{75Exh}	0.843	22, F_{Exh}^{w}	0.825
7	20, M_{Exh}	0.839	11, S_{Inh}	0.824
8	18, V_{65Exh}	0.815	15, V_{80Exh}	0.827
9	3, V_{90Inh}	0.807	12, V_{95Exh}	0.823
10	21, S_{Exh}	0.801	9, V_{Inh}^{w}	0.814
11	2, V_{95Inh}	0.791	14, V_{85Exh}	0.804
12	5, V_{70Inh}	0.798	6, V_{75Inh}	0.797
13	19, V_{Exh}^{w}	0.803	5, V_{70Inh}	0.802
14	12, V_{95Exh}	0.806	21, S_{Exh}	0.807
15	9, V_{Inh}^{w}	0.811	2, V_{95Inh}	0.814
16	7, V_{70Inh}	0.819	20, M_{Exh}	0.831
17	14, V_{85Exh}	0.817	1, ΔV_{Inh}	0.847
18	15, V_{80Exh}	0.820	16, V_{75Exh}	0.858
19	22, F_{Exh}^{w}	0.822	4, V_{85Inh}	0.877
20	10, M_{Inh}	0.821	18, V_{65Exh}	0.923
21	11, S_{Inh}	0.825	13, V_{90Exh}	0.984
22	8, V_{65Inh}	0.829	17, V_{70Exh}	1.034
23	23, F_{Inh}^{w}	0.830	3, V_{90Inh}	1.323

67 subjects were randomly selected as the training set, and the remaining seven subjects were considered as the test set. This procedure was repeated until a stable performance was achieved. Figure 1.13 shows the average accuracy of the resulting classifier for all classes over 500 interactions where it converges to 69.20%.

In the first few iterations, the average accuracy was overestimated because of overfitting or weak training; it converged to a realistic value of 69.2% as the iteration number increased. Table 1.8 shows the confusion matrix of the k-NN classifier with recall and precision parameters for each class. The table indicates modest prediction accuracy, which may have stemmed from the limited number of subjects involved in the study, which has a spoiling effect on training and test procedures, leading to only limited overall accuracy.

According to the last row of Table 1.8, the precision for most of the classes increases with higher COPD GOLD stage. This stems from the fact that COPD is a progressive disease, which implies more enhanced abnormal image and function features with

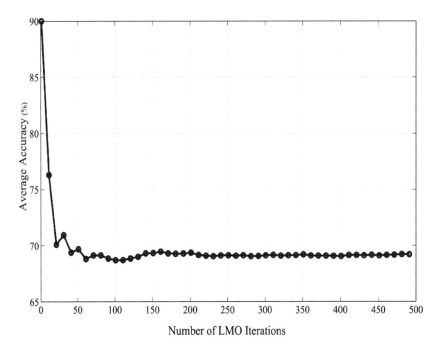

Figure 1.13 Variations of average accuracy of all classes for k-NN method, evaluated through the LMO method with $m = 7$ over 500 iterations. The average accuracy converges to 69.20%.

higher COPD GOLD stages. As mentioned earlier, COPD is associated with permanent damage to the lung; hence, it is critically important to diagnose the disease as early as possible. In order to increase the chance of diagnosis in early stages of COPD, an NB classifier was developed. The performance of this classifier will be compared to that of the k-NN classifier.

1.5.3 NB Classifier

The NB classifier is one of the most common classifiers that has been recently applied extensively in various machine learning applications. This classifier's performance

TABLE 1.8 Confusion Matrix of the Designed k-NN Classifier With Recall and Precision Parameters of Each Class

Actual	Predicted (%)					Recall for Each Class (%)
	Normal	GOLD 1	GOLD 2	GOLD 3	GOLD 4	
Normal	57.15	42.85	0	0	0	57.15
GOLD 1	27.75	65.86	6.39	0	0	65.86
GOLD 2	6.69	19.81	73.33	0.17	0	73.33
GOLD 3	0	0.12	22.43	63.74	13.71	63.74
GOLD 4	0	0	0	14.08	85.92	85.92
Precision for each class (%)	62.40	51.20	71.79	81.73	86.24	—

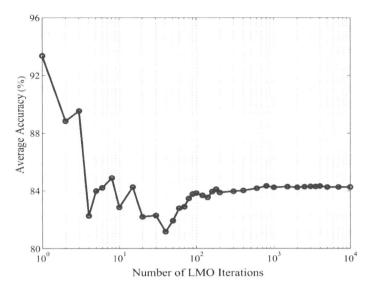

Figure 1.14   Variations of average accuracy of all classes in the NB method, evaluated by the LMO method with $m = 7$, over 10^4 iterations. The average accuracy converges to 84.18%.

(Adapted from [24])

has been investigated through many studies, confirming its efficiency in various applications [28]. NB is expected to be a proper choice in this COPD stage classification application, as it has proven effectiveness in scenarios where only a limited amount of training data and functionally independent features are available [29]. To develop this classifier in this investigation, the selected features were fed to the training procedure, and the LMO method, with $m = 7$, was utilized to evaluate the performance of the trained classifier. The LMO was repeated for 10^4 iterations for seven different combinations of 69 subjects. The classification procedure was repeated several times on the data set to ascertain the stability of the classifier performance. Figure 1.14 illustrates the variation of average accuracy over the 10^4 iterations and shows that it converged to a final value of 84.18%.

High oscillatory variations were observed in the beginning of the curve until ~40 iterations was reached. This is a consequence of overfitting or weak training. As the iterations increase, the average accuracy converges to a stable value. The confusion matrix is shown in Table 1.9, which reports the recall and precision values.

1.6 Discussion

In our proposed method, lung volumes and their variations were measured over the respiration cycles from CT images. The corresponding data were then utilized to extract image-based features that are used to assess the pulmonary system performance associated with COPD symptoms and indications. Moreover, the air-to-tissue ratio analysis was used to evaluate local air distribution within the lung.

TABLE 1.9　Confusion Matrix of the Designed NB Classifier With Recall and Precision Parameters of Each Class

Actual	Predicted (%)					Recall for Each Class (%)
	Normal	GOLD 1	GOLD 2	GOLD 3	GOLD 4	
Normal	87.03	12.16	0.81	0	0	87.03
GOLD 1	10.07	81.15	8.78	0	0	81.15
GOLD 2	0	3.16	86.91	9.93	0	86.91
GOLD 3	0	0	9.16	80.61	10.23	80.61
GOLD 4	0	0	0	14.78	85.22	85.22
Precision for each class (%)	89.63	84.12	82.25	76.54	89.28	—

The correlation of all the extracted features with clinical data was investigated. Table 1.3 illustrates that ΔV_{Inh} is more appropriate for normalization of the lung's air volume variations features because lung volumes are less influenced by air trapping in the end-inhalation phase in contrast to the end-exhalation phase. Results of the statistical study reported in Table 1.3 to Table 1.6 strongly support the hypothesis that the amount of air within the lung air voxels and their distribution throughout the lung are highly correlated with the results of PFT measurements. According to the data summarized in Table 1.4 and Table 1.5, V_{70Exh} is the most correlated feature with the severity of airflow obstruction through the lung, which is assessed by FEV_1 and $\dfrac{FEV_1}{FVC}$. The severity of airflow obstruction is an indication of COPD progression. Among all the lung's air distribution features in the inspiration phase, the V_{95Inh}, V_{90Inh}, and V_{85Inh} features show the most correlation with both FEV_1 and $\dfrac{FEV_1}{FVC}$ parameters. This indicates that COPD leads to increasing the percentage of the numbers of the lung air voxels with a high amount of air during the inspiration phase. The existence of the regions with a high concentration of air within the lung could be considered a sign of emphysema. In contrast, the V_{70Exh} and V_{75Exh} features demonstrated high correlations with FEV_1 and $\dfrac{FEV_1}{FVC}$. This means that COPD leads to a reduction in the percentage of lung air voxels with a low amount of air during the expiration phase. The inability to fully breathe out the air from the lung during expiration results in air trapping, where this is reflected in the lung's air distribution features, especially in V_{70Exh} and V_{75Exh}.

Mean and standard deviation values of the lung air distribution features in both the inhalation and the exhalation phase, summarized in Table 1.6, indicate that the percentage of voxels that contain a high concentration of air in the inspiration phase increases with COPD severity progression. Although this increase in the features corresponding to a high concentration of air, that is, V_{95Inh} and V_{90Inh}, is clearly discernible, it declines in the features corresponding to a low concentration of air, that is, V_{65Inh} and V_{70Inh}. Most of the lung air voxels contain a high amount of air during inhalation. As such, the value of the features that include a high concentration of air approaches 100% in the inhalation phase, and consequently no meaningful difference could be seen between the values of these features with respect to COPD severity progression. On the other hand, most of the lung air voxels lose their air content during expiration. As such, the value of features corresponding to a high concentration of air approaches 0% in the exhalation phase. However, as a result of air trapping in COPD, a considerable difference could be seen between the values of all the features of V_{65Exh} to V_{75Inh} corresponding to COPD patients with various GOLD stages. The V_{70Exh} and V_{75Exh} features have the highest correlation with FEV_1 and $\dfrac{FEV_1}{FVC}$ in comparison to other features because the features corresponding to low air concentration include almost all the regions that contain air within the lung; hence, the V_{70Exh} and V_{75Exh} features are capable of assessing air trapping.

According to the results obtained from both the SFS and the SBS method, the percentage of the number of voxels with a high concentration of air in the inhalation phase, the percentage of the number of voxels that include low concentration of air in the exhalation phase, lung air volume variations between inspiration and expiration normalized with respect to the lung's air volume in the inhalation phase, and mean and standard deviation values of V_{65Exh} to V_{95Inh} demonstrate the most discriminatory power among all the features. The obtained results of the correlation coefficients of the first, second, and third groups of features support the concluded discriminatory powers of the features. However, among all the features of the fourth group of features, V_{Exh}^w, M_{Exh}, and S_{Exh} demonstrate the most discriminatory power because they are capable of assessing the overall effects of air trapping within the lung.

The confusion matrix of the NB method in Table 1.9 shows that the average accuracy of the classifier in all classes is 84.18%, where the most and the least accuracy among all the classes belong to classes of normal subjects and COPD patients with GOLD stage 3, respectively. Furthermore, this confusion matrix demonstrates that the misclassifications occur only in association with neighboring classes. As such, according to the obtained results of the implemented classifier, this technique is capable of effectively diagnosing and determining reasonably accurately the stage of COPD based on GOLD criterion.

In order to evaluate the effectiveness of the extracted features and the performance of the developed classifiers, obtained results are compared with the results reported in Nimura et al. [26] as presented in Table 1.10. In Nimura et al. [26], the image-extracted features are computed mainly based on LAA% and its volumetric version, that is, the percentage of low-attenuation volume LAV% [30]. Moreover,

TABLE 1.10 Comparison of the Characteristics and Results of the Proposed Method and the Method Proposed in Nimura et al. [26]

| Method | Classifier | Used Features | | Number of Cases (COPD, Normal) | Validation Method | Overall Accuracy (%) |
		CT Images	PFT Measurements			
Proposed method	NB	✓	✗	69 (56, 13)	LMO, $m = 7$	84.18
	k-NN	✓	✗	69 (56, 13)	LMO, $m = 7$	69.20
Nimura et al. [26]	AdaBoost	✓	✓	49 (46, 3)	LMO, $m = 1$	53.10

shape-describing features of the diaphragm and blood vessels, lung volumes, and partial pressure of respiratory gases (from PFTs) were extracted. As explained earlier, since LAA% and LAV% are computed based on predetermined empirical threshold values, the obtained results are not satisfactory where such features are utilized. In that study, they tried to improve their results by utilizing the results of clinical tests and PFTs. While that approach was successful, the drawback of utilizing clinical tests and PFTs is that data pertaining to the clinical tests are not necessarily available in conjunction with image data.

Due to accurate analysis of the lung air voxels, the extracted features in the proposed method are more effective, as they demonstrate higher discriminatory power as confirmed by the results showing higher classification accuracy. The extracted features encapsulate two very important criteria of emphysema and air trapping in COPD. Moreover, the results indicate that the image-based features described here are highly correlated with the results of PFT measurements.

References

1. Lomborg B, ed. *Global Problems, Smart Solutions: Costs and Benefits*. Cambridge, England: Cambridge University Press, 2013.
2. Galbán CJ, Han MK, Boes JL, et al. Computed tomography-based biomarker provides unique signature for diagnosis of COPD phenotypes and disease progression. *Nat Med*. 2012;18(11):1711–1715.
3. Kauczor HU, Heussel CP, Fischer B, Klamm R, Mildenberger P, Thelen M. Assessment of lung volumes using helical CT at inspiration and expiration: comparison with pulmonary function tests. *Am J Roentgenol*. 1998;171(4):1091–1095.
4. Patroniti N, Bellani G, Manfio A, et al. Lung volume in mechanically ventilated patients: measurement by simplified helium dilution compared to quantitative CT scan. *Intensive Care Med*. 2001;30(2):282–289.
5. Iwano S, Okada T, Satake H, Naganawa S. 3D-CT volumetry of the lung using multidetector row CT. *Acad Radiol*. 2009;16(3):250–256.
6. Müller NL, Staples CA, Miller RR, and Abboud RT. Density mask: an objective method to quantitate emphysema using computed tomography. *Chest*. 1988;94(4):782–787.
7. Sieren JP, Newell JD, Judy PF, et al. Reference standard and statistical model for intersite and temporal comparisons of CT attenuation in a multicenter quantitative lung study. *Med Phys*. 2012;39(9):5757.
8. Hoffman EA, Lynch DA, Barr RG, van Beek EJR, Parraga G. Pulmonary CT and MRI phenotypes that help explain chronic pulmonary obstruction disease pathophysiology and outcomes. *J Magn Reson Imaging*. 2016;43(3):544–557.
9. Hayhurst MD, MacNee W, Flenley DC, et al. Diagnosis of pulmonary emphysema by computerised tomography. *Lancet*. 1984;324(8398):320–322.
10. Roth MD, Connett JE, D'Armiento JM, et al. Feasibility of retinoids for the treatment of emphysema study. *Chest*. 2006;130(5):1334–1345.
11. Gevenois PA, De Vuyst P, Sy M, et al. Pulmonary emphysema: quantitative CT during expiration. *Radiology*. 1996;199(3):825–829.
12. Madani A, Zanen J, de Maertelaer V, Gevenois PA. Pulmonary emphysema: objective quantification at multi–detector row CT—comparison with macroscopic and microscopic morphometry 1. *Radiology*. 2006;238(3):1036–1043.

13. Busacker A, Newell JD, Keefe T, et al. A multivariate analysis of risk factors for the air-trapping asthmatic phenotype as measured by quantitative CT analysis. *Chest.* 2009;135(1):48–56.

14. Jain N, Covar RA, Gleason MC, Newell JD, Gelfand EW, Spahn JD. Quantitative computed tomography detects peripheral airway disease in asthmatic children. *Pediatr Pulmonol.* 2005;40(3):211–218.

15. Newman KB, Lynch DA, Newman LS, Ellegood D, Newell JD. Quantitative computed tomography detects air trapping due to asthma. *Chest.* 1994;106(1):105–109.

16. Kanner RE, Hoffman E, Tashkin DP. The relationship between spirometry, air trapping and dyspnea in spiromics: a study of patients with COPD. In: *B43. COPD: Screening and Diagnostic Tools.* New York, NY: American Thoracic Society; 2014:A2978–A2978.

17. Cazzola M, Celli B, Dahl R, Rennard S. *Therapeutic Strategies in COPD.* Oxford, England: Clinical Publishing; 2005.

18. Choi S, Hoffman EA, Wenzel SE, et al. Quantitative computed tomographic imaging–based clustering differentiates asthmatic subgroups with distinctive clinical phenotypes. *J Allergy Clin Immunol.* 2017;140(3):690–700.

19. Moghadas-Dastjerdi H, Ahmadzadeh M, Samani A. Towards computer based lung disease diagnosis using accurate lung air segmentation of CT images in exhalation and inhalation phases. *Expert Syst Appl.* 2017;71:396–403.

20. Sadeghi Naini A, Lee T-Y, Patel RV, Samani A. Estimation of lung's air volume and its variations throughout respiratory CT image sequences. *IEEE Trans Biomed Eng.* 2011;58(1):152–158.

21. Roan E, aWaters CM. What do we know about mechanical strain in lung alveoli? *Am J Physiol Lung Cell Mol Physiol.* 2011;301(5):L625–L635.

22. Doherty DE. The pathophysiology of airway dysfunction. *Am J Med Suppl.* 2004;117(2):11–23.

23. Decramer M, Janssens W. Chronic obstructive pulmonary disease and comorbidities. *Lancet Respir Med.* 2013;1(1):73–83.

24. Moghadas-Dastjerdi H, Ahmadzadeh M, Karami E, Karami M, Samani A. Lung CT image based automatic technique for COPD GOLD stage assessment. *Expert Syst Appl.* 2017;85:194–203.

25. Flohr T, Ohnesorge B. Fundamentals of multislice CT scanning and its application to the periphery. In: Mukherjee D, Rajagopalan S, eds. *CT and MR Angiography of the Peripheral Circulation: Practical Approach With Clinical Protocols.* London, England: CRC Press; 2007:1.

26. Nimura Y, Kitasaka T, Honma H, et al. Assessment of COPD severity by combining pulmonary function tests and chest CT images. *Int J Comput Assist Radiol Surg.* 2013;8(3):353–363.

27. James G, Witten F, Hastie T, Tibshirani R. *An Introduction to Statistical Learning.* Vol. 103. New York, NY: Springer; 2013.

28. Caruana R, Niculescu-Mizil A. An empirical comparison of supervised learning algorithms. In: *Proceedings of the 23rd International Conference on Machine Learning—ICML '06.* Pittsburgh, PA; 2006:161–168.

29. Rish I. An empirical study of the naive Bayes classifier. In: *IJCAI 2001 Workshop on Empirical Methods in Artificial Intelligence.* Seattle, WA: Morgan Kaufmann; 2001;3(22):41–46.

30. Nagao J, Aiguchi T, Mori K, et al. A CAD system for quantifying COPD based on 3-D CT images. In: *International Conference on Medical Image Computing and Computer-Assisted Intervention.* Berlin, Germany: Springer; 2003:730–737.

2

Early Detection of Chronic Obstructive Pulmonary Disease: Influence on Lung Cancer Epidemiology

Amany F. Elbehairy and Ahmed Sadaka

Contents

2.1 Prevalence and Burden of Chronic Obstructive Pulmonary Disease and Lung Cancer

Lung cancer and chronic obstructive pulmonary disease (COPD) are two of the most common causes of morbidity and mortality worldwide. They are also among the most common smoking-related diseases. Despite the increasing efforts and strategies directed toward reducing tobacco smoking rates, COPD incidence and prevalence are still on the rise. In 2015, it has been estimated that the disease affected more than 174.5 million individuals worldwide and has been responsible for more than 3 million deaths. The disease is known to be one of the major causes of disability and poor quality of life [1]. This is reflected in an increasing economic burden with direct medical and indirect absenteeism costs. In the United States, the estimated annual direct costs of care for COPD are $32 billion and $20 billion as indirect costs [2]. In Europe, the total costs incurred by respiratory diseases reached more than €380, of which €48.4 is spent on COPD [3]. The larger share of the costs is usually attributed to hospitalizations, long-term oxygen therapy, and rehabilitation services in addition to workdays lost, which are directly proportional to the disease severity [2]. Another factor that comes into play when considering the burden of the disease is the common presence of comorbidities that are encountered across the different stages of severity of COPD [4]. In this regard, cardiovascular disease, pulmonary emboli, hypertension, metabolic syndrome, and lung cancer are frequent disease associations.

The presence of lung cancer as a comorbidity in COPD patients hospitalized for exacerbations is associated with increased costs as well as increased mortality [5]. With more than 234,000 newly diagnosed lung cancer patients, of which almost two out of three die, lung cancer is not only the deadliest smoking-related disease but also the leading cause of cancer-related mortality worldwide [6]. Lung cancer accounts for almost 13% of different types of cancers diagnosed in the United States (U.S.) and Europe and is associated with a low 5-year survival rate worldwide based on data from the CONCORD-2 trial [7]. The incidence and mortality rates of lung cancer do, however, show socioeconomic and gender inequalities in different countries. It was shown that despite decreasing incidence and deaths of lung cancer among males, the reverse is true for females in many countries [8]. In addition, there are reports of higher cancer incidence and mortality in developed countries [8]. It is important to note that the aforementioned disease trends need to be cautiously interpreted given the expected underdiagnosis and the fact that recording and reporting systems are neither equally robust nor standardized across different institutions and countries.

Taking into account the lack of disease-modifying treatments and the worlds's aging population, it is expected that a rising trend of both diseases may continue to dominate for at least a decade. It is thus imperative to have a deep understanding of the different links between tobacco smoke, COPD, and lung cancer development to improve the chances of limiting their economic burden and toll on the society.

2.2 COPD and Lung Cancer: Cross-Linking Pathophysiology

It is well known that tobacco smoking is a common causative factor for the development of both COPD and lung cancer. However, this historic relation was not discovered until 1912, when Isaac Adler first suggested a link between tobacco smoke exposure and lung cancer, a rather "rare disease" at that time [9]. Since then, there has been mounting evidence associating cigarette smoking to the increasing incidence of lung cancer [10]. Despite the inherently polar nature of COPD and lung cancer pathogenetic pathways, with respect to apoptosis, cell division, and vascularization, several mechanistic and epidemiological studies have shown a strong relation linking both diseases. Indeed, most of the patients diagnosed with lung cancer already have COPD. Epidemiological studies have confirmed that the latter is the most importat risk for the development of bronchogenic carcinoma. The presence of a common risk factor among both diseases predicts a shared pathogenetic process [10–12].

Skillrud et al. were the first to report an increased incidence of lung cancer in patients with COPD in the 1980s. Including 113 COPD patients and 114 controls (smokers without COPD) matched for age, sex, and smoking history, they reported a fourfold increased risk of lung cancer among patients with airflow obstruction [10]. Since then, this association has been reproduced in many studies while controlling for age and amount of smoke exposure [11–13]. The presence of radiological evidence of emphysema has also been found to be an independent risk factor for the development of lung cancer. Emphysema is associated with a two to three times increased risk of cancer development and even carries a worse prognosis compared with non-emphysematous patients [14–16]. Interestingly, when airflow obstruction and emphysema were included in a single regression model, only emphysema remained as an independent risk factor for lung cancer, suggesting that part of the risk attributed to spirometrically-defined COPD could be due to the presence of emphysema [15]. In this regard, a more recent study comparing the prevalence of lung cancer among current, former, and never smokers found that lung cancer prevalence in smokers (current or former) with emphysema was similar to that found in never smokers with emphysema (2.1% and 2.6%, respectively, $p = 0.61$) [17]. Thus, the current evidence proves the association between the obstructive airway disease and carcinogenesis. However, this is not a straightforward relationship due to COPD heterogeneity and the presence of multiple disease phenotypes.

COPD has been historically classified into two major phenotypes: emphysema and chronic bronchitis. Emphysema is secondary to an imbalance between proteolytic enzymes (mainly neutrophil elastase) and alpha-1 anti-trypsin (A1AT), ultimately leading to epithelial and endothelial cell apoptosis and CD4--CD8-driven inflammation. Chronic bronchitis is associated with an inflammatory process mainly affecting the large airways and is characterized by mucus hypersecretion, subepithelial fibrosis, and airway wall thickening. Although tobacoo smoking is a main leading factor of both COPD phenotypes as well as lung cancer, only 15% of those who smoke develop COPD, and 10% of patients diagnosed with lung cancer were nonsmokers in previous epidemiologic studies, suggesting an additional genetic component [18, 19]. Generally, the link between COPD and lung cancer remains obscure due to the different nature of both diseases. Various mechanisms have been proposed to explain the association between COPD and lung cancer (Figure 2.1). These mechanisms include genetic susceptibility, deoxyribonucleic acid (DNA) damage and repair, epigenetics, downregulation of specific micro-RNA (ribonucleic acid), expression of proinflammatory genes induced by hypoxia, tumor growth factor-B and integrins, telomere length and dysfunction, and immune adaptive responses [20–24].

2.2.1 Genetic Elements

The discrepancy between tobacco exposure and incidence of both COPD and lung cancer strongly suggests a genetic role in the pathogenesis. Although a large body of research has addressed the etiologic basis of COPD, only limited genetic factors have been proven to be associated with the disease [25]. A1ATD is considered the main sole

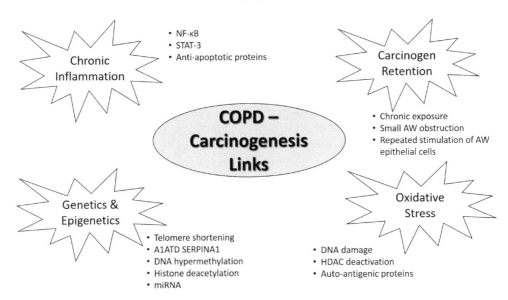

Figure 2.1 Factors linking COPD and lung cancer development. Abbreviations: A1ATD, alpha-1 antitrypsin deficiency; mi-RNA, micro-ribonucleic acid; AW, airway; HDAC, histone deacetylase; NF-κB, nuclear factor-κB; STAT-3, signal transducer and activator of transcription 3.

genetic cause of COPD and is secondary to a mutation in the SERPINA1 gene [26]. This results in an unchecked action of the neutrophil elastase in the lung parenchyma with destruction of the elastin fibers responsible for the elastic recoil of the lungs. The loss is irreversible because elastin fibers cannot be generated after adolescence. Obviously low levels of A1AT mean a decrease in the intracellular proapoptotic stimuli with more chance of tumorigenesis. The protease–antiprotease imbalance leaves neutrophil elastase action unchecked, which in turn is responsible for limiting the apoptotic role of TNF (tumor necrosis factor) [27, 28]. Those who are homozygous for A1ATD usually report no to little exposure to tobacco smoke due to early diagnosis and smoking restriction and also due to the relatively shorter life expectancy [29]. The reported lower lung cancer incidence, despite severe emphysema, could be attributed to the associated severe loss of lung tissue. On the other hand, A1ATD carriers (heterozygous) were shown to have at least a 70% increased risk of lung cancer even among never smokers [30].

Linkage and genome-wide analysis studies have identified different single nucleotide polymorphisms associated with both lung cancer and COPD. One of the important loci found to be commonly implicated is 15q25, encoding for nicotinic acetyl-choline receptors [31, 32]. It is via activation of these receptors, by nicotine in tobacco smoke, that airway epithelial cells show enhanced proliferative capacity and become more resistant to apoptosis [33, 34]. Additionally, epigenetic changes among COPD patients are thought to play an important role in tumorigenesis. These changes do not involve the DNA nucleotide sequence but rather affect gene regulatory segments through biochemical changes (e.g., hypermethylation and histone deacetylation), leading to activation or deactivation of genes. This results in increased expression of oncogenes (induce cell proliferation) and inactivation of the counteractive tumor suppressor gene function facilitating carcinogenesis progression [35]. DNA hypermethylation is one of the well-reported epigenetic changes in COPD associated with lung function decline, cell hyperplasia, squamous metaplasia, and carcinoma in situ [36]. Decreased histone deacetylation is another epigenetic alteration encountered in severe COPD [37]. Histone deacetylation causes chromatin coiling around histone complexes, offering less access for RNA polymerase action and completion of the transcription process and thus functionally silencing genes that could otherwise lead to oncogenesis. Furthermore, NF-κB (nuclear factor-κB), a proinflammatory marker, is upregulated in both lung cancer and COPD [37] and is responsible for upregulating oncogenes and antiapoptotic genes, adding further evidence linking the COPD and lung cancer development [38].

Finally, micro-RNAs (miRNAs), short noncoding single-stranded RNA segments, play a role in COPD/lung cancer pathogenesis. They control protein production through binding to mRNA strands, leading to their degradation and blocking of the translation process. Some of the miRNA molecules are important for suppressing tumor progression. Previous studies have shown reduced expression of these miRNA in COPD patients; this has been linked to increased mortality among COPD patients with lung cancer [39, 40].

2.2.2 Carcinogen Retention

Tobacco smoke contains over 4,000 chemicals, of which more than 70 are known to cause, initiate, or promote cancer and are called carcinogens. Of these, polycyclic aromatic hydrocarbons and the tobacco-specific nitrosamine 4-(methylnitrosamino)-1-(3-pyridyl)-1-butanone are likely to play major roles. COPD involves destruction of the lung parenchyma and airway inflammation, causing emphysema and chronic bronchitis, respectively. This invariably results in chronic airflow limitation, a hallmark feature of the disease. This not only is manifest as air trapping and poor clearance of secretions but also leads to chronic retention of airborne carcinogens. Persistent exposure to these carcinogens will create a continuous stimulus for the airway epithelial to undergo mesenchymal transformation and bronchoalveolar stem cell stimulation, which are two central components of the carcinogenesis process [21].

2.2.3 Oxidative Stress

Tobacco smoke is a complex mixture of chemicals, many of which have an oxidative capacity capable of promoting cellular damage. The vast number of free radicals ($>10^5$ organic radicals per puff) to which a smoker is exposed play an integral role in the oxidative damage to airway and alveolar epithelial cells [41, 42]. Tobacco smoke is not the only source of reactive nitrogen oxide species (RNOS) implicated in the oxidative stress; endogenous inflammatory mediators also lead to cellular apoptosis

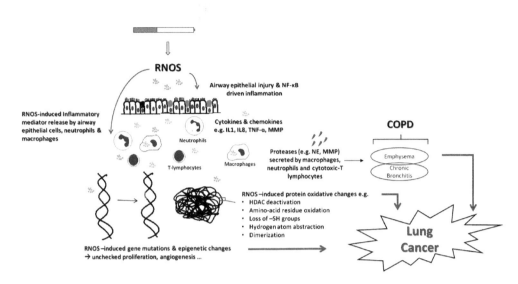

Figure 2.2   Role of oxidative stress induced by cigarette smoking and the associated inflammatory response in lung carcinogenesis. Abbreviations: RNOS, reactive nitrogen oxide species; NF-κB, nuclear factor-κB; IL, interleukin; TNF, tumor necrosis factor; MMP, matrix metalloproteinase; NE, neutrophil elastase; HDAC, histone deacetylase; COPD, chronic obstructive pulmonary disease.

and genotoxicity through DNA mutations, promoting carcinogenesis [43, 44]. RNOS can alter the structure and thus function of some proteins by changing their amino acid sequence. This can render some proteins autoantigenic, thus promoting inflammation [45]. Also, these changes are responsible for the deactivation of the histone deacetylase in COPD patients, further prolonging the inflammatory process as mentioned earlier [46] (Figure 2.2).

Aging is another important cross-linking mechanism between COPD and lung cancer, as both are diseases related to senescence. Patients with a COPD diagnosis are mostly above 40 years, with the prevalence significantly increasing with advancing age. Similarly, most of those diagnosed with lung cancer are age 65 or older. Aging is the result of two mechanisms: failure of the DNA repair mechanisms in the face of oxidative stress and shortening of telomeres (protective chromosomal nucleoprotein end caps) with every cell division that is not appropriately corrected by telomerase activity. In the normal order of things, shorter telomere length signals cell senescence–related apoptosis; however, heavily truncated telomeres also render coding DNA unstable and liable for mutations. Both aging-related mechanisms increase the risk of DNA mutations and carcinogenesis [24, 47].

2.2.4 Inflammatory Changes

Chronic systemic inflammation is estimated to affect 25% to 30% of COPD patients and is a predictor of comorbidities [48]. Given that most cancerous tissues display an inflammatory picture, with leukocytic infiltration, and that some inflammatory disease are associated with increased risk of malignancy, it is worth considering a strong linkage between the inflammatory pathways in COPD and the development of lung cancer. The process of malignant transformation and tumor progression is triggered by the persistent inflammation, which involves repeated cycles of tissue damage and repair [49]. This involves apoptosis, resulting in inflammatory cell recruitment, and tissue regeneration in which stem cells are recruited into the cell cycle with unstable DNA replicative activity susceptible to mutagenic hits from the inflammatory mediators and environmental carcinogens [50]. Unfortunately, some cells may escape the inherent protective mechanisms, accumulating genetic and epigenetic changes sufficient to cause different grades of carcinogenic changes. For example, polycyclic aromatic hydrocarbons are metabolized by Langerhans cells (found in the small airways of COPD patients in increased numbers) to carcinogenic intermediates [51, 52].

A key element in the intracellular signaling pathways in COPD is the transcription factor NF-κB, which upregulates inflammatory mediator expression and activates antiapoptotic proteins, thus increasing cell longevity and the associated risk of mutations and tumorigenesis [38, 53]. The production of NF-κB is also directly stimulated by RNOS found in tobacco smoke. Another proinflammatory signal transducer is the signal transducer and activator of transcription (STAT-3), which is also found to play a major role in COPD inflammation as well as carcinogenesis. Normally, STAT-3 is activated by phosphorylation for a short time span before being quickly dephosphorylated by protein phosphatases. However, in cancerous tissues, aberrant persistent protein activation occurs, where it induces transcription of multiple genes responsible for inhibiting apoptosis, increasing cell proliferation, angiogenesis, and evasion of the body immune system. These are central domains to the process of tumorigenesis [38].

Matrix metalloproteinases (MMPs) are proteolytic enzymes implicated in the tissue remodeling and degradation of extracellular matrix (ECM) components and thus have an important role in the development of emphysema in COPD patients. MMPs also lead to growth factor activation, in turn stimulating endothelial cell proliferation and angiogenesis [54], which are central processes in lung cancer development. Recent studies reveal that the expression of MMPs is extremely high in lung tumors compared with nonmalignant lung tissue. Theoretically, loosening the ECM makes it easier for malignant cells to spread locally and metastasize systemically [55]. Thus, MMPs, especially MMP-2, -9, and -7, may play crucial roles in invasion and metastasis of malignant tumors [56]. Furthermore, MMP inhibitors have recently been developed to prevent and treat invasion, metastasis, and angiogenesis of malignant tumors, including lung cancer.

2.3 Screening of Lung Cancer in COPD

2.3.1 Rationale

Lung cancer is the leading cause of death from malignant disease worldwide [57, 58] and specifically among COPD patients [59]. In fact, continued cigarette smoking

TABLE 2.1   COPD Lung Cancer Screening Score [60]

Variable	Points
BMI < 25 kg/m^2	1
Pack-year smoking history > 60	2
Age > 60 years	3
Presence of emphysema on LDCT scan	4
Total	10

poses an additional lung cancer risk in patients with preexisting COPD [60]. Thus, the priority of lung cancer preventive measures is smoking cessation, which can reduce the risk of lung cancer by 50% [61, 62].

Recently, screening of lung cancer among COPD patients using low-dose computed tomography (LDCT) of the chest has emerged as a technique to improve lung cancer diagnosis and burden. This technique has gradually moved from clinical trials to clinical practice. The results of many previous clinical trials all over the world have demonstrated beneficial role of using LDCT in terms of detecting lung cancer at an earlier stage [63–66]. There has been always a debate between the need for CT and its cost-effectiveness. Different criteria have been set to identify patients with COPD who would require LDCT to screen for lung cancer. In one study, independent predictors of lung cancer among COPD patients included disease severity (i.e. Global Initiative for Chronic Obstructive Lung Disease (GOLD) stage), age, body mass index (BMI), and diffusion capacity of the lung for carbon monoxide (D_LCO) [67]. The same group of investigators developed a score to predict lung cancer risk for patients with COPD: the COPD-specific score (COPD-LUCSS) (Table 2.1). The score ranges between 0 and 10 and is determined by pack-year smoking history > 60, age > 60, BMI < 25 kg/m^2, and presence of radiological emphysema [60]. Patients were stratified based on COPD-LUCSS score into two categories—low risk (0–6) and high risk (6–10)—with a 3.5-fold increase in lung cancer risk among patients in the high-risk category. Stratification of patients will help in deciding about the frequency of screening CT; with patients in the low-risk category requiring less frequent imaging and thus reducing associated costs and side effects.

The question that remains is, who are the patients who should be screened? Based on the National Lung Screening Trial (NLST), high-risk individuals included current or former (at least for 15 years) cigarette smokers between the ages of 55 and 74, with at least a 30-pack-years smoking history. On the other hand, the National Comprehensive Cancer Network screening recommendations are based on lower-level evidence, in individuals age 50 or older, with at least a 20 pack-year smoking history and one additional risk factor (e.g., family history of lung cancer, radon exposure, and occupational exposure to silica, cadmium, asbestos, arsenic, beryllium, chromium, diesel fumes, and nickel) [68]. The American College of Chest Physician follows a closely similar protocol with age criteria of 55 to 79 years and at least a 30-pack-year smoking history [69–73]. In 1993, the Early Lung Cancer Action Project (ELCAP) initiated a study of the early diagnosis of lung cancer in cigarette smokers

TABLE 2.2   Different Eligibility Criteria for LDCT Screening for Lung Cancer Among COPD [69–73]

Organization	Year Published	Smoking Status	Pack-Year Smoking History	Age (Years)
American Association for Thoracic Surgery	2012	Any active or former smoker	At least 30 → At least 20 →	55–79 50–79[a]
American Cancer Society[b]	2013	Active smoker or quit within the past 15 years	At least 30	55–74
American College of Chest Physicians	2013	Active smoker or quit within the past 15 years	At least 30	55–74
National Comprehensive Cancer Network	2015	Active smoker or quit within the past 15 years	At least 30 → At least 20 →	55–74 ≥50[c]
American College of Chest Physicians	2018	Active smoker or quit within the past 15 years	At least 30	55–77

[a]Age 50 to 79 years with a 20-pack-year smoking history and additional comorbidity that produces a cumulative risk of developing lung cancer ≥5% in 5 years.

[b]Exclusion criteria: life-limiting comorbid conditions, metallic implants or devices in the chest or back, and requirement for home oxygen supplementation.

[c]Additional risk factor: cancer history (survivors of lung cancer, lymphomas, head and neck cancer, or smoking-related cancers), family history of lung cancer, COPD or pulmonary fibrosis, radon exposure, or occupational exposure (silica, cadmium, asbestos, arsenic, beryllium, chromium, diesel fumes, and nickel).

with the use of annual screening with spiral CT [63, 74]. Using their earlier studies, they have provided more inclusive guidelines to include individuals 40 years of age and older with either a history of cigarette smoking, occupational exposure (to asbestos, beryllium, uranium, or radon), or exposure to secondhand smoke [75]. In this regard, the U.S. Preventive Services Task Force recommended that screening should not be offered to people who have substantial comorbid conditions with limited life expectancy [76]. Table 2.2 summarizes different recommendation guidelines for screening for lung cancer in COPD [69–73].

2.3.2 Significance and Effect on Lung Cancer Epidemiology

Screening for lung cancer among smokers with COPD will certainly result in early detection of cancer with potential positive outcomes. But weighing the risks and benefits when deciding about screening for lung cancer in COPD patients has always been an issue of discussion. Additionally, overdiagnosis in the presence of an indolent disease is always a theoretical concern. In one study by Patz et al. using a cohort from the NLST study [77], more than 18.5% of all lung cancers diagnosed by LDCT seemed to be indolent (i.e., risk of overdiagnosis). Another retrospective study has also identified potentially overdiagnosed lung cancer as slow-growing or indolent lesions [78]. Overdiagnosis will lead to a further risk of overuse of invasive techniques as well as overtreatment with the resultant rise in the financial burden on health systems.

Therefore, some suggest a more conservative "wait and see" approach [79]; however, physicians should be cautious using this approach, as the growth rate of some cases of indolent cancer can increase markedly from one scan to the next [80]. One more point is the risk of complications with multiple use of LDCT. The exposure to LDCT itself does not carry a significantly harmful radiation dose. However, with multiple screens over years, there is a nonnegligible risk of radiation-induced lung cancer. One study has suggested that 1 in every 2,500 persons screened with LDCT will develop radiation-induced cancer [81]. A more recent study concluded that one radiation-induced major cancer would be expected for every 108 lung cancers detected through screening [82]. This risk of radiation-induced lung cancer is unquestionably nonnegligible but may be considered acceptable considering the substantial mortality reduction associated with screening.

On the other bright side of the use of LDCT, in the ELCAP study, annual screening proved lung cancer diagnosis in almost 80% of smokers [83]. They have shown that over 80% of patients who have a lung cancer detected by CT screening can be cured, which means that these patients were diagnosed at early, curable stages of the disease. Early detection of lung cancer will improve patients' outcomes. In this regard, the NLST demonstrated that lung cancer screening with LDCT significantly reduces lung cancer mortality [84]. This supports the notion that screening high-risk COPD patients may be more advantageous than not and leads us to the fact that early detection of COPD can also be beneficial in identifying high-risk patients.

2.4 Early Detection of COPD

It is well known that COPD, *especially in its early stages*, is often not recognized by patients and is underdiagnosed by caregivers and consequently undertreated. For a long time, diagnosis of the disease relied mainly on the detection of fixed airflow obstruction on spirometry in symptomatic smokers who sought medical advice. Even though spirometry is the gold standard initial investigation, some studies reported that primary care physicians included spirometry in their assessment in only a minority of symptomatic smokers [85–88]. Spirometry is simple, reproducible and more importantly widely available. But its combination with symptoms, novel physiological tests, and imaging techniques yields better diagnosis even before the appearance of overt airflow obstruction on spirometry.

2.4.1 Clinical Presentation

Dyspnea is the most common symptom in patients with COPD, especially those with radiological emphysema. Unfortunately, patients with mild airflow obstruction may underestimate their disease, and the symptoms are not elicited until the respiratory system is stressed (e.g., during exercise). Other symptoms include chronic cough and phlegm production, which point to a diagnosis of chronic bronchitis rather than emphysema. Some patients report the combination of the three as their troublesome symptoms. Van Schayck et al. examined the role of cross-sectional case findings for subjects with a history of cigarette smoking who were at risk for developing COPD using a standardized symptoms questionnaire and spirometry [89]. Eighteen percent of the participants had airway obstruction, and when smokers were preselected based on respiratory symptoms, such as chronic cough, the percentage of smokers with airway obstruction increased to 48% among those over 60 years of age. The positive predictive value of having at least two respiratory symptoms, including cough, dyspnea, or wheezes, was 29%. In patients with all three symptoms, the prevalence of airflow obstruction was 35%. Therefore, it is recommended that pulmonary function testing be performed in all smokers with chronic respiratory symptoms. These results suggest that current or former smokers age 60 years or older and who have some respiratory symptoms should be screened for COPD by pulmonary function testing. Clearly, the diagnosis of COPD, especially in smokers with mild airflow obstruction, should not rely solely on spirometry, and the addition of further physiological tests (e.g., lung volume assessment and tests for small airway function) and imaging techniques (e.g., CT scan) is usually necessary.

2.4.2 Physiological Tests

Spirometry in the initial physiological test used to diagnose smokers with COPD. A fixed ratio of forced expiratory volume in 1 second over forced vital capacity (FEV_1/FVC) of less than 0.7 is diagnostic for large airway obstruction [90]. Caution should be taken to use only post-bronchodilator values. Also, the results must be compared to the reported lower limit of normal (LLN) values based on age, gender, and ethnicity to avoid over- or underdiagnosis in elderly and young individuals, respectively [91–95]. In this regard, a recent study showed that the combination of post-bronchodilator fixed ratio and LLN criteria together with FEV_1 values were strongly linked to relevant clinical outcomes [96]. Smokers with early COPD may have normal or near normal spirometry; thus, significant derangements can be missed. In this category of smokers, the addition of further physiological tests that assess specifically the function of small airways (<2 mm in diameter) might be beneficial.

The most famous measure of small airway dysfunction is reduced maximal mid-expiratory flow between 25% and 75% of FVC (FEF_{25-75}). Although it is an easy, widely available spirometric measure, it also shows wide variability, which may limit its use [97]. Instead, the use of another spirometric value (ratio between FEV in 3 seconds and 6 seconds, i.e., FEV_3/FVC_6) has been proposed as an alternative measure of small airway dysfunction and was found to be abnormal in 15% of a large data set of smokers with normal FEV_1/FVC (higher than LLN) [97, 98]. Today, there has been a renewed interest in using the old "nitrogen (N_2) washout" test in early detection of small airway disease, and the introduction of impulse oscillometry has also been extensively used in physiological studies to assess small airways [99, 100].

Furthermore, the use of graduated cardiopulmonary exercise testing in early stages of COPD may help uncover severe symptoms and hidden respiratory and cardiocirculatory derangements. Several previous physiological studies have shown

increased ventilatory requirements and respiratory mechanical abnormalities in
early COPD during symptom-limited incremental exercise when compared to age-
matched healthy non-smokers [101–104]. These abnormal findings may guide a clinician toward the need for further testing and follow-up even in smokers with normal
spirometry [105, 106]. The recent advances in physiological techniques help uncover
significant abnormalities in patients with COPD that are sometimes hidden using
simple spirometry. Collectively, this will help in early detection of COPD, which will
impact the early discovery of lung cancer among high-risk patients.

2.4.3 Chest Imaging

Although spirometry is the gold standard test used to diagnose COPD, the use of chest
imaging (mainly CT scan) has recently been expanded for both clinical and research
purposes. Thoracic imaging provides more sensitive and specific measurements that
potentially help to separate different COPD phenotypes. The use of CT in early diagnosis of COPD is evolving. With the use of advanced programming, radiologists are
currently able to identify structural and functional damage to the airways, alveoli,
and pulmonary vasculature before the appearance of overt spirometric abnormalities. CT enables visualization of structural derangements and hence anatomic localization of disease in contrast to spirometry, which is a more global measure. Visual
analysis can identify the overall degree of emphysema as well as emphysema subtypes
[107]. Additionally, emphysema can be accurately quantified using automated density
mask analysis via quantifying the low attenuating areas on inspiratory scan. Tissue
attenuation is measured by Hounsfield units (HU) on inspiratory images obtained at
total lung capacity (Figure 2.3). Thresholds of −910 HU and −950 HU have been used
to quantify mild and severe emphysema, respectively [108–110].

(a)   (b)

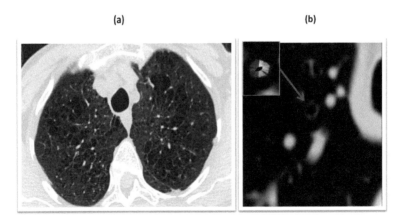

Figure 2.3 Computed tomography scans identifying structural abnormalities in an example patient with mild COPD. Panel (a) shows bilateral upper lobar centrilobular emphysema
that was quantified using density mask analysis. Panel (b) shows analysis of large airway
dimensions with the ability of measuring airway wall area and thickness.

In addition to the role of CT in early detection of emphysema, it can also identify COPD patients with airway-dominant disease. It is well known that small airways are the major site of obstruction on COPD, but this cannot be easily visualized on CT scans. Density mask analysis on expiratory scan is used to identify gas trapping, a marker of small airway remodeling and increased small airway resistance. The most accepted threshold for gas trapping, assessed on expiratory scans, is −856 HU, though other thresholds have also been used [111]. This measure of gas trapping using CT scan has been shown to correlate strongly with spirometrically measured airflow obstruction [112]. Larger airways can be easily identified on CT scans with the ability to measure airway wall thickness, airway wall area, and square roots of the wall areas of hypothetical airways with internal perimeters of 10 and 15 mm (Pi10 and Pi15, respectively) (Figure 2.3). CT measures of large airway abnormalities correlate with FEV_1 and bronchodilator responsiveness and are associated with subsequent lung function decline [113–115]. Previous studies have also confirmed abnormalities in these measurements in patients with only mild COPD and in smokers without COPD but with respiratory symptoms [103, 104, 116]. Collectively, the novel CT measures and programming tools have broadened its use in clinical practice and helped identify patients with COPD even before the appearance of spirometric abnormalities.

2.5 Can We Prevent Lung Cancer?

As outlined above, smoking is closely linked to the occurrence of lung cancer. As such, smoking cessation seems to be the most effective way to reduce the risk of lung cancer. Early smoking cessation may be associated with a better chance of lung tissue repair and minimize continuous exposure to carcinogens. A large longitudinal study by Anthonisen et al. showed that 33% of asymptomatic smokers with mild to moderate COPD had died of lung cancer after a 14.5-year follow-up [62]. They reported that all-cause mortality was significantly lower in a special smoking cessation intervention group than in the usual-care group, though the difference was not statistically significant. There were some suggestions that healthy diet rich in vegetables may help protect against lung cancer in both smokers and non-smokers. In fact, attempts to prevent lung cancer with vitamins or other treatments have not worked. For example, beta-carotene, a drug related to vitamin A, has been tested for the prevention of lung cancer. It did not reduce the risk of cancer. Surprisingly, in people who continued to smoke, beta-carotene increased the risk of lung cancer [117]. Given the important role of chronic inflammation in cancer development outlined earlier, the use of anti-inflammatory agents in lung cancer prevention has been the subject of many previous trials with different controversial results. There are some reports that regular use of inhaled corticosteroids may reduce the risk of lung cancer among former smokers with COPD [118, 119]; however, this was rejected by other studies [120, 121].

Lung cancer screening is one method for second-line cancer prevention with the most important primary end point being reducing cancer-related mortality. Screening for lung cancer among COPD patients will not help in the prevention of its occurrence but will help in its early identification and proper management. Furthermore, the use of LDCT will also identify smokers with emphysema (i.e., high-risk patients), who should be followed regularly by LDCT for the early detection of lung cancer. As some people have a genetic predisposition for lung cancer, people whose first-degree relatives have lung cancer could have a higher risk of developing lung cancer themselves and should be regularly screened.

2.6 Summary

Both COPD and lung cancer are major leading causes of morbidity and mortality worldwide and incur significant economic burden. Thus, early detection of both disease conditions is crucial and will have potential positive outcomes. The use of novel physiological tests (both at rest and during exercise) and new imaging tools can identify smokers with COPD even before overt airflow obstruction is manifested in spirometry. Early diagnosis of COPD will help identify high-risk patients (e.g., those with emphysema) and the best candidates who may require regular follow-up and screening for lung cancer using LDCT. Physicians should carefully determine smokers eligible for lung cancer screening using LDCT via reviewing recent guidelines and weighing risks versus benefits.

References

1. Collaborators GBDCRD. Global, regional, and national deaths, prevalence, disability-adjusted life years, and years lived with disability for chronic obstructive pulmonary disease and asthma, 1990–2015: a systematic analysis for the Global Burden of Disease Study 2015. *Lancet Respir Med.* 2017;5(9):691–706.
2. Guarascio AJ, Ray SM, Finch CK, Self TH. The clinical and economic burden of chronic obstructive pulmonary disease in the USA. *Clinicoecon Outcomes Res.* 2013;5:235.
3. Gibson GJ, Loddenkemper R, Sibille Y, Lundbäck B. *The European Lung White Book: Respiratory Health and Disease in Europe.* Sheffield, England: European Respiratory Society; 2013.
4. Chen W, FitzGerald JM, Sin DD, Sadatsafavi M. Excess economic burden of comorbidities in COPD: a 15-year population-based study. *Eur Respir J.* 2017;50(1).pii:1700393.
5. Tachkov K, Kamusheva M, Pencheva V, Mitov K. Evaluation of the economic and social burden of chronic obstructive pulmonary disease (COPD). *Biotechnol Biotechnol Equip* 2017;31(4):855–861.
6. Ferlay J, Soerjomataram I, Dikshit R, et al. Cancer incidence and mortality worldwide: sources, methods and major patterns in GLOBOCAN 2012. *Int J Cancer.* 2015;136(5):E359-86.
7. Allemani C, Weir HK, Carreira H, et al. Global surveillance of cancer survival 1995–2009: analysis of individual data for 25 676 887 patients from 279 population-based registries in 67 countries (CONCORD-2). *Lancet.* 2015;385(9972):977–1010.
8. Wong MC, Lao XQ, Ho K-F, Goggins WB, Shelly L. Incidence and mortality of lung cancer: global trends and association with socioeconomic status. *Sci Rep.* 2017;7(1):14300.
9. Adler I. *Primary Malignant Growths of the Lungs and Bronchi.* London, England: Longmans, Green, and Company; 1912.

10. Skillrud DM, Offord KP, Miller RD. Higher risk of lung cancer in chronic obstructive pulmonary disease. A prospective, matched, controlled study. *Ann Intern Med.* 1986;105(4):503–507.

11. Tockman MS, Anthonisen NR, Wright EC, Donithan MG. Airways obstruction and the risk for lung cancer. *Ann Intern Med.* 1987;106(4):512–518.

12. Kuller LH, Ockene J, Meilahn E, Svendsen KH. Relation of forced expiratory volume in one second (FEV1) to lung cancer mortality in the Multiple Risk Factor Intervention Trial (MRFIT). *Am J Epidemiol.* 1990;132(2):265–274.

13. Wilson DO, Weissfeld JL, Balkan A, et al. Association of radiographic emphysema and airflow obstruction with lung cancer. *Am J Respir Crit Care Med.* 2008;178(7):738–744.

14. Zulueta JJ. Emphysema and lung cancer. More than a coincidence. *Ann Am Thorac Soc.* 2015;12(8):1120–1121.

15. de Torres JP, Bastarrika G, Wisnivesky JP, et al. Assessing the relationship between lung cancer risk and emphysema detected on low-dose CT of the chest. *Chest.* 2007;132(6):1932–1938.

16. Kinsey CM, Estépar RSJ, Wei Y, Washko GR, Christiani DC. Regional emphysema of a non–small cell tumor is associated with larger tumors and decreased survival rates. *Ann Am Thorac Soc.* 2015;12(8):1197–1205.

17. Henschke CI, Yip R, Boffetta P, et al. CT screening for lung cancer: importance of emphysema for never smokers and smokers. *Lung Cancer.* 2015;88(1):42–47.

18. Young RP, Hopkins RJ, Christmas T, Black PN, Metcalf P, Gamble G. COPD prevalence is increased in lung cancer, independent of age, sex and smoking history. *Eur Respir J.* 2009;34(2):380–386.

19. Samet JM, Avila-Tang E, Boffetta P, et al. Lung cancer in never smokers: clinical epidemiology and environmental risk factors. *Clin Cancer Res.* 2009;15(18):5626–5645.

20. Durham AL, Adcock IM. The relationship between COPD and lung cancer. *Lung Cancer.* 2015;90(2):121–127.

21. Houghton AM, Mouded M, Shapiro SD. Common origins of lung cancer and COPD. *Nat Med.* 2008;14(10):1023.

22. Rooney C, Sethi T. The epithelial cell and lung cancer: the link between chronic obstructive pulmonary disease and lung cancer. *Respiration.* 2011;81(2):89–104.

23. Adcock IM, Caramori G, Barnes PJ. Chronic obstructive pulmonary disease and lung cancer: new molecular insights. *Respiration.* 2011;81(4):265–284.

24. Caramori G, Adcock IM, Casolari P, et al. Unbalanced oxidant-induced DNA damage and repair in COPD: a link towards lung cancer. *Thorax.* 2011;66(6):521–527.

25. Mannino DM, Buist AS. Global burden of COPD: risk factors, prevalence, and future trends. *Lancet.* 2007;370(9589):765–773.

26. Stoller JK, Aboussouan LS. α1-antitrypsin deficiency. *Lancet.* 2005;365(9478):2225–2236.

27. Rath PC, Aggarwal BB. TNF-induced signaling in apoptosis. *J Clin Immunol.* 1999;19(6):350–364.

28. Sun Z, Yang P. Role of imbalance between neutrophil elastase and alpha 1-antitrypsin in cancer development and progression. *Lancet Oncol.* 2004;5(3):182–190.

29. Tanash HA, Nilsson PM, Nilsson J-Å, Piitulainen E. Survival in severe alpha-1-antitrypsin deficiency (PiZZ). *Respiratory Res.* 2010;11(1):44.

30. Yang P, Sun Z, Krowka MJ, et al. Alpha1-antitrypsin deficiency carriers, tobacco smoke, chronic obstructive pulmonary disease, and lung cancer risk. *Arch Intern Med.* 2008;168(10):1097–1103.

31. Hung RJ, McKay JD, Gaborieau V, et al. A susceptibility locus for lung cancer maps to nicotinic acetylcholine receptor subunit genes on 15q25. *Nature.* 2008;452(7187):633.

32. Amos CI, Wu X, Broderick P, et al. Genome-wide association scan of tag SNPs identifies a susceptibility locus for lung cancer at 15q25. 1. *Nat. Genet.* 2008;40(5):616.

33. West KA, Brognard J, Clark AS, et al. Rapid Akt activation by nicotine and a tobacco carcinogen modulates the phenotype of normal human airway epithelial cells. *J Clin Invest.* 2003;111(1):81–90.

34. Schaal C, Chellappan SP. Nicotine-mediated cell proliferation and tumor progression in smoking-related cancers. *Mol Cancer Res.* 2014;12(1):14–23.

35. Sato M, Shames DS, Gazdar AF, Minna JD. A translational view of the molecular pathogenesis of lung cancer. *J Thorac Oncol.* 2007;2(4):327–343.

36. Sundar IK, Mullapudi N, Yao H, Spivack SD, Rahman I. Lung cancer and its association with chronic obstructive pulmonary disease: update on nexus of epigenetics. *Curr Opin Pulm Med.* 2011;17(4):279.

37. Ito K, Ito M, Elliott WM, et al. Decreased histone deacetylase activity in chronic obstructive pulmonary disease. *NEJM.* 2005;352(19):1967–1976.

38. Lee H, Herrmann A, Deng J-H, et al. Persistently activated Stat3 maintains constitutive NF-κB activity in tumors. *Cancer Cell.* 2009;15(4):283–293.

39. Pottelberge GRV, Mestdagh P, Bracke KR, et al. MicroRNA expression in induced sputum of smokers and patients with chronic obstructive pulmonary disease. *Am J Respir Crit Care Med.* 2011;183(7):898–906.

40. Takamizawa J, Konishi H, Yanagisawa K, et al. Reduced expression of the let-7 microRNAs in human lung cancers in association with shortened postoperative survival. *Cancer Res.* 2004;64(11):3753–3756.

41. Church DF, Pryor WA. Free-radical chemistry of cigarette smoke and its toxicological implications. *Environ Health Perspect.* 1985;64:111–126.

42. Pryor WA, Stone K. Oxidants in cigarette smoke radicals, hydrogen peroxide, peroxynitrate, and peroxynitritea. *Ann N Y Acad Sci.* 1993;686(1):12–27.

43. Kawanishi S, Ohnishi S, Ma N, Hiraku Y, Murata M. Crosstalk between DNA damage and inflammation in the multiple steps of carcinogenesis. *Int J Mol Sci.* 2017;18(8). pii: E1808.

44. Coussens LM, Werb Z. Inflammation and cancer. *Nature.* 2002;420(6917):860.

45. Kirkham PA, Caramori G, Casolari P, et al. Oxidative stress–induced antibodies to carbonyl-modified protein correlate with severity of chronic obstructive pulmonary disease. *Am J Respir Crit Care Med.* 2011;184(7):796–802.

46. Osoata GO, Yamamura S, Ito M, et al. Nitration of distinct tyrosine residues causes inactivation of histone deacetylase 2. *Biochem Biophys Res Commun.* 2009;384(3):366–371.

47. Morlá M, Busquets X, Pons J, Sauleda J, MacNee W, Agustí AGN. Telomere shortening in smokers with and without COPD. *Eur Respir J.* 2006;27(3):525–528.

48. Miller J, Edwards LD, Agusti A, et al. Comorbidity, systemic inflammation and outcomes in the ECLIPSE cohort. *Respir Med.* 2013;107(9):1376–1384.

49. Vakkila J, Lotze MT. Inflammation and necrosis promote tumour growth. *Nat Rev Immunol.* 2004;4(8):641.

50. Ferguson LR, Laing WA. Chronic inflammation, mutation and human disease. *Mutat Res.* 2010; 690(1–2):1–2.

51. Modi BG, Neustadter J, Binda E, et al. Langerhans cells facilitate epithelial DNA damage and squamous cell carcinoma. *Science.* 2012;335(6064):104–108.

52. Van Pottelberge GR, Bracke KR, Demedts IK, et al. Selective accumulation of langerhans-type dendritic cells in small airways of patients with COPD. *Respir Res.* 2010;11(1):35.

53. Di Stefano A, Caramori G, Oates T, et al. Increased expression of nuclear factor-κB in bronchial biopsies from smokers and patients with COPD. *Eur Respir J.* 2002;20(3):556–563.

54. Kessenbrock K, Plaks V, Werb Z. Matrix metalloproteinases: regulators of the tumor microenvironment. *Cell.* 2010;141(1):52–67.

55. Yao H, Rahman I. Current concepts on the role of inflammation in COPD and lung cancer. *Curr Opin Pharmacol.* 2009;9(4):375–383.

56. Curran S, Murray GI. Matrix metalloproteinases: molecular aspects of their roles in tumour invasion and metastasis. *Eur J Cancer.* 2000;36(13):1621–1630.

57. Spiro SG, Silvestri GA. One hundred years of lung cancer. *Am J Respir Crit Care Med.* 2005;172(5):523–529.

58. Shlomi D, Ben-Avi R, Balmor GR, Onn A, Peled N. *Screening for Lung Cancer: Time for Large-Scale Screening by Chest Computed Tomography.* Sheffield, England: European Respiratory Society; 2014.

59. Sin DD, Anthonisen NR, Soriano JB, Agusti A. Mortality in COPD: role of comorbidities. *Eur Respir J.* 2006;28(6):1245–1257.

60. de-Torres JP, Wilson DO, Sanchez-Salcedo P, et al. Lung cancer in patients with chronic obstructive pulmonary disease. Development and validation of the COPD Lung Cancer Screening Score. *Am J Respir Crit Care Med.* 2015;191(3):285–291.

61. Godtfredsen NS, Prescott E, Osler M. Effect of smoking reduction on lung cancer risk. *JAMA.* 2005;294(12):1505–1510.

62. Anthonisen NR, Skeans MA, Wise RA, Manfreda J, Kanner RE, Connett JE. The effects of a smoking cessation intervention on 14.5-year mortality: a randomized clinical trial. *Ann Intern Med.* 2005;142(4):233–239.

63. Henschke CI, McCauley DI, Yankelevitz DF, et al. Early Lung Cancer Action Project: overall design and findings from baseline screening. *Lancet.* 1999;354(9173):99–105.

64. Kaneko M, Eguchi K, Ohmatsu H, et al. Peripheral lung cancer: screening and detection with low-dose spiral CT versus radiography. *Radiology.* 1996;201(3):798–802.

65. Sone S, Takashima S, Li F, et al. Mass screening for lung cancer with mobile spiral computed tomography scanner. *Lancet.* 1998;351(9111):1242–1245.

66. Nawa T, Nakagawa T, Kusano S, Kawasaki Y, Sugawara Y, Nakata H. Lung cancer screening using low-dose spiral CT: results of baseline and 1-year follow-up studies. *Chest.* 2002;122(1):15–20.

67. de Torres JP, Marín JM, Casanova C, et al. Lung cancer in patients with chronic obstructive pulmonary disease: incidence and predicting factors. *Am J Respir Crit Care Med.* 2011;184(8):913–919.

68. Wood DE, Eapen GA, Ettinger DS, et al. Lung cancer screening. *J Natl Compr Canc Netw.* 2012;10(2):240–265.

69. Wender R, Fontham ET, Barrera E, et al. American Cancer Society lung cancer screening guidelines. *CA Cancer J Clin.* 2013;63(2):106–117.

70. Jaklitsch MT, Jacobson FL, Austin JH, et al. The American Association for Thoracic Surgery guidelines for lung cancer screening using low-dose computed tomography scans for lung cancer survivors and other high-risk groups. *J Thorac Cardiovasc Surg.* 2012;144(1):33–38.

71. Detterbeck FC, Mazzone PJ, Naidich DP, Bach PB. Screening for lung cancer: diagnosis and management of lung cancer: American College of Chest Physicians evidence-based clinical practice guidelines. *Chest.* 2013;143(5):e78S–e92S.

72. Wood DE. National Comprehensive Cancer Network (NCCN) Clinical Practice Guidelines for Lung Cancer Screening. *Thorac Surg Clin.* 2015;25(2):185–197.

73. Mazzone PJ, Silvestri GA, Patel S, et al. Screening for lung cancer: CHEST guideline and expert panel report. *Chest*. 2018;153(4):954-985.

74. Henschke CI, Naidich DP, Yankelevitz DF, et al. Early lung cancer action project: initial findings on repeat screenings. *Cancer*. 2001;92(1):153–159.

75. Henschke C, Yankelevitz D, Miettinen O. CT screening for lung cancer: survival upon stage I diagnosis. *N Engl J Med*. 2006;355:1763–1771.

76. Moyer VA. Screening for lung cancer: U.S. Preventive Services Task Force recommendation statement. *Ann Intern Med*. 2014;160(5):330–338.

77. Patz EF, Pinsky P, Gatsonis C, et al. Overdiagnosis in low-dose computed tomography screening for lung cancer. *JAMA Intern Med*. 2014;174(2):269–274.

78. Veronesi G, Maisonneuve P, Bellomi M, et al. Estimating overdiagnosis in low-dose computed tomography screening for lung cancer: a cohort study. *Ann Intern Med*. 2012;157(11):776–784.

79. Yankelevitz DF, Reeves AP, Kostis WJ, Zhao B, Henschke CI. Small pulmonary nodules: volumetrically determined growth rates based on CT evaluation. *Radiology*. 2000;217(1):251–256.

80. Lindell RM, Hartman TE, Swensen SJ, Jett JR, Midthun DE, Mandrekar JN. 5-year lung cancer screening experience: growth curves of 18 lung cancers compared to histologic type, CT attenuation, stage, survival, and size. *Chest*. 2009;136(6):1586–1595.

81. Bach PB, Mirkin JN, Oliver TK, et al. Benefits and harms of CT screening for lung cancer: a systematic review. *JAMA*. 2012;307(22):2418–2429.

82. Rampinelli C, De Marco P, Origgi D, et al. Exposure to low dose computed tomography for lung cancer screening and risk of cancer: secondary analysis of trial data and risk-benefit analysis. *BMJ*. 2017;356:j347.

83. Henschke CI, Yankelevitz DF, Smith JP, et al. CT screening for lung cancer: assessing a regimen's diagnostic performance. *Clin Imaging*. 2004;28(5):317–321.

84. The National Lung Screening Trial Research Team. Reduced lung-cancer mortality with low-dose computed tomographic screening. *N Engl J Med*. 2011;365(5):395–409.

85. Chapman KR, Tashkin DP, Pye DJ. Gender bias in the diagnosis of COPD. *Chest*. 2001;119(6):1691–1695.

86. Walters JA, Hansen E, Mudge P, Johns DP, Walters EH, Wood-Baker R. Barriers to the use of spirometry in general practice. *Aust Fam Phys*. 2005;34(3):201–203.

87. Walters JA, Hansen EC, Walters EH, Wood-Baker R. Under-diagnosis of chronic obstructive pulmonary disease: a qualitative study in primary care. *Resp Med*. 2008;102(5):738–743.

88. Nishi SP, Wang Y, Kuo Y-F, Goodwin JS, Sharma G. Spirometry use among older adults with chronic obstructive pulmonary disease: 1999–2008. *Ann Am Thorac Soc*. 2013;10(6):565–573.

89. Van Schayck C, Loozen J, Wagena E, Akkermans R, Wesseling G. Detecting patients at a high risk of developing chronic obstructive pulmonary disease in general practice: cross sectional case finding study. *BMJ*. 2002;324(7350):1370.

90. Vogelmeier CF, Criner GJ, Martinez FJ, et al. Global Strategy for the Diagnosis, Management, and Prevention of Chronic Obstructive Lung Disease 2017 Report. GOLD Executive Summary. *Am J Respir Crit Care Med*. 2017;195(5):557–582.

91. Güder G, Brenner S, Angermann CE, et al. GOLD or lower limit of normal definition? a comparison with expert-based diagnosis of chronic obstructive pulmonary disease in a prospective cohort-study. *Respir Res*. 2012;13(1):13.

92. Schermer TR, Smeele I, Thoonen B, et al. Current clinical guideline definitions of airflow obstruction and COPD overdiagnosis in primary care. *Eur Respir J*. 2008;32(4):945–952.

93. James E, Hansen J, Sun X, Wasserman K. Spirometric criteria for airway obstruction. *Chest*. 2007;131:349–355.
94. Joo MJ, Au DH, Fitzgibbon ML, McKell J, Lee TA. Determinants of spirometry use and accuracy of COPD diagnosis in primary care. *J Gen Int Med*. 2011;26(11):1272.
95. Quanjer PH, Stanojevic S, Cole TJ, et al. Multi-ethnic reference values for spirometry for the 3–95-yr age range: the global lung function 2012 equations. *Eur Respir J*. 2012; 40(6):1324–1343.
96. van Dijk W, Tan W, Li P, et al. Clinical relevance of fixed ratio vs lower limit of normal of FEV1/FVC in COPD: patient-reported outcomes from the CanCOLD cohort. *Ann Fam Med*. 2015;13(1):41–48.
97. Hansen JE, Sun X-G, Wasserman K. Discriminating measures and normal values for expiratory obstruction. *Chest*. 2006;129(2):369–377.
98. Dilektasli AG, Porszasz J, Casaburi R, et al. A novel spirometric measure identifies mild COPD unidentified by standard criteria. *Chest*. 2016;150(5):1080–1090.
99. Buist AS. Early detection of airways obstruction by the closing volume technique. *Chest*. 1973;64(4):495–499.
100. Crim C, Celli B, Edwards LD, et al. Respiratory system impedance with impulse oscillometry in healthy and COPD subjects: ECLIPSE baseline results. *Resp Med*. 2011;105(7):1069–1078.
101. Ofir D, Laveneziana P, Webb KA, Lam Y-M, O'Donnell DE. Mechanisms of dyspnea during cycle exercise in symptomatic patients with GOLD stage I chronic obstructive pulmonary disease. *Am J Respir Crit Care Med*. 2008;177(6):622–629.
102. Guenette JA, Chin RC, Cheng S, et al. Mechanisms of exercise intolerance in global initiative for chronic obstructive lung disease grade 1 COPD. *Eur Respir J*. 2014;44(5):1177–1187.
103. Elbehairy AF, Raghavan N, Cheng S, et al. Physiologic characterization of the chronic bronchitis phenotype in GOLD grade IB COPD. *Chest*. 2015;147(5):1235–1245.
104. Elbehairy AF, Ciavaglia CE, Webb KA, et al. Pulmonary gas exchange abnormalities in mild chronic obstructive pulmonary disease. Implications for dyspnea and exercise intolerance. *Am J Respir Crit Care Med*. 2015;191(12):1384–1394.
105. Di Marco F, Terraneo S, Job S, et al. Cardiopulmonary exercise testing and second-line pulmonary function tests to detect obstructive pattern in symptomatic smokers with borderline spirometry. *Respir Med*. 2017;127:7–13.
106. Elbehairy AF, Guenette JA, Faisal A, et al. Mechanisms of exertional dyspnoea in symptomatic smokers without COPD. *Eur Respir J*. 2016;48(3):694–705.
107. Lynch DA, Austin JH, Hogg JC, et al. CT-definable subtypes of chronic obstructive pulmonary disease: a statement of the Fleischner Society. *Radiology*. 2015;277(1):192–205.
108. Gould G, Redpath A, Ryan M, et al. Lung CT density correlates with measurements of airflow limitation and the diffusing capacity. *Eur Respir J*. 1991;4(2):141–146.
109. Gould GA, MacNee W, McLean A, et al. CT measurements of lung density in life can quantitate distal airspace enlargement—an essential defining feature of human emphysema. *Am Rev Respir Dis*. 1988;137(2):380–392.
110. Müller NL, Staples CA, Miller RR, Abboud RT. "Density Mask". *Chest*. 94(4):782–787.
111. Foreman MG, Zhang L, Murphy J, et al. Early-onset chronic obstructive pulmonary disease is associated with female sex, maternal factors, and African American race in the COPDGene Study. *Am J Respir Crit Care Med*. 2011;184(4):414–420.
112. Hersh CP, Washko GR, Estépar RSJ, et al. Paired inspiratory-expiratory chest CT scans to assess for small airways disease in COPD. *Resp Res*. 2013;14(1):42.

113. Hoesein FAM, de Jong PA, Lammers JW, et al. Airway wall thickness associated with forced expiratory volume in 1 second decline and development of airflow limitation. *Eur Respir J.* 2015;45(3):644–651.

114. Mohamed Hoesein FA, de Jong PA, Lammers JW, et al. Contribution of CT quantified emphysema, air trapping and airway wall thickness on pulmonary function in male smokers with and without COPD. *COPD.* 2014;11(5):503–509.

115. Kim V, Desai P, Newell JD, et al. Airway wall thickness is increased in COPD patients with bronchodilator responsiveness. *Resp Res.* 2014;15(1):84.

116. Bankier AA, De Maertelaer V, Keyzer C, Gevenois PA. Pulmonary emphysema: subjective visual grading versus objective quantification with macroscopic morphometry and thin-section CT densitometry. *Radiology.* 1999;211(3):851–858.

117. Omenn GS, Goodman GE, Thornquist MD, et al. Effects of a combination of beta carotene and vitamin A on lung cancer and cardiovascular disease. *N Engl J Med.* 1996;334(18):1150–1155.

118. Khan A, Agarwal R. Lung cancer chemoprevention with inhaled corticosteroids? *Am J Respir Crit Care Med.* 2007;176(11):1169; author reply 1169.

119. Parimon T, Chien JW, Bryson CL, McDonell MB, Udris EM, Au DH. Inhaled corticosteroids and risk of lung cancer among patients with chronic obstructive pulmonary disease. *Am J Respir Crit Care Med.* 2007;175(7):712–719.

120. van den Berg RM, van Tinteren H, van Zandwijk N, et al. The influence of fluticasone inhalation on markers of carcinogenesis in bronchial epithelium. *Am J Respir Crit Care Med.* 2007;175(10):1061–1065.

121. Calverley PM, Anderson JA, Celli B, et al. Salmeterol and fluticasone propionate and survival in chronic obstructive pulmonary disease. *N Engl J Med.* 2007;356(8):775–789.

3

Dual Energy Computed Tomography for Lung Cancer Diagnosis and Characterization

Victor Gonzalez-Perez, Estanislao Arana, and David Moratal

Contents

3.1 Introduction

Lung cancer is one of the world's leading causes of death, killing more than 1.2 million people every year [1]. Its impact is strongly linked to smoking, and although it is predicted to decrease in Western society, this decline has been slowed due to an increase of cases in women and the elderly [2].

If lung cancer is suspected, the first diagnostic test performed is a chest X-ray followed by a computed tomography scan with contrast of the chest and upper abdomen.

Recently, dual energy computed tomography (DECT) technology was introduced for the assessment of the benignity or malignancy of tumors both in lung lesions [3–5] and in other locations, such as the head and neck [6], bone metastases [7], pathological lymph nodes [8], thyroid carcinoma [9], or renal tumors [10].

DECT provides us with new tools for the quantitative analysis of images, such as the reconstruction of studies with the amount of iodine in each voxel, effective atomic number (Z), or spectral curves that reflect the absorption of a tissue under a monoenergetic photon beam in an energy range. As far as we know [9], the Z parameter was proposed to determine the benignity or malignancy of the lesion in the case of lung or thyroid cancer. With regard to lung lesions, the iodine uptake [3, 4] or spectral curves have been used [5] to distinguish malignant tumors from benign tumors.

The quantitative analysis of the tissues allowed by DECT could expand the clinical utility of CT beyond the benign–malignant differential diagnosis. Thus, in this chapter, we assess the relation of the quantitative parameters of the DECT with characteristics of the tumor staging, necrosis status, and the ability to differentiate adenocarcinoma (ADC) from squamous cell carcinoma.

3.1.1 Introduction to DECT

The concepts of DECT were postulated more than 30 years ago [11–13]. Only recent technical developments have allowed its implementation. Specifically, the simultaneous acquisition of different data sets with a low-energy and a high-energy tube and its coregistration presented an unsolvable technical issue [14].

The main concept of the DECT is based on the separation of a photon spectrum in two components of high and low energy [15]. The basic feature of the DECT is that it allows the differentiation of materials due to the different attenuation that each one of these spectrums represents [16]. In the solution implemented in our center, we use photon spectrums of 80 and 140 kVp. They consist of a continuous spectrum of *bremsstrahlung* radiation, with the overlying characteristic lines of the anode material (tungsten). The average energies are 56 and 76 keV, respectively.

These groups of images would separately present more noise than standard CT. Advanced reconstruction algorithms gather both sets of data and obtain a resulting image of a sole study with the combination of high contrast associated to the low energy and the low noise typical of high-energy acquisitions [17]. The dose provided by both X-ray spectrums is even smaller than the one used in a conventional CT scanner [18]. As well as standard CT, the DECT image is measured in Hounsfield units (HU).

Currently, DECT uses three technical solutions for the simultaneous data collection with two photon spectrums [14]:

1. Two X-ray tubes and their respective detectors are perpendicularly installed [19] so that the projections are taken with a difference of 90°. The postprocessing is performed after the reconstruction of the images of both acquisitions, with a convolution kernel [15].
2. A sole X-ray tube is used that quickly alternates the energy of the tube from 80 to 140 kVp. Each exposition lasts 0.5 ms. The detector is able to acquire each projection

separately so that once the process is finished, we obtain 1,000 projections of high energy and 1,000 projections of low energy. This switch of energy requires twice the rotary projections to obtain enough data for the reconstruction of the study.

3. A sandwich detector is used. If a material of a certain thickness is placed between two or more X-ray detectors, one directly over the other, the low-energy photons are better absorbed, and the photon spectrum that each detector obtains is different. Thus, the reconstruction with two different energies is allowed even though the tube delivers only a photon beam [20].

3.1.2 Quantitative Studies in DECT

In the energy range used in radiology, attenuation of the photons is due to the photoelectric effect and the Compton dispersion. The importance of these effects and of the coherent dispersion varies with the material and energy of the photons. There is a maximum photoelectric effect in the iodine to the energy of 33 keV (binding energy of the layer K). There are more photons of that energy in the low-energy X-ray beam [21], so the absorption will be higher in that spectrum, and the iodine can be readily identified. Thus, the algorithms of the postprocessing, with the different attenuation in the projections of high and low energy, provide us with quantitative information of the iodine present in a volume. In the case of lung cancer, we can measure the amount of iodine contrast that a lesion absorbs in mg/cm^3.

As the probability of the photoelectric effect depends on the atomic number of the material Z and the energy E of the photons proportionally to Z^3 and $1/E^3$, respectively, the algorithms of reconstruction are also able to calculate the Z of every voxel.

Thus, after an acquisition of DECT, we can reconstruct the following image studies: CT images at 80 and 140 kVp, the reconstruction from both projections that combines the high contrast of the low energy with the low level of noise typical of high energy, and an image that gives different levels of gray according to the absorbed amount of iodine and another that scales the gray level of voxels according to its effective atomic number. In addition, the DECT allows the reconstruction of virtual images that show how the CT image would be if taken with a monoenergetic spectrum.

3.1.2.1 Iodine Uptake Study
Regarding lung cancer, DECT lets us measure the amount of iodine contrast material that the lung tumor absorbs.

The algorithms show a large difference in the attenuation of the different energies used in the X-ray beams in their calculations. This attenuation can be caused by the Compton effect, coherent dispersion, or the photoelectric effect. As the photoelectric effect increases with the material atomic number and decreases with the energy, comparing the projections of high and low energy, the software can reconstruct the amount of contrast absorbed in a determined region [15].

The attenuation ratio obtained for two different energies can be obtained to discriminate between different materials. Thus, the processed images are density images for a pair of materials. Figure 3.1 shows an image obtained by means of DECT where

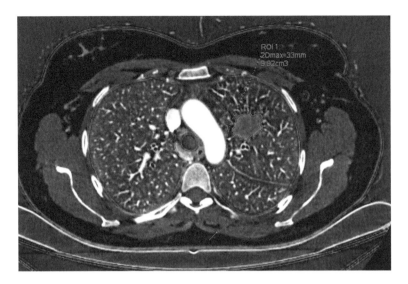

Figure 3.1　Virtual image reconstructed by means of DECT of the quantification of the amount of absorbed iodine contrast (mg/cm³) considering that the image is formed by the water–iodine pair. It shows the contoured lesion in an axial image.

the pair of materials, iodine and water [22], has been reconstructed and the gray level of each pixel quantifies the amount of iodine in mg/cm³. By contouring the lesion, we can obtain the absorbed iodine values.

3.1.2.2　Study of the Effective Atomic Number

Analogous to the quantification of the contrast material, the algorithms of reconstruction of DECT let us measure the effective atomic number Z of each voxel,

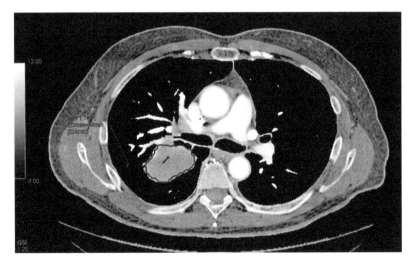

Figure 3.2　Virtual image reconstructed by means of DECT of the quantification of the effective atomic number.

comparing the projections of two different energies. In this case, the gray level of each pixel quantifies its value of the effective atomic number.

In Figure 3.2, we show a virtual image of the reconstruction of the Z on a lung cancer on the right lower lobe.

3.1.2.3 *Virtual Monochromatic Studies and Spectral Curves*

By means of DECT, the virtual images of the CT images can be reconstructed as obtained with monochromatic tube energy, as shown in Figure 3.3. For this purpose, the projections are assembled, and the mass attenuation coefficient of materials is used at certain energy [23].

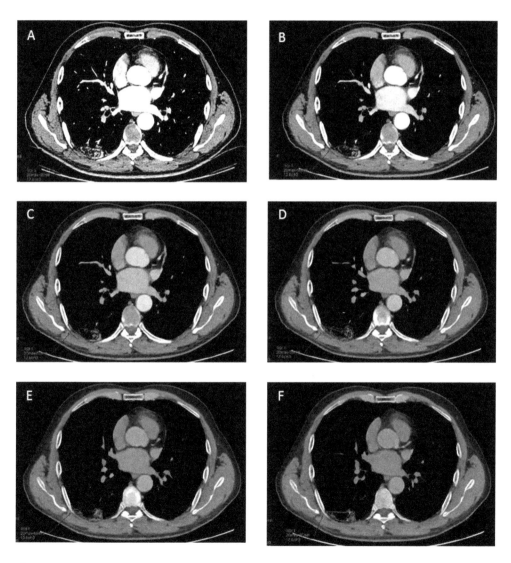

Figure 3.3   Reconstructed virtual monochromatic images. Top: A) 40 keV, B) 60 keV; center: C) 80 keV, D) 100 keV; bottom: E) 120 keV, F) 140 keV.

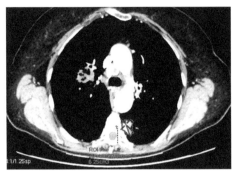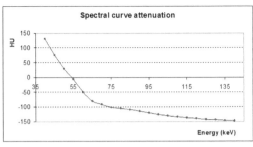

Figure 3.4 Left: Contoured lesion in conventional attenuation study. Right: Spectral curve of that lesion. The spots indicate the average of the attenuation value in HU of the tumor for each energy.

Several studies have shown that these monochromatic images can be useful for the improvement of image quality [24], to detect small lesions [25], for tumor discrimination [26], or to reduce artifacts caused by metallic structures [27].

The spectral curves show how the attenuation would be in terms of HU in the range of 40–140 keV. Figure 3.4 shows the spectral curve for the volume of a lung tumor. After the contouring, the algorithms reconstruct the attenuation according to the energy if the photon beam was of monochromatic energy.

The X-rays present a different attenuation in each material, depending on the energy. Thus, the attenuation coefficients that characterize a substance are gathered in the spectral curves, which could reflect characteristics, such as cellularity, tissue, density, and iodine concentration after the injection of contrast, and describe the tumor properties [6].

Several studies have parameterized these spectral curves to distinguish between benign and malignant lesions in the head and neck [6] and bone lesions [7].

3.2 Material and Methods

3.2.1 Study Population

The patients included in the study were referred to the Valencia Oncology Institute Foundation by other health care providers due to suspected lung cancer pathology. From July 2013 to January 2017, a total of 252 patients (170 men, 82 women) with 256 lesions were enrolled in this protocol, approved by the local institutional review board.

Patients were ages (average ± typical deviation) 65 ± 10 years (range 20–88 years). Concerning the smoking habits at the point of diagnosis, 40.3% smoked, 44.8% were ex-smokers, and 14.9% were nonsmokers.

No tumor was excluded due to its location or size. The average of the volume of the pulmonary findings in the sample was 3.12 cm³ (range 0.03–496 cm³). The average diameter in the largest axial image was 23 mm (range 4–335 mm).

The samples of the lesions were evaluated by histologic analysis by the Department of Pathological Anatomy of our foundation. In our group of patients, the technique used to take the sample was mostly by means of surgery (40.2%), fine-needle aspiration (30.4%), and surgical biopsy (19.1%). From the histopathological examination, most of the lesions were malignant (78.9%), the most frequent being lung ADC (59.4%).

Table 3.1 shows a complete summary of the description of the population and the technique used to evaluate the lung lesion as well as the main nature of present lesions.

TABLE 3.1   Patient Demographics and Clinical and Lesion Characteristics. Data: Average (Range) or Patient Number (Percentage of Total)

Variable	Number of Cases (Divided by the Total) or Average (Range)
Age	65 (20–88) years old
Sex:	
Male	170 (67.4%)
Female	82 (32.6%)
Size:	
Diameter	23 (4–335) mm
Volume	3.07 (0.03–496) cm^3
Diagnostic technique:	
Surgery	103 (40.2%)
Fine-needle aspiration	78 (30.4%)
Surgical biopsy	49 (19.1%)
Bronchoscopy	9 (3.5%)
Other techniques	15 (5.9%)
No data	2 (0.8%)
Histology:	
Benign	54 (21.1%)
Malignant	202 (78.9%)
Malignant lesions:	
ADC	120 (59.4%)
Metastasis	42 (20.8%)
Squamous carcinoma	25 (12.4%)
Other non–small cell lung cancer	2 (1.0%)
Small cell lung cancer	13 (6.4%)
Benign lesions:	
Chronic inflammation	18 (33.3%)
Nonspecified granuloma	4 (7.4%)
Carcinoid	3 (5.6%)
Mycobacterium tuberculosis	1 (1.9%)
Other benign tumors	7 (13.0%)
Other: stable for 3 years or more by imaging follow-up	21 (38.9%)

TABLE 3.2   Number of Patients per Stage. Data: Number of Patients (Percentage of Total)

Stage	Lung Cancer Group (200 Patients, 202 Malignant Lesions)
T	Total: 158 (78.2%)
T1a	47 (29.7%)
T1b	25 (15.8%)
T2a	45 (28.5%)
T2b	8 (5.1%)
T3	18 (11.4%)
T4	15 (9.5%)
N	Total: 160 (79.2%)
N0	91 (56.8%)
N1	14 (8.8%)
N2	36 (22.5%)
N3	19 (11.8%)
M	Total: 162 (80.2%)
M0	122 (75.3%)
M1a	6 (3.7%)
M1b	31 (19.1%)
MX	3 (1.9%)
TNMc	Total: 160 (79.2%)
IA	47 (29.4%)
IB	22 (13.8%)
IIA	10 (6.3%)
IIB	4 (2.5%)
IIIA	27 (16.9%)
IIIB	13 (8.1%)
IVA	6 (3.8%)
IVB	31 (19.4%)

Besides the histology described in Table 3.1, the presence of necrosis in 119 malignant tumors was registered, showing a prevalence of 40.3% for all the lesions of a malignant nature.

In the patient diagnosis, the stage of the patients with lung cancer was determined according to the seventh edition of the Tumor, Node, and Metastasis (TNM) Classification developed by the American Joint Committee on Cancer and the Union for International Cancer Control [28]. The results are shown in Table 3.2.

3.2.2 Characteristics of the DECT Scanner

Our center has a Discovery CT750HD DECT scanner model (GE Healthcare, Chicago, IL, USA) The solution used is called Gemstone Spectral Imaging (GSI), so we refer to its studies here as GSI studies.

At acquisition, the quick switch of kVp between the high and low energy of adjacent projections was used. These projections are almost simultaneous in the same localization, and thus they minimize the influence of the movement of the patient and his or her organs. So, in each rotation, two complete sets of projections are obtained [29].

Patients performed a DECT in inhalation during a normal cycle of breathing (non-deep). They were given iodine contrast (Iopamidol, 300 mg/mL; Bracco, Milan, Italy) at a rate of 4 mL/s through an antecubital vein. A complete chest GSI study was performed with a delay of 35 seconds after the injection of the contrast in the arterial phase, followed by a non-GSI chest and abdomen study of the venous phase 30 seconds after the arterial phase to determine the tumor stage. In our approximation, the parameters of DECT were quantified only in the arterial phase. Other studies have also evaluated these parameters in the venous phase [30].

The study of the arterial phase was held as a DECT with a kilovoltage switch between 80 and 140 kVp. The rest of the parameters were time of rotation of the tube (0.5 seconds), current of the tube (600 mA), pitch helicoidal (1.375), field of view (500 mm), collimation (40 mm), and slice thickness and range for axial images (2.5 mm).

For the study of the venous phase (no GSI), the parameters of acquisition were time of rotation of the tube (0.5 seconds), modulated current of the tube (SmartmA) with a noise ratio of 20 for the initial images of 5 mm, pitch helicoidal (1.375), field of view (500 mm), collimation (40 mm), and slice thickness and range for axial images (2.5 mm).

A protocol of acquisition with a computed tomography dose index (CTDIvol) was used for each phase of the DECT acquisition of 12.72 mGy. The value of the dose-length product was 280 ± 40 mGy/cm.

3.2.3 Quantitative Analysis Through DECT

Two radiologists contoured the lung lesions using an ADW4.4 workstation (GE Healthcare) and a semiautomatic method based on the HU window: If the lesion was in contact with the mediastinum, a window of 400 HU and a level of 40 HU were used, whereas a window of 1,000 HU and a level of -700 HU were used on isolated nodules. The lesion was contoured in every axial image, so the lung tumor was completely covered by this contour. Similar studies have assessed the contour of the lesion only on the image showing the largest diameter [3, 9] or using regions of interest (ROI) scarcely reproducible in the interior of the tumor [30].

By means of the GSI Viewer software (GE Healthcare), the obtained data were processed and visualized with the technique of switching the energy of the DECT scanner. Thus, the following studies were reconstructed from the original set of data:

- Attenuation in terms of HU
- Absorbed iodine (in mg/cm^3)
- Effective atomic number (dimensionless)
- The spectral curves with the HU of the volume of a tumor throughout the monochromatic energies reconstructed between 40 and 140 keV

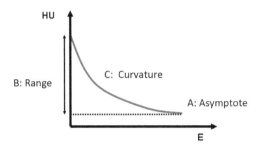

Figure 3.5 Parametrization of the spectral curve to an exponential. HU, Hounsfield units; E, energy.

The minimum, mean, and maximum values and the standard deviation of the HU, iodine, and Z absorption were collected. In order to quantify the different spectral curves, they were parameterized. Thus, the mean HU data of the complete lesion for each energy (40–140 keV in intervals of 5 keV) were fitted to an exponential [6]:

$$UH = A + Be^{\frac{C(kev)-40}{100}} \tag{1}$$

where A represents the asymptote with the trend of the HU values to high energy, B the range between the maximum and minimum value of HU, and C the slope of the curve, as shown in Figure 3.5:

Thus, the values A, B, and C of the curves were collected. In addition, the benignity of the adjustment was measured through the correlation coefficient R^2. The parameterization of the curves was performed through the MATLAB 2010a software (Mathworks Inc., Natick, MA, USA). A nonlinear least-squares adjustment method was used to adjust each curve to the model.

In total, 18 parameters were taken to assess the lesion. From now on, we will use L to refer to the lesion, and between brackets, we will refer to the studied parameter of lesion: A, B, and C for the parameterization of the spectral curves, HU for the values of the attenuation study; I for the values of the absorbed iodine study; and Z for the values of the study of the reconstruction of the effective atomic number. For HU, I, and Z, we will use the subindices min, mean, max, and σ to refer to minimum, mean, maximum, and standard deviation of each one, respectively. Thus, the maximum diameter of an axial image of the lesion and its volume are also assessed.

Table 3.3 summarizes all the analyzed parameters of the lesion in the different studies.

Similar studies have also evaluated the influence of other normalization structures for the quantification of DECT parameters [6]. Thus, to minimize the influence of body weight or blood flow on the contrast uptake, the DECT parameters of the

TABLE 3.3   Analyzed Parameters of DECT

Spectral Curves	Attenuation Study (HU)	Absorbed Iodine Study (I)	Effective Atomic Number Study (Z)
L(A)	$L(HU_{min})$	$L(I_{min})$	$L(Z_{min})$
L(B)	$L(HU_{mean})$	$L(I_{mean})$	$L(Z_{mean})$
L(C)	$L(HU_{max})$	$L(I_{max})$	$L(Z_{max})$
$L(R^2)$	$L(HU_\sigma)$	$L(I_\sigma)$	$L(Z_\sigma)$
	L(diameter)		
	L(volume)		

lesion were normalized by subtracting the ROI values of the paraspinal muscle [6] or obtaining a ratio to an ROI on the thoracic aorta [30].

The radiologist contoured the lesion in the attenuation study (HU) with a semiautomatic method. Then the studies of iodine uptake I and the effective atomic number Z were reconstructed, and the structures previously contoured in the HU study were coregistered. Then the studies of the spectral curves on the lesions were performed and parameterized by means of Matlab software.

The licensed statistical software package SPSS 20 (IBM, Somers, NY, USA) was used in the statistical analysis. A bivariate analysis was performed using the Mann-Whitney U test to distinguish tumor characteristics (benign or malignant lesion, ADC vs. SCC and necrotic status). Significance was set at $p = 0.05$, and Bonferroni adjustment was used to correct the significance level due to multiple comparisons. Receiver operating characteristic (ROC) curves were generated, and diagnostic capability was determined by calculating the area under the ROC curve (AUC). According to the AUC value [31], parameters can be considered poor (AUC < 0.6), fair (0.6 < AUC < 0.75), good (0.75–0.9), very good (0.9–0.97), and excellent (0.97–1) to differentiate between tumor characteristics.

An exploratory multivariate analysis was performed. Logistic regression models were built using a backward strategy; those variables that altered the effect by 10% when eliminated from the model were considered as confounders. The collinearity of the maximal models was evaluated and the significance level set at 5% [17].

3.3 Results

3.3.1 Differences Between Benign and Malignant Tumors

A bivariate analysis was performed to relate the parameters measured by DECT (Table 3.3) to the benignity or malignancy of the tumors confirmed by histopathological analysis.

Table 3.4 shows the results of the Mann-Whitney U test for the 18 former variables. We will modify the values considered statistically significant at $p = 0.05$ through

TABLE 3.4   **Diagnostic Capability of the DECT Variables for the Differentiation of Benign and Malignant Tumors**

Variable (Lesion)	p
L(A)	<0.001*
L(B)	0.19
L(C)	0.1
L(R^2)	<0.001*
L(HU_{min})	0.998
L(HU_{mean})	<0.001*
L(HU_{max})	<0.001*
L(HU_σ)	<0.001*
L(diameter)	<0.001*
L(volume)	<0.001*
L(I_{min})	0.002*
L(I_{mean})	0.014
L(I_{max})	<0.001*
L(I_σ)	0.003
L(Z_{min})	<0.001*
L(Z_{mean})	<0.001*
L(Z_{max})	0.092
L(Z_σ)	0.060

*Statistically significant $p < 0.0027$

Bonferroni correction, so those variables with a p value < 0.0027 (0.05/18) were considered statistically significant.

Table 3.5 shows the AUC parameter that describes the capability of these variables to differentiate between benign and malignant lesions as well as the range where it meets a confidence interval (CI) of 95%.

TABLE 3.5   **AUC Values for the Variables That Significantly Distinguish Between Benign and Malignant Tumors**

Variable	AUC ± standard deviation	CI 95%
L(A)	0.70 ± 0.04	0.621–0.774
L(R^2)	0.68 ± 0.04	0.608–0.759
L(HU_{mean})	0.70 ± 0.04	0.623–0.777
L(HU_{max})	0.73 ± 0.04	0.653–0.800
L(HU_σ)	0.67 ± 0.04	0.589–0.745
L(diameter)	0.72 ± 0.04	0.647–0.797
L(volume)	0.73 ± 0.04	0.660–0.808
L(I_{max})	0.68 ± 0.04	0.595–0.761
L(I_{min})	0.67 ± 0.04	0.576–0.742
L(Z_{min})	0.68 ± 0.04	0.592–0.762
L(Z_{mean})	0.68 ± 0.04	0.603–0.761

TABLE 3.6   Sensitivity and Specificity of the DECT Parameters in the Differentiation of Benign and Malignant Tumors

Variable	Sensitivity	Specificity	Threshold
L(A)	74.3	57.4%	>-114.60 HU
L(R^2)	61.2%	66.7%	>0.9976
L(HU$_{mean}$)	70.8%	66.7%	>-39.50 HU
L(HU$_{max}$)	62.9%	72.8%	>113.50 HU
L(HU$_\sigma$)	68.5%	65.8%	<101 HU
L(diameter)	68.3%	70.4%	>17.50 mm
L(volume)	72.3%	72.2%	>1.39 cm^3
L(I$_{max}$)	61.9%	64.8%	>86.5 mg/cm^3
L(I$_{min}$)	60.7%	62.6%	>-41 mg/cm^3
L(Z$_{min}$)	61.1%	72.1%	<1.66
L(Z$_{mean}$)	64.8%	66.7%	<9.20

The optimal threshold value for each one of these variables was assessed to calculate the sensitivity and specificity in the differentiation of benign and malignant lesions. Table 3.6 summarizes those values. We defined positive values as malignant cases and negative values as benign ones.

The volume of the lesion was the best variable for differentiating the benignity or malignancy of lung tumors: 72.3% of sensitivity and 72.2% of specificity for a threshold value of 1.39 cm^3.

Ancillary variables that were related to attenuation in terms of HU and volume and diameter of lesion correspond to conventional variables, also obtained on standard CT. In contrast, those related to the iodine uptake and the effective atomic number are exclusive to the DECT technique.

In view of these results, we highlight that a quantitative study through DECT of the mentioned variables does not add new possibilities to the diagnosis of the malignancy of lesions compared to conventional CT. Following is a multivariate analysis to evaluate a possible improvement in the diagnosis ability.

In the multivariate analysis, we introduced as covariates those parameters that have a value of $p < 0.05$ in the univariate analysis. Thus, in this case, the covariates were L(A), L(B), L(R^2), L(HU$_{mean}$), L(HU$_{max}$), L(HU$_\sigma$), L(volume), L(I$_{min}$), L(I$_{mean}$), L(I$_{max}$), L(I$_\sigma$), L(Z$_{min}$), and L(Z$_{mean}$). We excluded diameter as strongly correlated with the volume.

After performing a binary logistic relation with a backward method through the likelihood ratio, the model for the prediction of benignity concluded that L(I$_{max}$), L(I$_\sigma$), and L(Z$_{min}$) were statistically significant variables with a Nagelkerke value of $R^2 = 0.239$. The multivariate model presented a sensitivity of 74.0% and specificity of 72.2% for the correct classification of the benignity or malignancy of the lung findings. These values are barely better than those obtained from using the lesion volume as sole variable, so we can state that our quantitative analysis of DECT does not add more information than standard CT.

TABLE 3.7   Diagnosis Ability of the DECT Parameters for the Differentiation of TNMc I and II From TNMc III and IV

Variable (Lesion)	I and II vs. III and IV (83 vs. 77 Cases) p
L(A)	<0.001*
L(B)	<0.001*
L(C)	0.004
L(R^2)	<0.001*
L(HU_{min})	0.543
L(HU_{mean})	<0.001*
L(HU_{max})	<0.001*
L(HU_σ)	<0.001*
L(I_{min})	0.004
L(I_{mean})	<0.001*
L(I_{max})	0.689
L(I_σ)	<0.001*
L(Z_{min})	0.002*
L(Z_{mean})	<0.001*
L(Z_{max})	0.013
L(Z_σ)	<0.001*

*Statistically significant $p < 0.0031$

3.3.2 Stage Differentiation

In lung cancer staging, the most important division is located between the cases TNM I and II compared to TNM III and IV. This division also separates those patients who benefit from surgical treatment from those who will undergo other therapies. For this reason, we performed a Mann-Whitney U test to assess if any of the 16 studied variables (Table 3.3) could differentiate tumor stages I and II from stages III and IV. We did not include tumor volume or maximum diameter, as their values compromised TNM as well.

Table 3.7 shows the Mann-Whitney U test outcomes for that comparison. We will modify the statistically significant value $p = 0.05$ through Bonferroni correction: $0.05/16 = 0.0031$.

Tables 3.8 and 3.9 show the AUC, sensitivity–specificity, and optimal threshold values for the variables that significantly distinguish stages III and IV from stages I and II.

L(A) was the only variable with AUC $\geq$ 0.8. In Figure 3.6, we see the box-and-whisker diagram in the differentiation of both stage groups and their ROC curves.

We also evaluated this parameter L(A) for the prediction of the nodal involvement (stage N0 vs. N1, N2, and N3) and metastasis existence (M0 vs. M1). In both, L(A) presents a value of $p < 0.001$. In the prediction of the nodal involvement, L(A) had an AUC value of 0.80 ± 0.03 (confidence interval [CI] 95%: 0.763–0.867), with a sensitivity and specificity of 79.7% and 69.5%, respectively. For the metastatic diagnosis, L(A)

TABLE 3.8 Values of the AUC for the Variables That Distinguish TNMc I and II From TNMc III and IV

Variable	AUC ± Standard Deviation	CI 95%
L(A)	0.80 ± 0.03	0.736–0.872
L(B)	0.72 ± 0.04	0.639–0.796
L(R^2)	0.69 ± 0.04	0.618–0.780
L(HU_{mean})	0.79 ± 0.03	0.727–0.863
L(HU_{max})	0.70 ± 0.04	0.621–0.782
L(HU_σ)	0.72 ± 0.04	0.648–0.804
L(I_{mean})	0.72 ± 0.04	0.642–0.798
L(I_σ)	0.77 ± 0.03	0.703–0.845
L(Z_{min})	0.61 ± 0.04	0.523–0.696
L(Z_{mean})	0.79 ± 0.03	0.722–0.861
L(Z_σ)	0.71 ± 0.04	0.629–0.787

TABLE 3.9 Sensitivity and Specificity of the DECT Parameters in the Distinction Between TNMc I and II and TNMc III and IV

Variable	Sensitivity	Specificity	Threshold
L(A)	81.8%	71.8%	>47.4
L(B)	62.4%	70.1%	<173.0
L(R^2)	68.8%	61.9%	>0.9978
L(HU_{mean})	80.5%	70.6%	>−10 HU
L(HU_{max})	62.3%	68.2%	>164.5 HU
L(HU_σ)	68.2%	70.1%	<83.15 HU
L(I_{mean})	61.2%	71.4%	<22.2 mg/cm^3
L(I_σ)	61.2%	85.7%	<14.3 mg/cm^3
L(Z_{min})	35.7%	85.7%	<2.98
L(Z_{mean})	66.7%	81.8%	<9.05
L(Z_σ)	60.7%	67.5%	<0.77

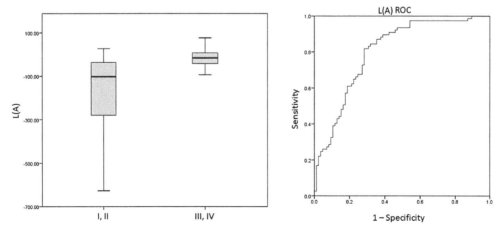

Figure 3.6 Box and whisker diagram (left) and ROC curve (right) in the differentiation of stages TNMc I and II and TNMc III and IV.

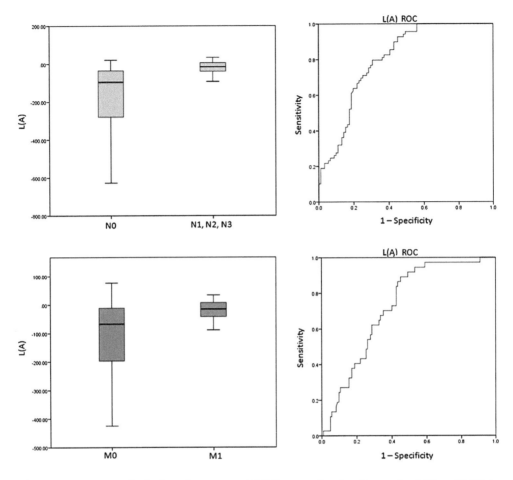

Figure 3.7 Box-and-whisker diagram and ROC curve for the diagnosis ability of L(A) in the prediction of regional affection (top) and distance affection (bottom).

presents a AUC of 0.72 ± 0.04 (CI 95%: 0.637–0.804) with a sensitivity of 89.5% and a specificity of 54.2% at the optimal detection threshold. Figure 3.7 shows the box diagram and the ROC curves to evaluate the diagnosis ability of L(A) on lymph nodes and metastatic involvement.

3.3.3 Differentiation Between ADC and Squamous Carcinoma

We analyzed the ability of DECT to distinguish between the two more common primary kinds of lung carcinoma in our sample: ADC and squamous carcinoma. The only variable that differentiated statistically significant was L(A), with $p = 0.002$. L(A) presented an AUC of 0.80 ± 0.03 (CI 95%: 0.733–0.867) with a sensitivity of 72.0% and a specificity of 61.7% in the optimal detection threshold. Figure 3.8 shows the box-and-whisker diagram and the ROC curve.

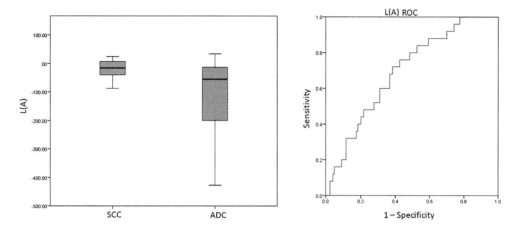

Figure 3.8   Box-and-whisker diagram and ROC curve for the diagnosis ability of L(A) in the differentiation of ADC in comparison to squamous carcinoma.

3.3.4 Necrosis Diagnosis

Table 3.10 summarizes the outcomes of Mann-Whitney U test in the differentiation of tumor necrotic status. In order to determine the statistically significant value, the Bonferroni correction was performed: $p = 0.05/18 = 0.0028$.

TABLE 3.10   Diagnostic Capability of the DECT Variables for the Distinction of Necrotic Tumors

Variable (lesion)	p
L(A)	<0.001*
L(B)	0.003
L(C)	0.110
L(R^2)	0.003
L(HU_{min})	0.470
L(HU_{mean})	<0.001*
L(HU_{max})	0.001*
L(HU_σ)	<0.001*
L(diameter)	<0.001*
L(volume)	<0.001*
L(I_{min})	0.127
L(I_{mean})	0.001*
L(I_{max})	0.900
L(I_σ)	<0.001*
L(Z_{min})	0.003
L(Z_{mean})	<0.001*
L(Z_{max})	0.184
L(Z_σ)	0.028

*Statistically significant $p < 0.0028$

Variables L(A), L(HU$_{mean}$), L(HU$_{max}$), L(HU$_\sigma$), L(diameter), L(volume), L(I$_{mean}$), L(I$_\sigma$), and L(Z$_{mean}$) clearly distinguished those tumors with necrotic regions from those without. Table 3.11 resumes the AUC values for these variables.

Figure 3.9 shows the box diagrams and the ROC for the variables that presented an AUC value > 0.75 (defined as "good" according to Zweig and Campbell [31]).

Table 3.12 shows sensitivity and specificity values of these variables qualified as good in the distinction of necrotic cases (defined as positive for the sensitivity specificity) in the cohort with lung carcinoma.

In the multivariate analysis for necrosis diagnosis by means of linear logistic regression, covariates with $p < 0.05$ were introduced into the equation: L(A), L(B), L(R^2), L(HU$_{mean}$), L(HU$_{max}$), L(HU$_\sigma$), L(diameter), L(volume), L(I$_{mean}$), L(I$_\sigma$), L(Z$_{min}$), L(Z$_{mean}$), and L(Z$_\sigma$).

TABLE 3.11   Diagnosis Capability of the DECT Variables for the Distinction of Necrotic Tumors

Variable	AUC ± standard deviation	CI 95%
L(A)	0.75 ± 0.05	0.664–0.839
L(HU$_{mean}$)	0.73 ± 0.05	0.635–0.817
L(HU$_{max}$)	0.68 ± 0.05	0.582–0.778
L(HU$_\sigma$)	0.70 ± 0.05	0.604–0.796
L(diameter)	0.70 ± 0.05	0.598–0.793
L(volume)	0.70 ± 0.05	0.611–0.803
L(I$_{mean}$)	0.69 ± 0.05	0.596–0.788
L(I$_\sigma$)	0.74 ± 0.05	0.649–0.834
L(Z$_{mean}$)	0.78 ± 0.04	0.699–0.865

TABLE 3.12   Sensitivity and Specificity of DECT in the Distinction of Necrotic Cases

Variable	Sensitivity	Specificity	Threshold
L(A)	84.8%	60.9%	>−79.49 HU
L(Z$_{mean}$)	89.1%	58.8%	<9.20

TABLE 3.13   Variables Statistically Significant on the Logistic Regression Model of Necrotic Tumors

Variable	β	Significance	Exp(β)	Exp(β) CI 95%
L(A)	0.008	0.003	1.008	0.1003–1.013
L(B)	0.134	0.161	1.144	0.948–1.380
L(R^2)	301.509	0.055	8.728 e^{130}	—
L(diameter)	−0.014	0.145	0.986	0.968–1.005
L(I$_{mean}$)	−1.092	0.138	0.335	0.079–1.421
Constant	−298.902	0.057	—	—

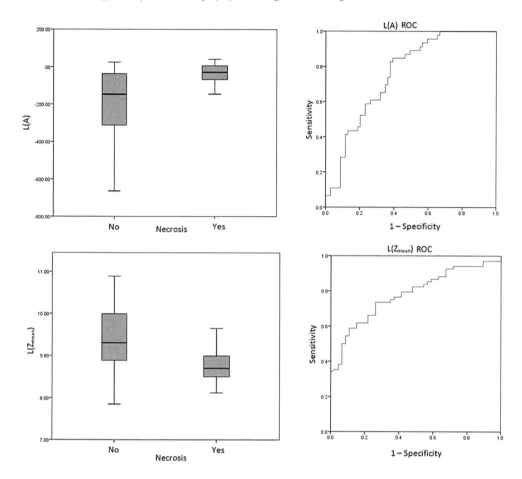

Figure 3.9 Box diagram and ROC of L(A) (top) and L(Z_{mean}) (bottom) for the differentiation of tumor necrosis.

L(A), L(B), L(R^2), L(diameter), and L(I_{mean}) were significant in the final model with $R^2 = 0.431$. Table 3.13 shows values of the logistic regression.

A threshold value on the logistic function at $p = 0.50$, a sensitivity of 71.7%, and a specificity of 74.6% for necrosis diagnosis were obtained.

3.4 Discussion

We studied iodine uptake, spectral curves, and effective atomic number parameters as well as the attenuation in terms of HU. Our initial hypothesis was that these parameters could characterize altered vasculature and relate it to tumor histology, malignancy, necrosis, and staging [32].

Relations between DECT variables and tumor vasculature have been published, such as those between iodine contrast absorbed by a lung tumor and its angiogenesis [33] and between tumor perfusion and iodine uptake quantified through the spectral curve slope and the difference of HU in the monoenergetic studies of 40 and 70 keV [34].

Reproducibility in biomedical research is an issue of concern to the scientific community [35]. In the current study, lesion contour was performed semiautomatically, on the whole lesion in axial images. This methodology was robust and obtained reproducible results. Thus, we found in a previous reproducibility analysis with our method [36] that the intraobserver reproducibility of the lung lesion presents an intraclass correlation coefficient (ICC) of 0.95 (CI 95%: 0.80–0.98) and for the interobserver an ICC of 0.92 (CI 95%: 0.70–0.98). Other, similar studies that placed ROIs arbitrarily on lesions [30] obtained better sensitivity and specificity. However, no reliability was specified, nor have subsequent studies replicated their findings.

3.4.1 Differentiation Between Benign and Malignant Tumors

In the distinction between benign and malignant tumors, conventional CT is highly sensitive for the detection of lung cancer, but its specificity is very limited. For example, a multicenter prospective study (356 cases) [37] has shown 98% of sensitivity and 58% of specificity when assessing the increase of HU units after injection of iodine contrast. This feature has also been evaluated [4] in DECT by virtually subtracting absorbed iodine contrast with sensitivity results of 92.0% and specificity results of 70.0%. A DECT study [38] that compared HU increase after contrast injection with a direct amount of the absorbed iodine in the lesion, placing an ROI in the interior of the lesion, obtained an AUC of 0.79 in both cases, although nodules smaller than 5 mm in diameter were excluded.

Our results are based on formerly published preliminary studies with a cohort of only 125 patients [36]. It has not been proven that exclusive DECT parameters are better than standard CT parameters, although they could distinguish statistically significant benign from malignant tumors. Thus, the best predictor of our benignity–malignancy study of the lesion was the volume of the lesion, with sensitivity and specificity values of 72.3% and 72.2%, respectively. Other studies that used DECT [5] have also concluded that parameters such as iodine concentration, slope of the spectral curve, and the 40-kV CT number distinguish significantly ($p < 0.05$) benign from malignant lesions.

It is worth mentioning some studies that have achieved excellent results using DECT parameters [3, 30]. Zhang et al. [30], after the evaluation of 63 patients (37 malignant and 26 benign) concluded that iodine concentration values and slopes of the spectral curves, analyzed in ROIs placed in homogeneous areas of the lung nodule, presented AUCs of 0.89 and 0.96 in the arterial phase, respectively, and 0.96 and 0.89 in the venous phase. They showed a sensitivity of 93.8% and a specificity of 85.7% for the iodine uptake in the venous phase. Hou et al. [3] stated that an HU increase after contrast injection, iodine concentrations, and slope of the spectral curve distinguished significantly between lung cancer and inflammatory lesions. Sensitivity-specificity values of 86%–100% were obtained, using the normalized iodine concentration to the aorta at the venous phase and contouring the ROIs in the central and peripheral regions of the lesion. We highlight that those results are based on nonreproducible ROIs.

More current work analyzed a larger spectrum of lesions than others, which deal only with cases of pneumonia versus squamous carcinoma and lung ADC [3, 5, 30]. Varied histologies in our sample could also explain our lower diagnostic accuracy. The size and volume of the lung lesions also present a wider variation in our population than in other studies, some are more stringent in their inclusion criteria [3, 4], whereas others have not even reported theirs [5]. The present approach has some advantages. The semiautomatic contouring presented excellent reproducibility, and no case was excluded from the sample due to the geometry or anatomic location of a tumor, whereas other, similar studies included only peripheral lesions [30]. Our DECT measurements were obtained from the whole volume, whereas other studies used ROI contours on only an axial image [3, 9].

3.4.2 Tumor Stage

Schmid-Bindert et al. [39] found a moderate correlation between maximum standardized uptake value on lesions with positron emission tomography (PET) and maximum absorption of iodine with DECT for tumor histology. The correlation was better in non–small cell lung cancer than in small cell lung cancer, which could be explained by tumor differences in angiogenesis. However, the correlation was worse when maximum iodine uptake of the lesion was compared with lymph node involvement.

Lymph node staging is the most important finding in nonmetastatic patients, as N2–N3 excludes surgery. Contrast-enhanced CT and PET are used for the depiction of lymph nodes; PET achieves greater accuracy [40], with sensitivity and specificity [41] of 85% and 91%, respectively.

The conventional study of regional and distant invasion is based on nodes and/or metastases imaging. In our case, we did not study lymph nodes; rather, we tried to distinguish among different lung tumor phenotypes that tend to extend. Another study [42] with a similar methodology assessed the ratio of attenuation of the 3D contour of the lesion in the arterial phase compared to the venous phase (A/D). That study concluded that A/D corresponds to lymphatic permeation, vascular invasion, and pleural involvement.

3.4.3 Tumor Differentiation

Earlier studies [5] have found that iodine concentration, slope of the spectral curves, and the CT number at 40 kV significantly distinguished ($p < 0.05$) between squamous cell lung carcinoma and ADC. It is hypothesized that ADC has a rich and homogeneous capillarity with more angiogenesis than squamous carcinoma, and a smaller presence of hemorrhagic and necrotic zones [43]. Squamous cell carcinoma grows more slowly and has more fragile capillaries that break more easily. Thus, it is related to more cases of necrosis and less iodine contrast absorption than ADC [44]. We highlight that our univariate analysis, L(A), showed an AUC of 0.80, whereas in other studies with multivariate analysis where texture analysis was used [45], the best result was obtained for a model with five parameters, with an AUC of 0.72 for a sample of patients (62 ADC and 90 squamous cell carcinoma) on a validation data set.

3.4.4 Characterization of Tumor Necrosis

As a tumor grows, necessary nutrients can decrease in its core and develop necrotic regions that modify its perfusion. Li et al. [46] concluded that necrotic tumors have less perfusion. Our results, based on preliminary studies [47], show a smaller uptake of iodine contrast through the $L(Z_{mean})$ parameter (since contrast does not reach necrotic zones) as well as a larger asymptotic value of the spectral curves L(A) parameter in the necrotic cases.

References

1. Howlader N, Noone AM, Krapcho M, et al., eds. SEER Cancer Statistics Review, 1975–2013. *Natl Cancer Inst.* 2016;1992–2013.
2. Palshof T, Jakobsen E. Lungecancerarsrapport 2011 (2010). *Dansk Lunge Cancer Gruppe.* http:\\www.lungecancer.dk.
3. Hou WS, Wu HW, Yin Y, Cheng JJ, Zhang Q, Xu JR. Differentiation of lung cancers from inflammatory masses with dual-energy spectral CT imaging. *Acad Radiol.* 2015;22(3):337–344.
4. Chae EJ, Song J-W, Seo JB, Krauss B, Jang YM, Song K-S. Clinical utility of dual-energy CT in the evaluation of solitary pulmonary nodules: initial experience. *Radiology.* 2008;249(2):671–681.
5. Wang G, Zhang C, Li M, Deng K, Li W. Preliminary application of high-definition computed tomographic gemstone spectral imaging in lung cancer. *J Comput Assist Tomogr.* 2014;38(1):77–81.
6. Srinivasan A, Parker RA, Manjunathan A, Ibrahim M, Shah GV, Mukherji SK. Differentiation of benign and malignant neck pathologies: preliminary experience using spectral computed tomography. *J Comput Assist Tomogr.* 2013;37(5): 666–672.
7. Dong Y, Zheng S, Machida H, et al. Differential diagnosis of osteoblastic metastases from bone islands in patients with lung cancer by single-source dual-energy CT: advantages of spectral CT imaging. *Eur J Radiol.* 2015;84(5):901–907.
8. Tawfik AM, Razek AA, Kerl JM, Nour-Eldin NE, Bauer R, Vogl TJ. Comparison of dual-energy CT-derived iodine content and iodine overlay of normal, inflammatory

and metastatic squamous cell carcinoma cervical lymph nodes. *Eur Radiol.* 2014; 24(3):574–580.

9. Li M, Zheng X, Li J, Yang Y, et al. Dual-energy computed tomography imaging of thyroid nodule specimens: comparison with pathologic findings. *Invest Radiol.* 2012; 47(1):58–64.

10. Graser A, Becker CR, Staehler M, et al. Single-phase dual-energy CT allows for characterization of renal masses as benign or malignant. *Invest Radiol.* 2010;45(7): 399–405.

11. Di Chiro G, Brooks RA, Kessler RM, et al. Tissue signatures with dual-energy computed tomography. *Radiology.* 1979;131(2):521–523.

12. Genant HK, Boyd D. Quantitative bone mineral analysis using dual energy computed tomography. *Invest Radiol.* 1977;12(6):545–551.

13. Millner MR, McDavid WD, Waggener RG, Dennis MJ, Payne WH, Sank VJ. Extraction of information from CT scans at different energies. *Med Phys.* 1979;6(1): 70–71.

14. Kang M-J, Park CM, Lee C-H, Goo JM, Lee HJ. Dual-energy CT: clinical applications in various pulmonary diseases. *RadioGraphics.* 2010;30(3):685–698.

15. Johnson TRC, Fink C, Schönberg, SO, Reiser MF. *Dual Energy CT in Clinical Practice.* Berlin, Germany: Springer-Verlag; 2011:3–10.

16. Johnson TRC, Krauss B, Sedlmair M, et al. Material differentiation by dual energy CT: initial experience. *Eur Radiol.* 2007;17(6):1510–1517.

17. Holmes DR, Fletcher JG, Apel A, et al. Evaluation of non-linear blending in dual-energy computed tomography. *Eur J Radiol.* 2008;68(3):409–413.

18. Apel A, Fletcher JG, Fidler JL, et al. Pilot multi-reader study demonstrating potential for dose reduction in dual energy hepatic CT using non-linear blending of mixed kV image datasets. *Eur Radiol.* 2011;21(3):644–652.

19. Flohr TG, McCollough CH, Bruder H, et al. First performance evaluation of a dual-source CT (DSCT) system. *Eur Radiol.* 2006;16(2):256–268.

20. Fornaro J, Leschka S, Hibbeln D, et al. Dual- and multi-energy CT: approach to functional imaging. *Insights Imaging.* 2011;2(2):149–159.

21. Bushberg JT. The AAPM/RSNA physics tutorial for residents: X-ray interactions. *RadioGraphics.* 1998;18(2):457–468.

22. Silva AC, Morse BG, Hara AK, Paden RG, Hongo N, Pavlicek W. Dual-energy (spectral) CT: applications in abdominal imaging. *RadioGraphics.* 2011;31(4): 1031–1046.

23. Hsieh J, Fan J, Chandra N, Chandrall P, Kulpins M. A reconstruction technique for dual-energy X-ray computed tomography. In: *Proceedings of the First International Conference on Image Formation in X-Ray Computed Tomography.* 2010:10–13.

24. Kato Y, Sano H, Katada K, et al. Application of three-dimensional CT angiography (3D-CTA) to cerebral aneurysms. *Surg Neurol.* 1999;52(2):113–121.

25. Lv P, Lin XZ, Chen K, Gao J. Spectral CT in patients with small HCC: investigation of image quality and diagnostic accuracy. *Eur Radiol.* 2012;22(10): 2117–2124.

26. Lee SH, Hur J, Kim YJ, Lee HJ, Hong YJ, Choi BW. Additional value of dual-energy CT to differentiate between benign and malignant mediastinal tumors: an initial experience. *Eur J Radiol.* 2013;82(11):2043–2049.

27. Bamberg F, Dierks A, Nikolaou K, Reiser MF, Becker CR, Johnson TRC. Metal artifact reduction by dual energy computed tomography using monoenergetic extrapolation. *Eur Radiol.* 2011;21(7):1424–1429.

28. Egner JR. AJCC Cancer Staging Manual. *JAMA.* 2010;304(15):1726.

29. Zhang D, Li X, Liu B. Objective characterization of GE Discovery CT750 HD scanner: Gemstone spectral imaging mode. *Med Phys.* 2011;38(3):1178–1188.

30. Zhang Y, Cheng J, Hua X, et al. Can spectral CT imaging improve the differentiation between malignant and benign solitary pulmonary nodules? *PLoS One.* 2016;11(2):e0147537.

31. Zweig MH, Campbell G. Receiver-operating characteristic (ROC) plots: a fundamental evaluation tool in clinical medicine. *Clin Chem.* 1993;39(4):561–577.

32. Giatromanolaki A, Koukourakis M, O'Byrne K, et al. Prognostic value of angiogenesis in operable non-small cell lung cancer. *J Pathol.* 1996;179:80–88.

33. Jiang NC, Han P, Zhou CK, Zheng JL, Shi HS, Xiao J. Dynamic enhancement patterns of solitary pulmonary nodules at multi-detector row CT and correlation with vascular endothelial growth factor and microvessel density. *Chin J Cancer.* 2009;28(2):164–169.

34. Chen X, Xu Y, Duan J, Li C, Sun H, Wang W. Correlation of iodine uptake and perfusion parameters between dual-energy CT imaging and first-pass dual-input perfusion CT in lung cancer. *Medicine (Baltimore).* 2017;96(28): e7479.

35. Collins FS, Tabak LA. NIH plans to enhance reproducibility. *Nature.* 2014; 505(7485):612–613.

36. González-Pérez V, Arana E, Barrios M, et al. Differentiation of benign and malignant lung lesions: dual-energy computed tomography findings. *Eur J Radiol.* 2016;85(10): 1765–1772.

37. Swensen SJ, Viggiano RW, Midthun DE, et al. Lung nodule enhancement at CT: multicenter study. *Radiology.* 2000;214(1):73–80.

38. Reiter MJ, Winkler WT, Kagy KE, Schwope RB, Lisanti CJ. Dual-energy computed tomography for the evaluation of enhancement of pulmonary nodules ≤3 cm in size. *J Thorac Imaging.* 2017;32(3):189–197.

39. Schmid-Bindert G, Henzler T, Chu TQ, et al. Functional imaging of lung cancer using dual energy CT: how does iodine related attenuation correlate with standardized uptake value of 18FDG-PET-CT? *Eur Radiol.* 2012;22(1):93–103.

40. Reed CE, Harpole DH, Posther KE, et al. Results of the American College of Surgeons Oncology Group Z0050 Trial: the utility of positron emission tomography in staging potentially operable non-small cell lung cancer. *J Thorac Cardiovasc Surg.* 2003;126(6):1943–1951.

41. Gould MK, Kuschner WG, Rydzak CE, et al. Test performance of positron emission tomography and computed tomography for mediastinal staging in patients with non-small-cell lung cancer: a meta-analysis. *Ann Intern Med.* 2003;139(11):879–892.

42. Ito R, Iwano S, Shimamoto H, et al. A comparative analysis of dual-phase dual-energy CT and FDG-PET/CT for the prediction of histopathological invasiveness of non-small cell lung cancer. *Eur J Radiol.* 2017(95):186–191.

43. Dagnon K, Heudes D, Bernaudin J-F, Callard P. Computerized morphometric analysis of microvasculature in non-small cell lung carcinoma. *Microvasc Res.* 2008;75(1):112–118.

44. Padera TP, Stoll BR, Tooredman JB, Capen D, Di Tomaso E, Jain RK. Cancer cells compress intratumour vessels. *Nature.* 2004;427(6976):695.

45. Wu W, Parmar C, Grossmann P, et al. Exploratory study to identify radiomics classifiers for lung cancer histology. *Front Oncol.* 2016;6:71.
46. Li Y, Yang ZG, Chen TW, Chen HJ, Sun JY, Lu YR. Peripheral lung carcinoma: correlation of angiogenesis and first-pass perfusion parameters of 64-detector row CT. *Lung Cancer.* 2008;61(1):44–53.
47. González-Pérez V, Arana E, Cruz J, et al. Assessing tumor necrosis in lung cancer with dual energy CT quantitative imaging. *Radiotherapy Oncol.* 2017;123(suppl 1): S916–S917.

4

X-Ray Dark-Field Imaging of Lung Cancer in Mice

Deniz A. Bölükbas and Darcy E. Wagner

Contents

4.1 Introduction

Lung diseases are one of the leading causes of morbidity and mortality worldwide. Lung cancer, in particular, accounts for 1.6 million deaths per year in the world [1]. It is by far the most common cause of cancer-related deaths for both genders (Figure 4.1). There are no particular symptoms or signs for lung cancer detection at an early stage. Therefore, most patients are diagnosed at an advanced stage of the disease when treatment options are limited. The 5-year survival rate of patients with lung cancer at diagnosis is only around 15% [2]. However, when diagnosed at an early stage, lung cancer has a much better prognosis with 5-year survival rates up to 70% [3]. The most common risk factors are cigarette smoking or secondhand exposure, environmental exposures to carcinogens (e.g., asbestos, radon), and comorbidities such as human immunodeficiency virus infection, idiopathic pulmonary fibrosis, chronic obstructive pulmonary disease, and tuberculosis [4].

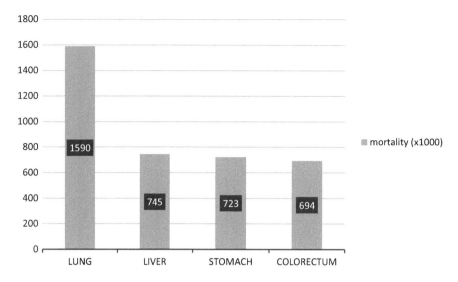

Figure 4.1 Estimated number of cancer deaths from the most common sites worldwide in 2012 [1].

4.1.1 Lung Cancer Classification

Lung cancer is classified in two subtypes: small cell lung cancer (SCLC) and non–small cell lung cancer (NSCLC). NSCLC accounts for 85% of all cases and is further categorized as adenocarcinoma, squamous cell carcinoma, and large cell carcinoma of the lung (Figure 4.2) [5]. The most common subtype in both genders, adenocarcinoma of the lung, often arises at the peripheral regions of the lung and has a slower growth rate. Therefore, chances of detecting adenocarcinoma prior to its metastasis

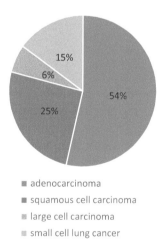

Figure 4.2 Major subtypes of lung cancer with their percent incidence rates [2].

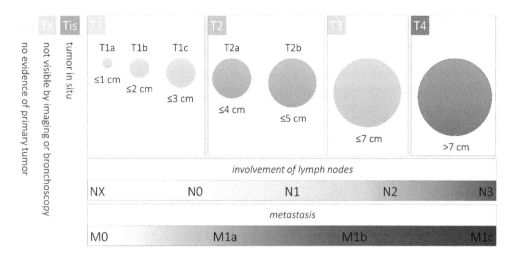

Figure 4.3 TNM classification of lung cancer (eighth edition) [9]. NX, regional lymph nodes cannot be assessed; N0, no involvement of lymph nodes; N1, tumor in ipsilateral peribronchial and/or ipsilateral hilar lymph nodes and intrapulmonary nodes; N2, tumor in ipsilateral mediastinal and/or subcarinal lymph nodes; N3, tumor in contralateral mediastinal, contralateral hilar, ipsilateral, or contralateral scalene or supraclavicular lymph nodes; M0, no distant metastasis; M1a, intrathoracic metastasis; M1b, single extrathoracic metastasis; M1c, multiple extrathoracic metastasis.

are higher [6]. Both squamous cell carcinoma and large cell carcinoma of the lung tend to arise at the proximal regions of the lung and are strongly correlated with cigarette smoking [7]. SCLC is also strongly associated with cigarette smoking and arises from neuroendocrine cells in the lung; it has the highest metastasis and lowest survival rates among all four subtypes [8].

The prognosis and handling of the disease are determined according to the size and invasion of the cancer cells. Current lung cancer staging is based on the eighth edition of the Tumor, Node and Metastasis (TNM) Classification (see Figure 4.3 and Table 4.1) [9]. Lung tumors are classified according to their size as follows: T1: tumors smaller than 3 cm; T2: tumors smaller than 5 cm; T3: tumors smaller than 7 cm; or T4: tumors larger than 7 cm. Lung cancer is diagnosed mostly at stage IV with metastasis [10]. Metastasis of lung cancer cells occurs via invasion of lymphatic and/or blood vessels. While the most common invasion site is the bone [11], depending on their type, lung cancer cells have additional preferential invasion sites as well. SCLC often metastasizes to the liver or the brain, adenocarcinoma often metastasizes to the brain, while squamous cell carcinoma invades the thoracic wall [10]. At earlier stages, lung tumors can be resected surgically. However, at later stages with accompanying metastasis, treatment involves systemic therapy with cytotoxic and/or molecularly targeted agents and palliative radiotherapy [11].

Additionally, the lung is an extremely common site for invasion of extrathoracic malignancies, that is, secondary lung tumors arising from metastasis [12]. In fact, the majority of pediatric tumors in the lung are secondary lung tumors [13]. These tumors originate mostly from breast, colon, kidney, uterus, and head and neck cancers.

TABLE 4.1   Staging of Lung Cancer According to the TNM Classification, Eighth Edition*

Stage	T	N	M
Occult carcinoma	TX	N0	M0
0	Tis	N0	M0
IA1	T1a	N0	M0
IA2	T1b	N0	M0
IA3	T1c	N0	M0
IB	T2a	N0	M0
IIA	T2b	N0	M0
IIB	T1a,b,c	N1	M0
	T2a,b	N1	M0
	T3	N0	M0
IIIA	T1a,b,c	N2	M0
	T2a,b	N2	M0
	T3	N1	M0
	T4	N0	M0
	T4	N1	M0
IIIB	T1a,b,c	N3	M0
	T2a,b	N3	M0
	T3	N2	M0
	T4	N2	M0
IIIC	T3	N3	M0
	T4	N3	M0
IVA	Any T	Any N	M1a
	Any T	Any N	M1b
IVB	Any T	Any N	M1c

*Adapted from Rami-Porta et al. [9].

4.1.2 Lung Cancer Diagnosis

The most common symptoms of lung cancer are cough, dyspnea, hemoptysis, weight loss, and anorexia [14]. Patients at high risk, that is, patients older than 40 years with risk factors and symptoms, first undergo chest radiography. Unless a clear diagnosis can be identified using chest radiography, the patients may undergo computed tomography and/or positron emission radiography [4]. If suspicion of lung cancer is high, the patient continues with a diagnostic evaluation: (1) tissue diagnosis, (2) staging, and (3) functional evaluation.

Ninety percent of lung cancer cases are symptomatic at presentation [14]. Primary assessment of a patient with suspected lung cancer starts with a history and physical examination; complete blood count; checking alkaline phosphatase, hepatic transaminase, and calcium levels; clinical chemistry analysis for electrolytes, blood urea nitrogen, creatinine; and chest radiography [15].

Conventional chest radiography is the most routinely used method for imaging the lung. Screening trials for early detection of lung cancer first began in the 1950s with chest X-rays and sputum cytology, but these attempts led to no improvement in overall survival rates compared with control subjects [16]. These failures could be attributed to the limitations of conventional chest radiography. Despite the fact that it is fast and low cost, the average size of missed lung lesions in chest radiographs is 1.6 cm [17], and the detection sensitivity is less than 50% for tumors of ~1.9 cm in size [18]. Therefore, conventional X-ray radiography is not a suitable technique for early diagnosis of lung cancer [19].

4.1.3 Potential Adverse Effects Due to CT Imaging

For chest radiographs that are not clear for diagnosis, computed tomography (CT) is employed to obtain more detailed images. However, CT exposes the patients to very high ionizing radiation doses (see Table 4.2) and can aggravate the disease. In experimental models investigating the effects of ionizing radiation, alterations in *CDKN1A* and *GADD45A* gene expression levels in a human myeloid leukemia cell line has been reported after receiving 20- to 500-mGy radiation doses [20]. Both *CDKN1A* and *GADD45A* genes play a role in cell cycle and proliferation pathways. In another study, alterations in protein synthesis pathways were also reported after irradiation of cancer cells [21]. Similarly, differences in the adaptive responses between healthy versus tumor cells have been reported by others [22]. The level of radiation injury depends on a variety of factors, such as total radiation dose, dose rate, delivery as a single or fractionated dose, internal or external exposure, and the amount of tissue exposed [23].

Adverse effects of radiation are also present in the lung, such as alterations in animal survival or tumor growth. Acute pneumonitis is the most common complication postirradiation and results in a permanent state of radiation-induced fibrosis in the lungs [24]. In experimental models, these effects have been investigated by exposing mice to radiation by using microcomputed CT (micro-CT) imaging [25]. Micro-CT allows for high-resolution imaging of the lungs and is one of the most commonly

TABLE 4.2 Radiation Doses From Select Medical Imaging Applications Versus Background Radiation*

Examination	Radiation Dose (mGy)	Time to Accumulate Similar Background Dose
Radiography:		
Chest	0.1	10 days
Computed tomography:		
Chest	7.0	2 years
Pulmonary embolism	10.0	3 years
Nuclear medicine:		
Lung ventilation/perfusion	2.0	8 months

*Effective radiation doses, proposed by the International Commission on Radiation Protection, are taken and adapted from Lin [29].

used techniques to image pulmonary pathologies in small animals [26]. For example, in the study by Miller et al. [24], 11 Gy of ionizing radiation was shown to induce significant increases in the lung density of mice, which is comparable to the doses received in radiation therapy of lung tumors [27]. In the study by Rodt et al. [25], various micro-CT protocols were performed on mice, and the accumulated radiation was assessed at the end of the study. They showed that the radiation dose from micro-CT scans varied between 170 and 280 mGy, which could potentiate noteworthy interactions with the experimental plans. Likewise, longitudinal studies with comparatively low dose but repetitive radiation could possibly have adverse effects on tumor growth in experimental studies. Various studies suggest caution for adverse effects of radiation while interpreting the study results [28].

4.1.4 Animal Models of Lung Cancer

The most common animal models for lung cancer are based in mice [30]. In these models, it is similarly of high importance to detect lung nodules as early as possible to be able to track disease progression and responses to potential therapies: morphological changes in these nodules on treatment should be monitored over time [31]. Noninvasive imaging of experimental animals allows for repetitive examinations of the tissues in longitudinal studies [32]. One major advantage of monitoring disease progression/regression is that each animal can serve as its own control, and the need for additional animals for various time points is minimized. Such an approach would not only enable early screening of lung nodules but also provide information regarding resistance acquired over time to the therapies applied. However, this requires an imaging modality with high sensitivity and minimal side effects.

Novel noninvasive imaging approaches that allow for earlier detection, coupled with new treatment options aimed at early stage lung cancer detection, are urgently needed. Recent reports demonstrate encouraging findings with novel X-ray dark-field imaging for early detection of lung nodules in mice with lung cancer [33, 34].

In this chapter, we discuss applications of this technology for imaging of lung (diseases) and in particular lung cancer in small animals with its future perspectives and potential challenges.

4.2 Radiographic Approaches and X-Ray Dark-Field Imaging

4.2.1 Conventional Radiography

Chest radiography first evolved at the end of the 19th century shortly after Roentgen's discovery of X-rays. At that time, tuberculosis accounted for 15% of all deaths in the world and played a notable role in rapid implementation and development of X-ray imaging of the lung [35]. One of the pioneers of chest radiography, Francis

Williams, thought that the path to cure tuberculosis was through early detection of the disease. Tuberculosis was often diagnosed at an advanced stage when the patients could no longer be cured. Williams first described the use of X-rays for diagnosis of early tuberculosis in patients in 1896. Ever since, X-ray examination of the chest has been the most commonly used medical imaging technique in the world [36].

X-rays are electromagnetic waves with wavelengths in the region of an angstrom (10^{-10} m) [37]. When an X-ray passes through an object, the X-ray's amplitude and phase are altered depending on the atomic composition and arrangement of the material [38]. Conventional X-ray imaging is based on obtaining contrast through local differences in absorption across the cross section of an object [39]. This approach is particularly useful where structures that absorb the X-rays strongly (e.g., bones) are located in weakly absorbing environments.

About 90% of misdiagnoses in lung cancer occur with chest radiography, where transmission images are solely evaluated [40]. Overlooked lung cancer cases can be due to observer errors, tumor characteristics, or technical considerations. Previous studies demonstrate that the average size of missed carcinomas is quite variable, for example, 16 mm in Austin et al. [41], 25 mm in Monnier-Cholley et al. [42], and 18.1 mm in Wu et al. [43]. The threshold visibility in conventional X-ray imaging is defined at 3 mm; that is, only objects larger than 3 mm in thickness can be visualized with this modality [44]. Yet, if the margins of the object are at an angle to the X-ray beam line, this sensitivity decreases progressively. Another aspect that directly affects the visibility is the location of the object. The efficiency is higher with objects that are located near or within the air-containing parenchyma and not blinded by overlying structures.

4.2.2 Interferometric Radiography

Interestingly, the interactions between the matter and the X-rays while they pass through the specimen also result in interference and refraction of the beam (see Figure 4.4). As an alternative approach, generating image contrast from these alterations are categorized as interferometric methods [38]. Phase-contrast X-ray imaging is based on detection and quantification of these phase changes in the X-rays during the traverse [38, 45, 46]. This phase change of the X-rays per unit path length is much higher than the X-ray amplitude itself; therefore, the image contrast obtained by these changes is much stronger than the image contrast generated by mere X-ray amplitude.

4.2.3 X-Ray Dark-Field Imaging

X-ray dark-field imaging, on the other hand, relies on quantification of small-angle scattering of the X-rays during the traverse [39, 47]. In this technology, the signal is obtained by small-angle scattering of X-rays passing through structures that are

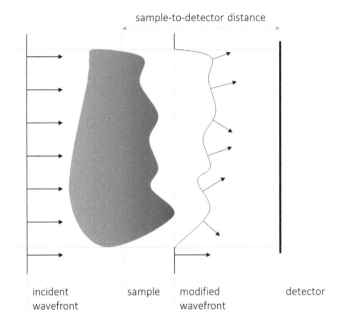

sample-to-detector distance

incident   sample   modified   detector
wavefront   wavefront

Figure 4.4   X-ray wave front before and after traversing a specimen.

below the spatial resolution of the imaging system. Hence, with X-ray dark-field imaging, one can not only acquire complementary data but also detect information that normally is below the resolution limit for conventional X-ray imaging [48]. Particularly in soft-tissue imaging, where the absorption contrast is significantly weak, X-ray phase-contrast and dark-field imaging can generate additional insights on the structural conditions of the tissue. In regions where structures with similar absorption cross sections are present, conventional X-ray imaging lacks sensitivity. Further, due to the ease of strong contrast obtained by phase-contrast and dark-field imaging, the radiation doses exerted on the specimen can be minimized.

Interferometric methods vary in their experimental setups, illuminating radiation requirements, and their signal acquisition. A common feature, though, is that these techniques require a highly parallel and monochromatic X-ray beam source with restricted spatial and temporal coherence lengths [39, 49, 50]. Due to the technical challenges associated with implementing X-ray beam sources with such parameters, routine use of these X-ray imaging modalities in the clinics or industry has been limited. In 2005, Weitkamp et al. [51] first demonstrated that two gratings can be used for differential phase-contrast imaging from polychromatic X-rays of brilliant synchrotron sources. Following this in 2006, Pfeiffer et al. [39] showed an alternative approach to retrieve quantitative phase images with polychromatic X-ray sources of low brilliance and dark-field scatter images using conventional X-ray tube sources [47] by exploiting the Talbot-Lau interferometer. His team proved that addition of a third grating to the system resulted in successful adaptation of this technique to X-ray sources of low brilliance [39]. Using a source grating G0, a phase grating G1, and an analyzer absorption grating G2 (Figure 4.5), they were able to achieve

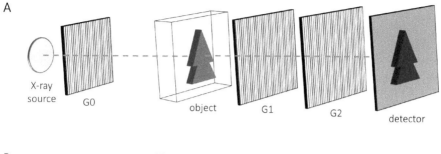

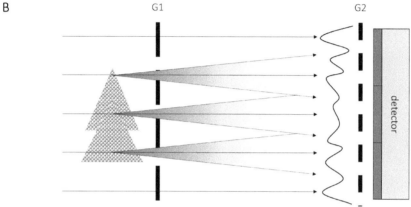

Figure 4.5 Grating-interferometric X-ray radiography. (A) Schematic representation of the X-ray radiography setup with the X-ray source; G0, G1, and G2 gratings; specimen; and the detector. (B) Representation of dark-field signal obtained by small-angle scattering of the X-rays traversing the specimen.

dark-field scatter images of high quality. This major achievement allowed for acquisition of adequate X-rays with conventional polychromatic laboratory sources and led to a more frequent use of grating-based imaging in preclinical models for biomedical applications [48].

So far, X-ray dark-field radiography has been used to visualize microcalcifications in mammography [52, 53], bone microstructures [54], and pulmonary disorders in mice [33, 34, 55–57]. While imaging of the lung, breast, and bones have been the main sites of interest for dark-field imaging, new applications are expected to arise [48].

4.3 Pulmonary Applications of X-Ray Dark-Field Imaging

The first dark-field radiography with a conventional polychromatic laboratory X-ray source was demonstrated in 2013 by Bech et al. [58] to visualize mouse lungs in vivo. His team demonstrated that grating-based multicontrast X-ray imaging was able to visualize mouse organs in vivo with differential contrasts (Figure 4.6). While the conventional transmission image provided suitable information about the bones (Figure 4.6A), phase-contrast images acquired by refraction of the X-rays

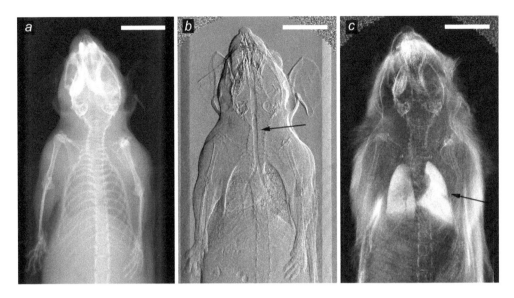

Figure 4.6 Grating-based multicontrast X-ray images of a mouse in vivo. (A) Conventional transmission image. (B) Phase-contrast image. (C) Dark-field image [58].

revealed higher contrast in structures such as the trachea (pointed at Figure 4.6B). Interestingly, dark-field images acquired from small-angle scattering of the X-rays revealed a strong contrast in the lungs (pointed at Figure 4.6C). This is due to the fact that small-angle scattering occurs significantly at the air–tissue interfaces in the

TABLE 4.3 X-Ray Dark-Field Visualization of the Lung in Various Models

Year	X-Ray Source	Model	Species	Breathing	Level	Reference
2000	Synchrotron radiation	Healthy lung	M	–	In vivo	[66]
2005	Synchrotron radiation	Healthy lung	M, Rb	–	In vivo	[67]
2010	Synchrotron radiation	Healthy lung	M	–	In vivo	[68]
2011	Synchrotron radiation	Pneumonitis	R	+	In vivo	[69]
2012	Compact synchrotron X-ray source	Emphysema	M	–	Ex vivo	[60]
2013	Polychromatic X-ray source	Healthy lung	M	+	In vivo	[58]
2013	Polychromatic X-ray source	Emphysema	M	–	Ex vivo	[55]
2014	Polychromatic X-ray source	Lung cancer	M	–	Ex vivo	[70]
2014	Polychromatic X-ray source	Emphysema	M	+	In vivo	[57]
2015	Polychromatic X-ray source	Emphysema, lung fibrosis	M	+	In vivo	[63, 71]
2016	Polychromatic X-ray source	Pneumothorax	M*	–	In vivo	[72]
2017	Polychromatic X-ray source	Lung cancer	M	+	In vivo	[33, 34]
2017	Polychromatic X-ray source	Healthy lung	P	–	In vivo	[73]
2017	Polychromatic X-ray source	Healthy lung	H	–	In vivo	[74]
2018	Polychromatic X-ray source	Pneumothorax	P	–	In vivo	[65]
2018	Polychromatic X-ray source	Lung inflammation	M	+	In vivo	[64]

Abbreviations: M, mouse; Rb, rabbit; R, rat; M*, mouse (neonate); P, pig; H, human (cadaver).

lung. This study indicated a potential applicability of X-ray dark-field imaging for visualization of lung diseases.

Since then, various studies have shown that dark-field imaging can detect detailed, structural information of the lung, such as the number and size of the alveoli (see Table 4.3) [55, 59–62]. In early studies by Hellbach et al. [56], the dark-field signal of the lung was found to be proportional to the size of the alveoli. Further, in the publication by Yaroshenko et al. [63], the dark-field signal was reported to decrease with decreasing number of alveoli. In follow-up studies, X-ray dark-field imaging was demonstrated to be capable of detecting lung diseases in in vivo experimental models, such as pulmonary fibrosis [63], emphysema [57], pulmonary inflammation [64], and pneumothorax [65]. Encouragingly, for detection of end-stage pulmonary fibrosis induced in mouse lungs, dark-field imaging was found to be significantly more sensitive to fibrotic changes in the lung than conventional X-ray imaging (Figure 4.7). Thus, X-ray dark-field imaging could be of potential use for earlier detection for pulmonary fibrosis [63].

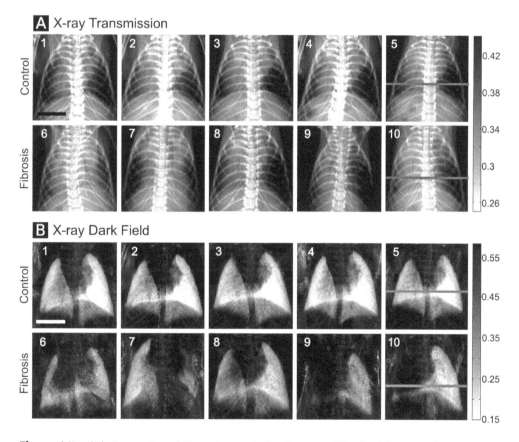

Figure 4.7   (A) Conventional X-ray transmission images of five healthy mice (1–5, top row) in comparison to five mice with pulmonary fibrosis (6–10, bottom row). (B) X-ray dark-field images of the same animals. Scale bar = 5 mm [63].

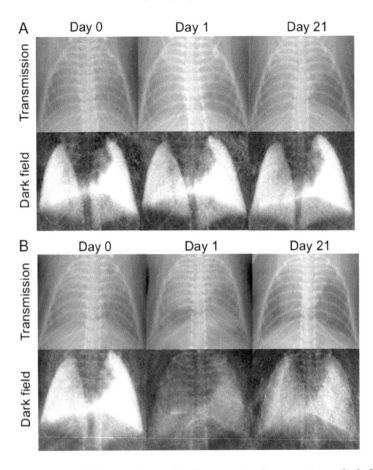

Figure 4.8 Conventional chest radiography (transmission) versus X-ray dark-field images acquired from (A) PBS-treated healthy and (B) elastase-treated inflamed lungs before (day 0) and after (day 1 and day 21) treatment [64].

More recently, Hellbach et al. [64] exploited X-ray dark-field imaging for monitoring the progression and resolution of elastase-induced acute lung inflammation in mice in vivo. Their findings show that dark-field radiography has substantial improvement over conventional transmission images for detection of inflammation-driven acute, bilateral infiltrates (Figure 4.8).

4.4 X-Ray Dark-Field Imaging of Lung Cancer in Murine Models

The dark-field signal decreases with increasing small-angle scattering in the object [45, 47, 49]. Normal lung tissue has a low dark-field signal caused by the strong scattering of its multiple air–tissue interfaces [75, 76]. However, tumor tissue is rather homogeneous and solid (i.e., less airspace), which leads to less small-angle scattering in comparison to the surrounding lung tissue (see Figure 4.9). Meinel et al. [70] were

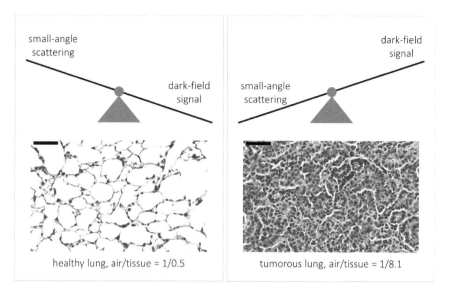

small-angle scattering

dark-field signal

dark-field signal

small-angle scattering

healthy lung, air/tissue = 1/0.5

tumorous lung, air/tissue = 1/8.1

Figure 4.9 The correlation between dark-field signal and small-angle scattering of X-rays traversing a specimen. Hematoxylin (violet, cell nuclei) and eosin (pink, proteins) staining of healthy versus tumorous lungs from mice. Scale bar = 50 µm.

the first to try visualizing lung cancer by grating-based imaging by using a prototype phase-contrast small-animal scanner equipped with a conventional polychromatic X-ray source. In brief, an excised lung with multiple tumors from a $Kras^{LA1}$ transgenic mouse, 6 months after activation of the oncogene, was imaged ex vivo. The tumors were characterized by decreased transmission signal and increased dark-field signal. In this study, no additional tumors other than the ones visible in the transmission image were visualized on the dark-field image.

The study by Scherer et al. [33] was the first to evaluate the efficacy of X-ray dark-field imaging for detection of lung nodules in vivo. In this setup, $Kras^{LA2}$ transgenic mice [77] with multiple primary lung tumors at different stages were anesthetized and imaged with a compact small-animal dark-field scanner. The conventional and dark-field images obtained from the scans were compared, and the lesions were histologically validated. In addition, the diagnostic value of dark-field imaging was evaluated by experts in a reader study: the transmission and dark-field images acquired were analyzed for tumor detection by three experienced readers in a blinded manner.

Large tumors were equally visible in both transmission and dark-field images. Interestingly, several small tumors that were apparent in dark-field images were not detected in the transmission images. Hence, this study demonstrated clearly that X-ray dark-field imaging is significantly superior to conventional X-ray radiography for detection of small lesions in tumorous mouse lungs in vivo. This was further pronounced in tomographs reconstructed from the conventional and dark-field images [34]. Strikingly, some small lesions that were readily detectable in dark-field images were missed in the reader study.

A

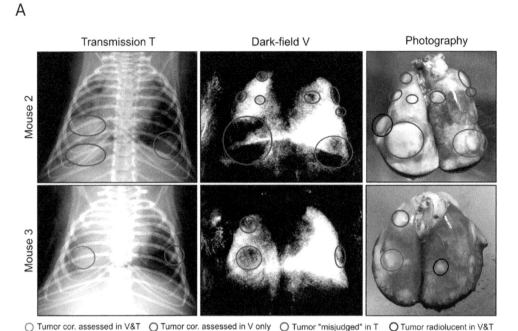

B

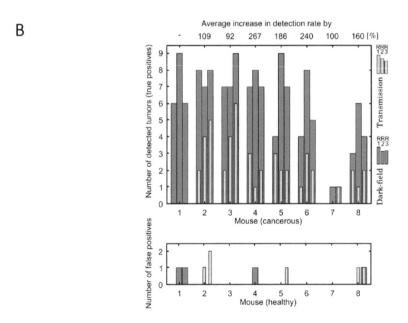

Figure 4.10 X-ray dark-field imaging of lung tumors in mice in vivo. (A) Comparison of conventional transmission image versus dark-field image obtained in reference to photographical images of the fixed tumorous mouse lungs. (B) Lung tumor detection rates (top panel) and false positives (lower panel) from the blinded randomized reader study [33].

Therefore, these early proof-of-principle studies in mice indicate that dark-field imaging may allow for early diagnosis of lung tumors that could be overlooked in conventional radiographs.

4.5 Computer-Aided Diagnosis of Pulmonary Diseases

Computer-aided diagnosis (CADx) strategies in pulmonary applications of X-ray dark-field radiography has been limited. A study by Einarsdóttir et al. [71] covers development of a CADx scheme for classification of emphysematous and fibrotic mouse lungs. Their approach comprised three stages: automatic lung segmentation, extraction of both intensity and shape features of the segmented lung, and classification of healthy, emphysematous or fibrotic lungs based on a linear support vector machine.

To our knowledge, there has been no study investigating diagnosis of lung cancer in rodents using CADx schemes in X-ray dark-field radiography. However, recent reports on other imaging modalities where CADx approaches were utilized for early diagnosis of lung cancer have encouraging findings [78–81]. Future attempts for developing a CADx strategy for small nodule detection in X-ray dark-field radiography will be an important advance for lung cancer detection.

4.6 Future Perspectives and Translational Challenges

Although preclinical data suggest the potential for earlier detection of lung cancer with X-ray dark-field imaging in mouse models as compared to conventional X-ray imaging, further advances are required to bring this technology for routine use in the clinics. Commercialized models will need to encompass units such as readily available, compact X-ray sources and detectors that are adequate to generate meaningful data in larger species. X-ray dark-field imaging of the lung can benefit from tomographical acquisition of the data as well. However, for both 2D and 3D imaging purposes, the scan time and the radiation dose implied needs to be reduced [82]. The report by Gromann et al. [73] offers encouraging findings where they could acquire dark-field chest radiography of a pig lung by 70 kV of source power in 40 seconds, resulting in an 80-μGy radiation dose. In addition, recent attempts of X-ray dark-field imaging of a human cadaver chest showed that dark-field radiography is capable of detecting lung edema. This is the first report where multicontrast X-ray images from a human cadaver chest were obtained and thus acts as a milestone for translation of dark-field radiography [74]. Clinical applications of similar setups for diagnosis of rheumatoid arthritis in human finger joints have already been reported by Tanaka et al. [83] and Momose et al. [84]. Additional clinical considerations aim at exploitation of dark-field imaging in mammography [85, 86].

The development of new strategies where X-ray dark-field imaging is coupled with conventional diagnostic imaging modalities (e.g., magnetic resonance imaging or positron emission tomography) may help enrich the readout for lung cancer screening and classification. Further, automating these units with lung function assessment systems might help improve image acquisition, and the lung function measurements would serve as additional reference points.

There are many other potential applications for X-ray dark-field imaging related to lung cancer detection and monitoring of therapeutic efficacy. Future studies should explore whether X-ray dark-field imaging can be used to identify the type and/or origin of the tumor. Contrast agents could be developed for X-ray dark-field imaging that allow for detection of the aggressiveness of the cancer cells. In recent studies, microbubbles were evaluated as contrast agents for dark-field radiography [61, 62, 87]. Using specifically targeted microbubbles could additionally allow for functional readouts in vivo, such as early detection of acquired resistance against applied therapeutics and thereon targeted drug delivery with loaded microbubbles. One other potential application of the technique could be to use X-ray dark-field imaging for immediate evaluation of biopsies or surgical resections. Current practice often requires time- and labor-intensive histological processing and evaluation of the resections. In trauma or during surgery, this could lead to fast and effective lifesaving decisions.

4.7 Summary

Lung cancer is by far the most common cause of cancer-related deaths with 1.6 million mortalities worldwide. The disease is often diagnosed at its advanced stages with an average 5-year survival rate of 15%. Reports show that lung cancer diagnosed at an early stage without metastasis can be controlled much more efficiently, with 5-year survival rates reaching up to 70%. Chest radiography is the most common technique to evaluate pulmonary disorders. However, conventional X-ray imaging is not sufficient to detect small tumors at the early stages of lung cancer due to technical limitations and observer errors. Grating-based X-ray dark-field imaging has emerged as an alternative technology to image pulmonary disorders, such as emphysema or pulmonary fibrosis, in mouse models in vivo. In particular, X-ray dark-field radiography was shown to be significantly superior for detection of small lung nodules in comparison to conventional chest radiography. While these findings encourage its further implementation for early detection of lung cancer in clinics, there are limitations for its translation to the bedside, some of which are summarized in Table 4.4.

TABLE 4.4   Brief Comparison of Conventional X-Ray Versus Dark-Field Imaging of the Lung

Features	Comparison
Availability	Conventional is much more common
Radiation	Conventional has less radiation exposure
Scan time	Conventional is much faster
Large lesion detection	No significant difference in performance
Small lesion detection	Dark field is significantly superior
Human scale	Only one report in dark-field imaging for human lungs

Therefore, further progress in the field is required for X-ray dark-field imaging before it reaches the clinics and be used for diagnosis of lung cancer.

References

1. Ferlay J, Soerjomataram I, Dikshit, et al. Cancer incidence and mortality worldwide: sources, methods and major patterns in GLOBOCAN 2012. *Int J Cancer.* 2015;136:E359–E386.
2. Gridelli C, Rossi A, Carbone DP, et al. Non-small-cell lung cancer. *Nat Rev Dis Primers.* 2015;1:15009.
3. Henschke CI, McCauley DI, Yankelevitz DF, et al. Early Lung Cancer Action Project: overall design and findings from baseline screening. *Lancet.* 1999;354:99–105.
4. Latimer KM, Mott TF. Lung cancer: diagnosis, treatment principles, and screening. *Am Fam Phys.* 2015;91(4):250-6.
5. Spira A, Ettinger DS. Multidisciplinary management of lung cancer. *New Engl J Med.* 2004;250:379–392.
6. Zappa C, Mousa SA. Non-small cell lung cancer: current treatment and future advances. *Trans Lung Cancer Res.* 2016;5:288.
7. Kenfield SA, Wei EK, Stampfer MJ, Rosner BA, Colditz GA. Comparison of aspects of smoking among the four histological types of lung cancer. *Tob Control.* 2008;17:198–204.
8. Park KS, Liang MC, Raiser DM, et al. Characterization of the cell of origin for small cell lung cancer. *Cell Cycle.* 2011;10:2806–2815.
9. Rami-Porta R, Asamura H, Travis WD, Rusch VW, Lung cancer—major changes in the American Joint Committee on Cancer eighth edition cancer staging manual. *CA Cancer J Clin.* 2017;67:138–155.
10. Popper HH. Progression and metastasis of lung cancer. *Cancer Metastasis Rev.* 2016;35:75–91.
11. Tamura T, Kurishima K, Nakazawa K, et al. Specific organ metastases and survival in metastatic non-small-cell lung cancer. *Mol Clin Oncol.* 2015;3:217–221.
12. Seo JB, Im J-G, Goo JM, Chung MJ, Kim M-Y. Atypical pulmonary metastases: spectrum of radiologic findings. *Radiographics.* 2001;21:403–417.
13. Dishop MK, Kuruvilla S. Primary and metastatic lung tumors in the pediatric population: a review and 25-year experience at a large children's hospital. *Arch Pathol Lab Med.* 2008;132:1079–1103.
14. Collins LG, Haines C, Perkel R, Enck RE. Lung cancer: diagnosis and management. *Am Fam Phys.* 2007;75:56–63.
15. Rivera MP, Mehta AC, Wahidi MM. Establishing the diagnosis of lung cancer: diagnosis and management of lung cancer: American College of Chest Physicians evidence-based clinical practice guidelines. *Chest.* 2013;143:e142S–e165S.
16. Spiro SG, Silvestri GA. One hundred years of lung cancer. *Am J Respir Crit Care Med.* 2005;172:523–529.
17. Fardanesh M, White C. Missed lung cancer on chest radiography and computed tomography. *Semin Ultrasound CT MR.* 2012;33:280–287.
18. Freedman MT, Lo SC, Seibel JC, Bromley CM. Lung nodules: improved detection with software that suppresses the rib and clavicle on chest radiographs. *Radiology.* 2011;260:265–273.

19. Oken MM, Hocking WG, Kvale PA, et al. Screening by chest radiograph and lung cancer mortality: the Prostate, Lung, Colorectal, and Ovarian (PLCO) randomized trial. *JAMA*. 2011;306:1865–1873.

20. Amundson SA, Lee RA, Koch-Paiz CA, et al. Differential responses of stress genes to low dose-rate γ irradiation1 1 DOE Grant ER62683. *Mol Cancer Res*. 2003;*1*:445–452.

21. Braunstein S, Badura ML, Xi Q, Formenti SC, Schneider RJ. Regulation of protein synthesis by ionizing radiation. *Mol Cell Biol*. 2009;29:5645–5656.

22. Amundson SA, Do KT, Fornace AJ. Induction of stress genes by low doses of gamma rays. *Radiat Res*. 1999;152:225–231.

23. Day RM, Barshishat-Kupper M, Mog SR, et al. Genistein protects against biomarkers of delayed lung sequelae in mice surviving high-dose total body irradiation. *J Radiat Res*. 2008;49:361–372.

24. Miller G, Dawson D, Battista J. Computed tomographic assessment of radiation induced damage in the lung of normal and WR 2721 protected LAF1 mice. *Int J Radiat Oncol Biol Phys*. 1986;12:1971–1975.

25. Rodt T, Luepke M, Boehm C, et al. Phantom and cadaver measurements of dose and dose distribution in micro-CT of the chest in mice. *Acta Radiol*. 2011;52:75–80.

26. Clark D, Badea C. Micro-CT of rodents: state-of-the-art and future perspectives. *Phys Med Eur J Med Phys*. 2014;30:619–634.

27. Timmerman R, Paulus R, Galvin J, et al. Stereotactic body radiation therapy for inoperable early stage lung cancer. *JAMA*. 2010;303:1070–1076.

28. Willekens I, Buls N, Lahoutte T, et al. Evaluation of the radiation dose in micro-CT with optimization of the scan protocol. *Contrast Media Mol Imaging*. 2010;5:201–207.

29. Lin EC. Radiation risk from medical imaging. *Mayo Clin Proc*. 2010;85:1142–1146.

30. Meuwissen R, Berns A. Mouse models for human lung cancer. *Genes Dev*. 2005;19:643–664.

31. Bölükbas DA, Meiners S. Lung cancer nanomedicine: potentials and pitfalls. *Nanomedicine (Lond)*. 2015;10:3203–3212.

32. O'Farrell A, Shnyder S, Marston G, Coletta P, Gill J. Non-invasive molecular imaging for preclinical cancer therapeutic development. *Br J Pharmacol*. 2013;169:719–735.

33. Scherer K, Yaroshenko A, Bölükbas DA, et al. X-ray dark-field radiography—in-vivo diagnosis of lung cancer in mice. *Sci Rep*. 2017;7:402.

34. Gromann LB, Scherer K, Yaroshenko A, et al. First experiences with in-vivo x-ray dark-field imaging of lung cancer in mice. *SPIE Med Imaging*. 2017;10132:101325L–101325L-6.

35. Greene R Fleischner Lecture. Imaging the respiratory system in the first few years after discovery of the X-ray: contributions of Francis H. Williams, M.D. *Am J Roentol*. 1992;159:1–7.

36. Gurney J. Why chest radiography became routine. *Radiology*. 1995;195:245–246.

37. Als-Nielsen J, McMorrow D. X-rays and their interaction with matter. In: *Elements of Modern X-Ray Physics*. New York, NY: John Wiley & Sons; 2011:1–28.

38. Momose A, Takeda T, Itai Y, Hirano K. Phase-contrast X-ray computed tomography for observing biological soft tissues. *Nat Med*. 1996;2:473–475.

39. Pfeiffer F, Weitkamp T, Bunk O, David C. Phase retrieval and differential phase-contrast imaging with low-brilliance X-ray sources. *Nat Phys*. 2006;2:258–261.

40. del Ciello A, Franchi P, Contegiacomo A, Cicchetti G, Bonomo L, Larici AR, Missed lung cancer: when, where, and why? *Diagn Interv Radiol*. 2017;23:118.

41. Austin J, Romney B, Goldsmith L. Missed bronchogenic carcinoma: radiographic findings in 27 patients with a potentially resectable lesion evident in retrospect. *Radiology*. 1992;182:115–122.

42. Monnier-Cholley L, Arrivé L, Porcel A, et al. Characteristics of missed lung cancer on chest radiographs: a French experience. *Eur Radiol*. 2001;11:597–605.

43. Wu M-H, Gotway M, Lee T, et al. Features of non-small cell lung carcinomas overlooked at digital chest radiography. *Clin Radiol*. 2008;63:518–528.

44. Delrue L, Gosselin R, Ilsen B, Van Landeghem A, de Mey J, Duyck P. Difficulties in the interpretation of chest radiography. In: *Comparative Interpretation of CT and Standard Radiography of the Chest*. New York, NY: Springer; 2011:27–49.

45. Keyriläinen J, Bravin A, Fernández M, Tenhunen M, Virkkunen P, Suortti P. Phase-contrast X-ray imaging of breast. *Acta Radiol*. 2010;51:866–884.

46. Momose A. Recent advances in X-ray phase imaging. *Jpn J Appl Phys*. 2005;44:6355.

47. Pfeiffer F, Bech M, Bunk O, et al. Hard-X-ray dark-field imaging using a grating interferometer. *Nat Mater*. 2008;7:134–137.

48. Yaroshenko A, Hellbach K, Bech M, et al. Grating-based X-ray dark-field imaging: a new paradigm in radiography. *Curr Radiol Rep*. 2014;2:57.

49. Chapman D, Thomlinson W, Johnston R, et al. Diffraction enhanced x-ray imaging. *Phys Med Biol*. 1997;42:2015.

50. Mayo S, Davis T, Gureyev T, et al. X-ray phase-contrast microscopy and microtomography. *Optics Express*. 2003;11:2289–2302.

51. Weitkamp T, Diaz A, David C, et al. X-ray phase imaging with a grating interferometer. *Optics Express*. 2005;13:6296–6304.

52. Stampanoni M, Wang Z, Thüring T, et al. The first analysis and clinical evaluation of native breast tissue using differential phase-contrast mammography. *Invest Radiol*. 2011;46:801–806.

53. Anton G, Bayer F, Beckmann MW, et al. Grating-based darkfield imaging of human breast tissue. *Z Med Phys*. 2013;23:228–235.

54. Thüring T, Guggenberger R, Alkadhi H, et al. Human hand radiography using X-ray differential phase contrast combined with dark-field imaging. *Skeletal Radiol*. 2013;42:827–835.

55. Yaroshenko A, Meinel FG, Bech M, et al. Pulmonary emphysema diagnosis with a preclinical small-animal x-ray dark-field scatter-contrast scanner. *Radiology*. 2013;269:427–433.

56. Hellbach K, Yaroshenko A, Meinel FG, et al. In vivo dark-field radiography for early diagnosis and staging of pulmonary emphysema. *Invest Radiol*. 2015;50:430–435.

57. Meinel FG, Yaroshenko A, Hellbach K, et al. Improved diagnosis of pulmonary emphysema using in vivo dark-field radiography. *Invest Radiol*. 2014;49:653–658.

58. Bech M, Tapfer A, Velroyen A, et al. In-vivo dark-field and phase-contrast x-ray imaging. *Sci Rep*. 2013;3:3209.

59. Malecki A, Eggl E, Schaff F, et al. Correlation of x-ray dark-field radiography to mechanical sample properties. *Microsc Microanal*. 2014;20:1528–1533.

60. Schleede S, Meinel FG, Bech M, et al. Emphysema diagnosis using X-ray dark-field imaging at a laser-driven compact synchrotron light source. *Proc Natl Acad Sci*. 2012;109:17880–17885.

61. Velroyen A, Bech M, Malecki A, et al. Microbubbles as a scattering contrast agent for grating-based x-ray dark-field imaging. *Phys Med Biol*. 2013;58:N37.

62. Velroyen A, Bech M, Tapfer A, et al. Ex vivo perfusion-simulation measurements of microbubbles as a scattering contrast agent for grating-based x-ray dark-field imaging. *PLoS One*. 2015:10:e0129512.

63. Yaroshenko A, Hellbach K, Yildirim AO, et al. Improved in vivo assessment of pulmonary fibrosis in mice using x-ray dark-field radiography. *Sci Rep.* 2015;5:17492.

64. Hellbach K, Meinel FG, Conlon TM, et al. X-ray dark-field imaging to depict acute lung inflammation in mice. *Sci Rep.* 2018;8:2096.

65. Hellbach K, Baehr A, De Marco F, et al. Depiction of pneumothoraces in a large animal model using x-ray dark-field radiography. *Sci Rep.* 2018;8:2602.

66. Zhong Z, Thomlinson W, Chapman D, Sayers D. Implementation of diffraction-enhanced imaging experiments: at the NSLS and APS. *Nucl Instrum Methods Phys Res Sect A Accelerators Spectrometers Detectors Assoc Equipment.* 2000;450:556–567.

67. Kitchen MJ, Lewis RA, Yagi N, et al. Phase contrast X-ray imaging of mice and rabbit lungs: a comparative study. *Br J Radiol.* 2005;78:1018–1027.

68. Kitchen MJ, Paganin DM, Uesugi K, et al. X-ray phase, absorption and scatter retrieval using two or more phase contrast images. *Optics Express.* 2010;18:19994–20012.

69. Connor DM, Zhong Z, Foda HD, et al. Diffraction enhanced imaging of a rat model of gastric acid aspiration pneumonitis. *Acad Radiol.* 2011;18:1515–1521.

70. Meinel FG, Schwab F, Yaroshenko A, et al. Lung tumors on multimodal radiographs derived from grating-based X-ray imaging—a feasibility study. *Phys Med.* 2014;30:352–357.

71. Einarsdóttir H, Yaroshenko A, Velroyen A, et al. Computer-aided diagnosis of pulmonary diseases using x-ray darkfield radiography. *Phys Med Biol.* 2015;60:9253.

72. Hellbach K, Yaroshenko A, Willer K, et al. Facilitated diagnosis of pneumothoraces in newborn mice using x-ray dark-field radiography. *Invest Radiol.* 2016;51:597–601.

73. Gromann LB, De Marco F, Willer K, et al. In-vivo X-ray dark-field chest radiography of a pig, *Sci Rep.* 2017;7:4807.

74. Noel PB, Willer K, Fingerle AA, et al. First experience with x-ray dark-field radiography for human chest imaging (conference presentation). *SPIE Med Imaging.* 2017; 10132:1.

75. Kitchen MJ, Lewis R, Morgan M, et al. Dynamic measures of regional lung air volume using phase contrast x-ray imaging. *Phys Med Biol.* 2008;53:6065.

76. Kitchen MJ, Paganin D, Lewis R, Yagi N, Uesugi K, Mudie S. On the origin of speckle in x-ray phase contrast images of lung tissue. *Phys Med Biol.* 2004;49:4335.

77. Johnson L, Mercer K, Greenbaum D, et al. Somatic activation of the K-ras oncogene causes early onset lung cancer in mice. *Nature.* 2001;410:1111–1116.

78. El-Baz A, Beache GM, Gimel'farb G, et al. Computer-aided diagnosis systems for lung cancer: challenges and methodologies. *Int J Biomed Imaging.* 2013;942353:1–46.

79. Doi K. Computer-aided diagnosis in medical imaging: historical review, current status and future potential. *Comput Med Imaging Graph.* 2007;31:198–211.

80. Farag AA, El-Baz A, Gimel'farb GG, Falk F, Hushek SG. Automatic detection and recognition of lung abnormalities in helical CT images using deformable templates. In: Barillot C, Haynor DR, Hellier P, eds. *Medical Image Computing and Computer-Assisted Intervention—MICCAI 2004.* Berlin, Germany: Springer; 2004:856–864.

81. Ye X, Lin X, Dehmeshki J, Slabaugh G, Beddoe G. Shape-based computer-aided detection of lung nodules in thoracic CT images. *IEEE Trans Biomed Eng.* 2009;56:1810–1820.

82. Horn F, Leghissa M, Kaeppler S, et al. Implementation of a Talbot-Lau interferometer in a clinical-like c-arm setup: a feasibility study. *Sci Rep.* 2018;8:2325.

83. Tanaka J, Nagashima M, Kido K, et al. Cadaveric and in vivo human joint imaging based on differential phase contrast by X-ray Talbot-Lau interferometry. *Z Med Phys.* 2013;23:222–227.

84. Momose A, Yashiro W, Kido K, et al. X-ray phase imaging: from synchrotron to hospital. *Philos Trans R Soc Lond A*. 2014;372:20130023.

85. Koehler T, Daerr H, Martens G, et al. Slit-scanning differential x-ray phase-contrast mammography: proof-of-concept experimental studies. *Med Phys*. 2015;42:1959–1965.

86. Arboleda C, Wang Z, Koehler T, et al. Sensitivity-based optimization for the design of a grating interferometer for clinical X-ray phase contrast mammography. *Optics Express*. 2017;25:6349–6364.

87. Millard TP, Endrizzi M, Everdell N, et al. Evaluation of microbubble contrast agents for dynamic imaging with x-ray phase contrast. *Sci Rep*. 2015;5:12509.

5

Lung Cancer Screening Using Low-Dose Computed Tomography

Alison Wenholz and Ikenna Okereke

Contents

5.1 Introduction

The American Cancer Society estimates that there were 155,870 lung cancer deaths in 2017. In the same year, there were 40,610 deaths from breast cancer, 26,730 deaths from prostate cancer, and 50,260 deaths from colorectal cancer [1]. Lung cancer kills more people yearly than breast cancer, prostate cancer, and colorectal cancer combined. Out of all cancer deaths in the United States, lung cancer is the cause of one out of four deaths. Lung cancer ranks as the second most prevalent cancer behind breast cancer in women and prostate cancer in men. Lung cancer does not present with symptoms such as persistent cough, hemoptysis, worsening shortness of breath, and chest pain until the cancer is in relatively advanced stages [2]. The absence of definitive symptoms correlates with the late stage of diagnosis of lung cancer.

In 2017, there were 222,500 new cases of lung cancer in the United States. There are approximately 415,000 people in the United States who are currently living with lung cancer [3]. The incidence of lung cancer has been declining since the 1980s in men but only since the early 2000s in women [1]. The decline in lung cancer in the United States is due in large part to the decline of cigarette smoking. Cigarette smoking is the leading cause of death by preventable disease in the United States. It is also the leading cause of lung cancer and a known cause of cardiovascular disease, chronic obstructive pulmonary disease (COPD), bladder cancer, and a long list of other cancers [4]. From 1965 to 2015, the number of American adult smokers has declined from 42% to 16.8% [4]. Despite this downward trend, it is estimated that there are 36.5 million adult smokers in the United States. Cigarette smoking causes an estimated 480,000 premature deaths each year. Even though the incidence of lung cancer in the United States is decreasing, it is still the leading cause of cancer deaths each year.

5.2 Current Outcomes

In 60% of patients diagnosed with small cell lung cancer, the disease has already progressed to stage IV. Non–small cell lung cancer is diagnosed at stage IV in 50% of patients [2]. The prognosis of lung cancer is poor because it is diagnosed in the advanced stages. The mean survival after diagnosis is only 9 months, and the 5-year survival rate is 15% [5]. Breast cancer is currently diagnosed as stage I in 40% of patients [6]. This is due primarily to the comprehensive screening program that exists in the United States with annual mammograms for women. The majority of prostate cancer is currently diagnosed at stage I. This rate of early diagnosis is, once again, due in part to a screening program that exists for prostate cancer. The American Cancer Society recommends that beginning at age 50, men who are at average risk of prostate cancer have a conversation with their primary care provider about prostate-specific antigen (PSA) testing and make an informed decision about whether to be tested based on their personal values and preferences. The widespread use of the PSA blood test has decreased because the test overinflated the diagnosed rate of prostate cancer. Colorectal cancer is currently diagnosed at a localized stage in 39% of patients. This is due to colonoscopy screening beginning at the age of 50. Colonoscopy allows physicians to detect and remove precancerous and cancerous lesions [1]. Current screening methods are effective at detecting breast cancer, prostate cancer, and colorectal cancer in their early stages. Compared to breast cancer, prostate cancer, and colorectal cancers, lung cancer is diagnosed at a much later stage because there is a lack of implemented screening. A widespread screening modality for lung cancer could increase the number of lung cancer cases detected at earlier, curable stages, thereby decreasing mortality.

5.3 Screening Trials

5.3.1 National Lung Screening Trial

Lung cancer screening programs are designed to detect and diagnose lung cancer in high-risk patients who are asymptomatic at a stage where curing the disease is more likely. In 1960, the Northwest London Mass Radiography Service was the first screening test designed for lung cancer. The study utilized a biannual chest X-ray and sputum cytology in 55,000 male smokers. In 1970, the Memorial Sloan-Kettering Cancer Center, Johns Hopkins, and the Mayo Clinic all instituted screening programs utilizing chest X-ray and sputum cytology. All four studies determined that sputum cytology was unnecessary and that screening with chest X-ray did not significantly alter mortality rates compared to the control group [7].All four studies had population biases skewed toward white males.

The National Lung Screening Trial (NLST) was a major change in the paradigm and ideas associated with lung cancer screening. Prior to the results of the NLST, there were only very few screening programs in the United States, and lung cancer screening was not reimbursed by Medicare and private insurance companies. The NLST was a randomized controlled trial that began accruing patients in 2002. The trial randomized high-risk patients to receive either yearly chest X-rays or low-dose helical computed tomography (CT) scans for lung cancer screening. The NLST enrolled approximately 54,000 current and former cigarette smokers who were between 55 and 74 years old [8]. The participants were required to have a minimum cigarette smoking history of 30 pack-years. Individuals who were former smokers had to have quit smoking within 15 years before the trial began. The participants were randomly assigned to the chest X-ray group or the low-dose computed tomography (LDCT) group. Each group had one screening test for 3 consecutive years. A chest X-ray was considered positive for a lung nodule if it showed a noncalcified lung nodule. An LDCT was considered positive if it had at least one noncalcified lung nodule greater or equal to 4 mm. At the end of 3 years, 6.9% of patients who had chest X-rays only and 24.2% of patients who had LDCTs only were positive for a lung nodule. There was a 1.1% cancer detection rate in the LDCT group. Furthermore, there was a 20% reduction in mortality in the LDCT group compared to the chest X-ray group. Additionally, the all-cause mortality was reduced by 6.7% [8] in the LDCT group. This was the first randomized screening trial that showed improvements in both disease-specific mortality and all-cause mortality [8] with screening using LDCT. The 3-year follow-up in the NLST may not have been long enough to account for the lead time of all cancers detectable by LDCT. Additional time is needed because tumor growth rates are variable. About 25% of nonbronchioalveolar non–small cell lung cancer tumors would have lead times of at least 5 years. Using the data collected in the NLST, 320 individuals require screening to save one life from lung cancer. This compares favorably to screening mammography, in which approximately 600 women need to be screened to save one life from breast cancer [8].

5.3.2 Overdiagnosis

A positive diagnosis of cancer that would not have progressed to cause symptoms or increase patient mortality is known as overdiagnosis. Overdiagnosis may occur because the cancer is biologically indolent and would have never grown large enough or cause symptoms before other factors in a patient's life caused mortality. Overdiagnosis also occurs in situations in which a patient is found to have a lung nodule that ultimately is not cancer. This mode of overdiagnosis is much more common. In these cases, patients may undergo unnecessary surveillance imaging, invasive diagnostic interventions, or unneeded surgical resection. The probability that lung cancer detected by LDCT in the NLST study was an overdiagnosis was 18.5% [9]. Patients who are diagnosed with lung cancer by LDCT may ultimately undergo invasive diagnostic procedures and surgical resection when their tumors may be clinically insignificant [9]. The *New York Times* published an article about the risk of overdiagnosis of lung cancer using LDCT. The article concluded that the invasive follow-up to a positive screening test is no longer trivial in patients over the age of 65 and that patients should have autonomy in the decision-making process to start screening [10]. The benefits of increased diagnosis of stage I lung cancer resulting in a decreased mortality rate outweigh the risk of overdiagnosis.

5.3.3 Inclusion Criteria

Inclusion criteria for lung cancer screening are current smokers who have a 30-pack-year cigarette smoking history and are between the ages of 55 and 77 years. The inclusion criteria also include former smokers with a 30-pack-year history who quit within the past 15 years. Smokers with COPD, compared to smokers with normal lung function, have up to a sixfold increased risk of developing lung cancer. This makes COPD the greatest risk factor for lung cancer in smokers [11]. Approximately 80%–90% of lung cancer occurs in tobacco smokers, but only 10%–15% of chronic smokers develop lung cancer [4]. The inclusion criteria for LDCT scans were established using the NLST's high-risk criteria.

5.4 Screening Technique

A low-dose protocol for computed tomography was determined to lower the patient's exposure to ionizing radiation. The CT technical parameters are important in achieving lower radiation exposure to adults compared to a traditional thoracic CT scan. This is important because radiation exposure is one potential risk associated with using CT scans as the screening method for lung cancer. Also, high-risk individuals will require yearly CT scans for an extended period of time, potentially decades [12]. An increase in the number of people exposed to radiation from CT screening could increase the radiation-induced cancers in the population. The middle-aged population that is screened primarily using LDCT is also the population at highest risk for radiation-induced lung cancer. The effective radiation dose estimates the participant dose of radiation that can be compared with other medical radiation procedures. Conservatively, the effective dose is 1.6 mSv for men and 2.1 mSv for women [12]. The annual population radiation dose at sea level, from all sources including the environment, averages 3 mSv. Annual LDCT causes an excess radiation risk of 0.85% in smoking females for developing lung cancer and 0.23% in smoking males (see Table 5.1).

$$CT_{\text{effective dose}} = k \times \text{dose length product [16]}$$

where dose length product = CT dose index$_{\text{volume}}$ × scan length and $k = 0.014$ mSv/mGy-cm [16].

TABLE 5.1   Risk of Radiation Exposure in Variable Circumstances

Source of Radiation	Average Dose
Low-dose CT [13]	1.5 mSv
Flying an airplane for 2 weeks [14]	3.024 mSv
Mammogram [13, 15]	0.4 mSv
Chest X-ray [13]	0.1 mSv
Standard chest CT [13]	7 mSv
Standing outside at sea level [14]	3 mSv annually

5.5 Lung Cancer Screening Results

In the NLST, 24.2% of all LDCTs were determined to be positive for a lung nodule, but only 3.6% of the positive LDCT screens resulted in a diagnosis of lung cancer, resulting in a positive predictive value <4%. A higher positive predictive value was seen in the Nederlands-Leuvens Longkanker Screenings Onderzoek (NELSON) trial by using a two-step process during the interpretation of the patient's nodule size. Lung nodules <5 mm were negative, those >10 mm were positive, and those ranging from 5 to 10 mm were indeterminate and underwent follow-up CT scan. The NELSON trial achieved a sensitivity of 94.6%, a specificity of 98.3%, a positive predictive value of 35.7%, and negative predictive values of 99.9% [17]. For every 1,000 individuals, nine stage I non–small cell lung cancers will be detected, but 235 false-positive nodules will also be detected [18, 19].

5.6 Implementation

The implementation of lung cancer screening requires considerable cooperation between specialties and the incorporation of current technology. Lung cancer screening implementation must be addressed in both civilian and veteran populations. The ultimate goals are to improve the diagnosis and management of early-stage lung cancer when it is responsive to curative resection and to reduce lung cancer mortality. These goals are best obtained by coupling LDCT screening with proactive smoking cessation programs. The screening program requires a multidisciplinary team including radiologists, thoracic surgeons, pulmonologists, nurse navigators, and pathologists. The screening program must also be tightly incorporated with institutional lung cancer treatment programs. The programs must be able to track individual patients and their screening results. The tracking aids primary care physicians in recalling individuals with positive screens and alerting them of their follow-up exams. Provider education and adoption of screening recommendations must be agreed on within the health care team. Patient education is crucial for the success of effective lung cancer screening. Individuals from disadvantaged backgrounds are more likely to have misconceptions about their individual risk of lung cancer, the benefits of surgical resection, and lung cancer mortality. The implementation of an effective lung cancer screening program across all socioeconomic classes will require multiple strategies to educate the public in these diverse groups. A current technological implementation advantageous to health care providers is the integration of electronic medical records, which can be utilized to find patients and alert primary care providers of high-risk patients who would benefit from lung cancer screening. Lung cancer screening that starts in the primary care physician's office has a higher probability of a successful outcome because the patients are seen in the early stage of disease. In addition to educating the civilian population, lung cancer screening requires special attention in the veteran population. One study found an increased rate of detection of lung cancer after implementation of a lung cancer screening program in a single Veterans Administration (VA) medical center. Lung cancers diagnosed after enactment of this program were more likely to be detected at an earlier stage than stage IV [5]. Implementation of a screening program at a veterans center differs from civilian medical centers for several reasons. There is minimal cost to the veterans receiving a screening CT scan. For this reason, the VA study was able to enroll a large number of veterans who met the criteria for screening. In addition, because of an extensive electronic medical record system, veterans who met the inclusion criteria were identified during their annual visits with primary care providers. This identification of patients allowed for the opportunity to counsel them about lung cancer screening and helped to increase enrollment. However, the rate of lung cancer may be higher in the veteran population than in the general population due to smoking history, so it is imperative to implement lung cancer screenings nationwide [5].

5.7 What to Do with the Results

The Lung Imaging Reporting and Data System (LungRADS) is a system deigned to classify the findings from LDCT scans for lung cancer [20] (see Table 5.2).

The primary treatment for stage I and II non–small cell lung cancer is surgical resection. At these stages, surgical resection has the best outcome for long-term survival. The 5-year survival rate for stage I non–small cell lung cancer after surgical resection is 60%–80% and 50%–60% for stage II non–small cell lung cancer after surgical resection. For stage III non–small cell lung cancer, surgical resection is combined with chemotherapy in patients who have resectable tumors. For unresectable tumors in stage III, chemotherapy is combined with radiation therapy [21]. LungRADS can be used to assess the next stage in management in patients screened with LDCT. Depending on the tumor stage in a positive result, chemotherapy, radiation, and surgery are available as treatment options.

5.8 Minimally Invasive Thoracic Surgery

Minimally invasive thoracic surgery is beneficial to patients because it decreases postoperative pain for the patient. Performing the surgery thoracoscopically or with robotic assistance minimizes surgical incisions and reduces trauma to tissues. This results in shorter hospital stays, reduced blood loss, decreased pain, and less scarring. Since the late 1990s, video-assisted thoracic surgery (VATS) has been utilized,

TABLE 5.2 LungRADS Classification System [20]

Category	Character	Malignancy Potential	Type of Nodule	Management
1	Negative	<1%	No lung nodules Nodule favoring benign (complete calcification, fat-containing nodules)	Continue annual screening with LDCT
2	Benign appearance	<1%	Solid nodule <6 mm, new nodule <4 mm Subsolid nodule <6 mm on baseline screening Ground glass nodule <20 or >20 mm and unchanged	Continue annual screening with LDCT
3	Probably benign	1–2%	Solid nodule >6 to <8 mm at baseline or new nodule 4 to <6 mm Subsolid nodule >6 mm total diameter with solid component <6 mm Ground glass nodule >20 mm on baseline	6-month follow-up with LDCT
4A	Suspicious	5–15%	Solid nodule >8 to <15 mm at baseline Subsolid nodule >6 mm with total solid 6 mm to <8 mm Endobronchial nodule	3-month follow-up with LDCT
4B	Suspicious	>15%	Solid nodule >15 mm, new or growing >8 mm Subsolid nodule with solid component >8 mm	Chest CT with or without contrast, positron emission tomography (PET)/CT, and/or tissue sampling depending on probability of malignancy
4X	Suspicious	>15%	Category 3 or 4 nodules with features suspicious of malignancy including spiculations, ground glass nodules that double in size in a year, or enlarged lymph nodes	Chest CT with or without contrast, PET/CT, and/or tissue sampling depending on probability of malignancy

particularly for early-stage lung cancers. One study analyzed the perioperative parameters in patients who underwent lobectomy by either an open approach or a VATS approach, and the consensus was that VATS major lung resection is favorable and results in shorter hospital stay and reduced overall costs [22]. According to a retrospective, multi-institutional database analyses of nearly 4,000 patients who underwent either open lobectomy or VATS lobectomy, VATS lobectomy was significantly superior to an open approach in hospital costs, length of stay, and risk of adverse events [22]. The only disadvantage of VATS procedure is a longer operating time, but recently most centers that have active minimally invasive programs have experienced similar operative times as the surgeon experience level has increased. Minimally invasive thoracic surgery is the optimal choice for patients undergoing a lobectomy if technically possible.

5.9 Effects of Implementation

Screening with LDCT has been shown to reduce lung cancer mortality by about 20% compared to standard chest X-ray among high-risk adults. Currently, the most frequent stage of diagnosis of lung cancer is stage IV. This is a significantly more advanced stage of diagnosis compared to breast, colorectal, and prostate cancers, all of which are most frequently diagnosed in early stages. Private insurers have made coverage of annual LDCT scans in high-risk patients mandatory. Under the Affordable Care Act, Medicare covers LDCT but requires counseling and shared decision making with a physician before reimbursement for the scan. Without insurance, an LDCT scan has a median charge of $241 [23]. This is significantly less than the cost of treating end-stage lung cancer, which can cost up to $25,000 during the initial months after diagnosis [24, 25]. In 2015, the United States spent $13.4 billion treating lung cancer [3]. One study followed patients for 47 months after they were diagnosed with lung cancer and concluded that the average treatment cost was $282,000 per person [25]. Annual LDCT screening for lung cancer in high-risk patients reduces the financial burden on patients exponentially by diagnosing lung cancer in its early stages. The therapeutic number needed to treat (NNT) is the number of patients who need to be screened to save one life from the disease. The NNT is 2000 for breast cancer, but the NNT for lung cancer is only 217. Effects of implementation would significantly reduce the financial burden associated with treating stage IV lung cancer, and the low NNT signifies the effectiveness of LDCT scans in reducing the mortality rate of lung cancer [26].

5.10 Computer-Aided Diagnosis

Computer aided diagnosis (CAD) is a technology designed to decrease observational oversights and the false-negative rates of physicians interpreting medical images, such as low-dose helical CT scans [27]. CAD is used in conjunction with a CT scan and automatically detects lung nodules on the CT [28]. One study found that LDCT detected 75 patients who had nodules suspicious of lung cancer, and CAD found an additional three suspicious nodules. CAD is not as sensitive with nodules close to the pleural surface, but it has better accuracy in the mediastinum [29].

5.11 Conclusion

Implementing lung cancer screenings using LDCT scans is an effective, noninvasive way to diagnose lung cancer in its earliest stages. Lung cancer has one of the highest mortality rates of solid organ tumors. Unlike breast, prostate, and colon cancers, lung cancer is usually not diagnosed until very advanced stages. LDCT scans reduce the amount of ionizing radiation by 70% compared to the standard CT scan. In the NLST, the largest screening trial for lung cancer, LDCT outperformed chest X-ray by 60% as an early detection method. While overdiagnosis is a potential harm with using LDCT, the benefits outweigh the risks. Implementing LDCT scans in patients with a high risk of developing lung cancer will require a multidisciplinary team working together to achieve the best prevention. Primary care providers need to alert their patients if they are at a high risk for developing lung cancer, and this can be aided by electronic medical records and a nurse navigator. These patients can be referred for their annual scans and work with pulmonologists, thoracic surgeons, and pathologists if needed. Patient education about LDCT screening is essential to increase the number of patients screened for early detection. LDCT is a cost-effective, highly sensitive and specific test for lung cancer. Annual screenings of high-risk patients using LDCT is a noninvasive, effective way to catch lung cancer early and reduce the high mortality rates associated lung cancer.

References

1. American Cancer Society. Cancer facts and figures. Available at: https://www.cancer.org/research/cancer-facts-statistics/all-cancer-facts-figures/cancer-facts-figures-2017.html. Accessed December 7, 2017.
2. Hammerschmidt S, Wirtz H. Lung cancer: current diagnosis and treatment. *Dtsch Arztebl Int*. 2009;106(49):809–820.
3. American Lung Association. Lung cancer fact sheet. Available at: http://www.lung.org/lung-health-and-diseases/lung-disease-lookup/lung-cancer/resource-library/lung-cancer-fact-sheet.html. Accessed December 7, 2017.
4. Centers for Disease Control and Prevention. Trends in current cigarette smoking among high school students and adults, United States, 1965–2014. Available at: https://www.cdc.gov/tobacco/data_statistics/tables/trends/cig_smoking/index.htm. Accessed December 7, 2017.
5. Okereke I, Bates M, Jankowich M, et al. Effects of implementation of lung cancer screening at one Veterans Affairs Medical Center. *Chest*. 2016; 150(5):1023–1029.
6. Eisemann N, Waldmann A, Katalinic A. Epidemiology of breast cancer – current figures and trends. *Geburtshilfe Frauenheilkunde*. 2013;73(2):130–135.
7. Sharma D, Newman T, Aronow W. Lung cancer screening: history, current perspectives, and future directions. *Arch Med Sci*. 2015;11(5):1033–1043.
8. Aberle DR, Abtin F, Brown K. Computed tomography screening for lung cancer: has it finally arrived? Implications of the National Lung Screening Trial. *J Clin Oncol*. 2013;31(8):1002–1008.
9. Patz E, Pinsky P, Gatsonis C, et al. Overdiagnosis in low-dose computed tomography screening for lung cancer. *JAMA Int Med*. 2014;174(2):269–274.
10. Span P. On Medicare and assessing the value of lung cancer screening. Available at: https://www.nytimes.com/2015/05/12/health/on-medicare-and-assessing-the-value-of-lung-cancer-screening.html. Accessed December 10, 2017.
11. Durham A, Adcock I. The relationship between COPD and lung cancer. *Lung Cancer*. 2015;90(2):121–127.
12. Kazerooni E, Austin J, Black W, et al. ACR–STR practice parameter for the performance and reporting of lung cancer screening thoracic computed tomography (CT). *J Thorac Imaging*. 2014;29(5):310–316.

13. Radiological Society of North America and American College of Radiology. Radiation dose in X-Ray and CT exams: patient safety. Available at: https://www.radiologyinfo.org/en/info.cfm?pg=safety-xray. Accessed December 7, 2017.

14. Mertens C, Meier M, Brown S, et al. NAIRAS aircraft radiation model development, dose climatology, and initial validation. *Space Weather*. 2013;11(10):603–635.

15. O'Connor M, Li H, Rhodes D, et al. Comparison of radiation exposure and associated radiation-induced cancer risks from mammography and molecular imaging of the breast. *Med Phys*. 2010;37(12):6187–6198.

16. Caroline C. Lung cancer screening with low dose CT. *Radiol Clin North Am*. 2014;52(1):27–46.

17. Gutierrez A, Suh R, Abtin F. Lung cancer screening. *Semin Interv Radiol*. 2013;30(2):114–120.

18. Gopal M, Abdullah S, Grady J, et al. Screening for lung cancer with low-dose computed tomography: a systematic review and meta-analysis of the baseline findings of randomized controlled trials. *J Thorac Oncol*. 2010;5(8):1233–1239.

19. Dajac J, Kamdar J, Moats A, et al. To screen or not to screen: low dose computed tomography in comparison to chest radiography or usual care in reducing morbidity and mortality from lung cancer. *Cureus*. 2016;8(4):e589.

20. Morgan M. Lung-RADS radiology reference article. Available at: https://radiopaedia.org/articles/lung-rads. Accessed December 8, 2017.

21. Lemjabbar-Alaoui H, Hassan O, Yang Y, et al. Lung cancer: biology and treatment options. *Biochim Biophys Acta*. 2015;1856(2):189–210.

22. Novello S, Asamura H, Bazan J, et al. Early stage lung cancer: progress in the last 40 years. *J Thorac Oncol*. 2014;9(10):1434–1442.

23. Radiology Business. LDCT lung cancer screening: an actuarial affirmation. Available at: http://www.radiologybusiness.com/topics/policy/low-dose-ct-tool-whose-time-has-come-lung-cancer-screenings. Accessed December 8, 2017.

24. Cipriano L, Romanus D, Earle C, et al. Lung cancer treatment costs, including patient responsibility, by stage of disease and treatment modality, 1992–2003. *Value Health*. 2011;14(1):41–52.

25. Dieguez G, Ferro C, Pyenson B. Milliman Research Report: A Multi-Year Look at the Cost Burden of Cancer Care. Retrieved from http://us.milliman.com/uploadedFiles/insight/2017/cost-burden-cancer-care.pdf.

26. Walker G, NNT Group. CT scans to screen for lung cancer. Available at: http://www.thennt.com/nnt/ct-scans-to-screen-for-lung-cancer. Accessed December 8, 2017.

27. Castellino R. Computer aided detection (CAD): an overview. *Cancer Imaging*. 2005;5(1):17–19.

28. Paulraj T, Chellliah K. Computer-aided diagnosis of lung cancer in computed tomography scans: a review. *Curr Med Imaging Rev*. 2017:13. doi:10.2174/1573405613666617011155017.

29. Abe Y, Hanai K, Nakano M, et. al. A computer-aided diagnosis (CAD) system in lung cancer screening with computed tomography. *Anticancer Research*. 2005;25:483–8.

6

Computer-Aided Diagnosis of Lung Nodules: Systems for Estimation of Lung Cancer Probability and False-Positive Reduction of Lung Nodule Detection

Mizuho Nishio

Contents

6.1 Introduction

A total of 1,685,210 new cancer cases and 595,690 cancer deaths were projected to occur in the United States in 2016 [1]. Among men, cancers of the prostate, lung, and colorectum accounted for about 44% of newly diagnosed cancers, and among women, cancers of the breast, lung, and colorectum accounted for half of newly diagnosed cancers. For men and women, 117,920 and 106,470 new lung cancers were projected to occur, respectively. Concerning cancer-related mortality, lung cancer was the leading cause of cancer deaths in the United States in 2016. For men and women, 85,920 and 72,160 cancer deaths were projected to be attributable to lung cancers, respectively. It was speculated that more than one-quarter of all cancer deaths were caused by lung cancers. Although there have been notable improvements in survival over the past three decades for most cancers, lung and pancreatic cancers have shown the least improvement in the United States [1]. This low survival rate of lung cancers is partly because more than one-half of the cases are diagnosed at an advanced stage.

Computed tomography (CT) is a useful diagnostic tool for lung cancers even if radiation exposure of CT is low [2]. Several observational studies have shown that, to detect early-stage lung cancers, low-dose CT is more sensitive than chest radiography [3]. Based on the observational studies, the National Lung Screening Trial (NLST) was conducted as a randomized trial in order to determine whether screening with low-dose CT, as compared with chest radiography, would reduce mortality from lung cancer among high-risk persons [4]. Results from the NLST show that, compared with chest radiography, lung cancer screening with low-dose CT significantly reduced lung cancer mortality among heavy smokers; the relative reduction in mortality from lung cancer was 20% in a low-dose CT screening group. Based on these results and recommendations by the U.S. Preventive Services Task Force, lung cancer screening is being implemented in the United States, where high-risk subjects will receive a yearly low-dose CT scan. Contrary to these results of the NLST, false positives in CT screening can be problematic. Over all three rounds of CT screening by the NLST, the rate of positive screening tests was 24.2%, and 96.4% of the positive results were false positives [4]. These false positives can result in unnecessary follow-up CT, fluorodeoxyglucose positron emission tomography (PET), and invasive procedures, such as bronchoscopy or surgical resection, raising concerns about the increased radiation exposure or surgery risks for the patient [5].

When lung cancer screening with low-dose CT is performed, radiologists must check for the presence of lung nodules detectable in the CT images. And, if lung nodules are detected, radiologists must estimate the risk of lung cancers and determine the management strategy for the detected nodules. Based on the evaluation of the radiologists, some nodules will be followed by CT, and the other nodules will be investigated by fluorodeoxyglucose PET and/or invasive procedures. Because of the high rate of false positives in CT screening, an unprecedented amount of CT scans will be produced, and radiologists will have to evaluate these CT images for performing nodule follow-up. To perform reasonable management of detected lung nodules and reduce false positives, the Lung Imaging Reporting and Data System

(Lung-RADS) has been recently proposed [6]. Lung-RADS defines a clear procedure to decide on a follow-up strategy based on nodule-specific characteristics, such as nodule type, size, and growth.

Computer-aided diagnosis (CAD) refers to software that helps clinicians diagnose disease, and CAD goes beyond just image processing to provide specific information about the disease [7–34]. Roughly, CAD is divided into the following two types: (1) the software that detects lesions (CADe, or computer-aided detection) and (2) the software that classifies lesions (CADx, or computer-aided diagnosis). Because the appearance of lung nodules varies according to its type, detection of lung nodules on CT images and estimation of lung cancer probability for detected lung nodules have become major challenges, often involving methodologies of various levels. CAD has the potential to optimize clinicians' workload, and CADe and CADx of lung nodules can make radiologists' evaluation efficient and effective. For example, a previous study showed that, as a second reader, CADe might be useful for the detection of missed lung cancers in CT screening by assisting radiologists in the interpretation of CT images [35]. As suggested in CADe, it is expected that CADx will be useful for reducing false positives in lung cancer CT screening.

Considering the clinical work flow in the CT screening of lung cancers, image processing by CAD of a lung nodule is divided into several steps. An example of these steps is shown in Figure 6.1. In most cases, image processing by CAD of lung nodules includes lung segmentation, nodule detection, nodule segmentation, and estimation of lung cancer probability. However, some of these steps can be excluded, and substeps can be added. For example, some systems of CADx do not perform lung segmentation, and false-positive reduction is added to the step of nodule detection in CADe. In many cases, CADe requires image preprocessing, lung segmentation, and nodule detection, and CADx requires image preprocessing, nodule segmentation, and estimation of lung cancer probability.

Machine learning is frequently used in CAD systems. When training data are given, machine learning produces the function that matches the training data. For example, it is assumed that training data of CADx consist of $\{x, y\}$, where x represents image data of a lung nodule and y is the label of x (y represents whether x is lung

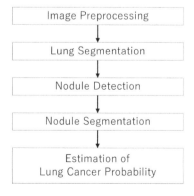

Figure 6.1 Diagram of image processing in CAD of a lung nodule.

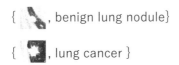

Figure 6.2 Example of training data in CADx of lung nodules.

cancer). Representative training data $\{x, y\}$ of CADx are shown in Figure 6.2. For CADx of a lung nodule, by using the training data, machine learning produces the function that requires the input x and outputs the estimation of lung cancer probability of x. Generally, for CAD of lung nodules, machine learning is used in CADx for calculating the probability of lung cancer and used in CADe for determining whether the image data contain lung nodules.

In the conventional type of CAD using machine learning, the image data x are converted to a one-dimensional (1D) vector that represents the image data x. This conversion process is often called feature extraction, and the 1D vector is called a feature vector. There are many ways to convert image data into a feature vector. In the past, radiologists recorded the nodule-related features and inputted the nodule features and clinical findings into CAD systems, and the CAD systems outputted the disease-specific information by use of the information obtained from radiologists. In this type of CAD of a lung nodule, the following features are frequently used: nodule size, nodule type, spicula, circularity, proportion of ground glass opacity, proportion of calcification, and so on [9]. However, in a clinical setting, it is difficult for radiologists to input clinical findings and nodule features into CAD systems. Therefore, in most recent CAD systems, the feature extraction is automatically performed using a handcrafted algorithm. For extracting features, nodule segmentation is frequently used, and features such as nodule size and circularity are extracted based on the results of nodule segmentation [24]. If nodule segmentation is not performed, texture analysis of lung nodules is performed by using the region of interest (volume of interest) of the lung nodule and handcrafted algorithms, such as the gray-level co-occurrence matrix and local binary pattern [15, 20].

Recently, deep learning and the deep convolutional neural network (DCNN) have been utilized for many types of CAD [10, 12, 27, 28, 33, 34, 36, 37]. As shown in the previous discussion, the conventional type of CAD requires feature extraction. However, deep learning does not always require such image processing. Litjens et al. [10] reviewed the studies of applying deep learning to medical image analysis. They summarized more than 300 contributions of deep learning and provided concise overviews of the medical application of deep learning for several domains, such as neurology, pulmonology, digital pathology, and so on. Several studies proposed the DCNN-based CAD of lung nodules. For example, Teramoto et al. [12] proposed CADe of lung nodules in which DCNN was used for false-positive reduction in PET/CT images. The results of Ciompi et al. [33] show that DCNN was useful for CADx in classifying lung nodules into six types (solid, nonsolid, part solid, and so on).

To develop CAD systems of lung nodules, training data of lung nodules are required. Several public data sets are suitable for the development of the CAD of lung nodules. Here, two data sets are introduced. The first is the LUNGx data set [38–40]. LUNGx

Challenge was conducted as part of the 2015 SPIE Medical Imaging Conference. LUNGx Challenge provided CT images to participants as an opportunity for them to compare their CADx algorithms to those of others using the same data sets. Details of LUNGx Challenge are available in the following sections and in prior publications [39, 40]. The second is the LUNA16 data set [41, 42]. LUNA16 is a completely open challenge for CAD of lung nodules. The goal of LUNA16 is to provide an opportunity for participants to test their algorithm on a common database with a standardized evaluation protocol. The data set is constructed for studying and developing CADe of lung nodules. The purposes of the LUNA16 data set is twofold: one is CADe of lung nodules, and the other is false-positive reduction of CADe. LUNA16 was organized by using a large public LIDC-IDRI data set [43].

The purpose of the current study was the following two points: (1) development of CADx for classification between lung cancer and benign lung nodule on CT images by using the LUNGx data set and (2) development of a false-positive reduction system for CADe by using the LUNA16 data set. In these types of CAD applications, nodule segmentation was frequently used in the previous studies. However, in the current study, nodule segmentation was not performed. The current study hypothesized that nodule segmentation was not necessary for these types of CAD applications. In addition, this study evaluated whether DCNN could be useful for CAD of lung nodules without feature extraction.

6.2 Materials and Methods

The current study used anonymous data from the public data sets. Therefore, approval by an institutional review board or informed consent obtained from patients was not necessary in Japan.

6.2.1 CADx of Lung Nodules

In this section, CADx of lung nodules was developed that performed the classification between lung cancer and benign lung nodules and estimated the probability of lung cancer. For the development of CADx of lung nodules, the LUNGx data set was used in the current study [38–40]. Two types of CADx were developed: one is the conventional type of CADx using feature extraction and machine learning, and the other is CADx with DCNN. In both types, nodule segmentation was not performed, and feature extraction was not used in the latter.

6.2.1.1 LUNGx Data Set
LUNGx Challenge provided 60 test sets of chest CT images with 10 calibration sets. In addition, the location of lung nodule and diagnosis of the lung nodule are also available. Visit the LUNGx Challenge website (https://wiki.cancerimagingarchive.net/display/Public/SPIE-AAPM+Lung+CT+Challenge) for the list of the nodules. Organizers of LUNGx clarified that the lung nodules in the calibration sets were not necessarily

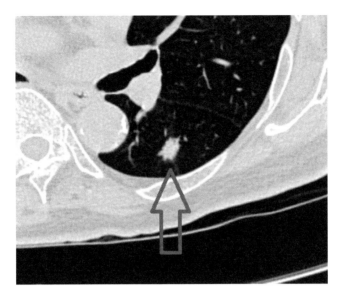

Figure 6.3   Representative example of lung cancer (LUNGx). The arrow shows lung cancer.

representative of the difficulty level in the test sets. The test sets were used in the present study to train the CADx system and to evaluate its performance. The following patient information and technical parameters of CT scan were obtained from Digital Imaging and Communication in Medicine data of the test sets [20]. In the test sets, the patients consisted of 23 men and 37 women (age, 60.0 ± 13.7 years [mean ± standard deviation]; age range, 18–84 years). The parameters of the CT scans were as follows: tube current, 240–500 mA; tube current-exposure time product, 200–325 mAs; tube potential, 120 or 140 kV; matrix size, 512 × 512; and slice thickness, 1 mm. Contrast-enhanced CT was performed for 46 of the 60 patients. The CT images included the whole lungs. In LUNGx Challenge, 73 nodules revealed in the test sets were evaluated; these nodules were also assessed in the present study. Among the 73 lung nodules, 36 nodules were lung cancer, and 37 nodules were benign. Examples of lung cancer and benign lung nodules are shown in Figures 6.3 and 6.4, respectively.

6.2.1.2 Conventional Type of CADx

The outline of the conventional type of CADx is shown in Figure 6.5. First, the CT images of lung nodules were loaded, and the CT images, including lung nodule, were cropped from the whole CT images. Then nodule features were extracted from the cropped CT images. In this type of CADx, feature extraction was performed by radiologists or handcrafted algorithms. In the former, patient age, patient sex, and nodule size obtained by radiologists were used in the current study. In the latter, histograms of CT density and of local binary patterns were obtained by the use of handcrafted algorithms. Then a classifier of CADx was built by utilizing machine learning, labels of lung nodules, and feature vectors that were obtained in the feature extraction step. As machine learning, a support vector machine and a random forest were used in

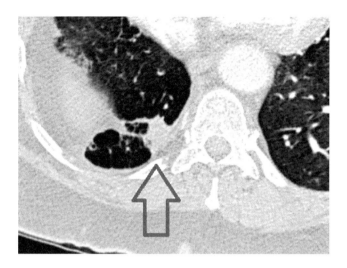

Figure 6.4 Representative example of benign lung nodule (LUNGx). The arrow shows benign lung nodule.

the current study [44, 45]. Finally, the probability of lung cancer was calculated by the classifier, for each lung nodule. For implementing this type of CADx, python-3.5 (http://www.python.org), scikit-learn (http://scikit-learn.org), and scikit-image (http://scikit-image.org) were used in the current study.

6.2.1.2.1 Image Preprocessing. The CT images of LUNGx Challenge were loaded, and its voxel size was converted to $1 \times 1 \times 1$ mm. In each lung nodule, because the position of the center of the lung nodule was available, the CT images, including the lung nodule, were cropped from the axial CT image with the region of interest located at the center of lung nodule. Refer to the list of the nodules on the LUNGx Challenge website for the position of the center of the lung nodule. The size of the region of interest was set to 64×64 mm (64×64 pixels). The cropped CT images were used as inputs to CADx, and feature extraction was performed from these cropped CT images.

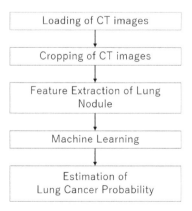

Figure 6.5 Diagram of the conventional type of CADx.

6.2.1.2.2 Radiological and Clinical Findings.   Nodule size, patient age, and patient sex are available for each nodule and each patient in the LUNGx data set, which can be obtained from a prior publication [20]. Based on the chest CT scan of LUNGx, nodule size was measured by board-certified radiologists who had 6 and 9 years of experience as chest radiologists. The cropped CT images of lung nodules are represented by these three items. Clinically, this information is important for differentiating between benign lung nodule and lung cancer. Although smoking history is also important as a clinical finding for differentiating lung nodules, it is not available in LUNGx. Algorithms of machine learning classified the lung nodules based on the three items.

6.2.1.2.3 Histogram of CT Density.   The pixel value of CT images is represented as CT density, and its value generally ranges from −1,000 to 1,000 Hounsfield units. Histograms of CT density can be used for evaluating the distribution of CT density in lung nodules. Because the distribution of CT density is different between lung cancer and benign lung nodules [46], it is expected that the histogram of CT density is useful for CADx of lung nodules. The histogram of CT density is frequently calculated after nodule segmentation is performed. However, the histogram was calculated without nodule segmentation in the current study. The number of histogram bins is represented by B_c, and the bins cover the range of CT density from −1,000 to 1,000 Hounsfield units.

6.2.1.2.4 Histogram of Local Binary Pattern.   Local binary pattern was originally proposed by Ojala et al. [47, 48] as a grayscale invariant measure for characterizing local structure in a 3×3 neighborhood. As an example of computing local binary pattern in a 3×3 neighborhood, a local CT image (see Figure 6.6) is used here. In the original local binary pattern, the center pixel and its surrounding 8 pixels are used. Based on value of the center pixel, the values of the surrounding 8 pixels are binarized, and the binarization results and the corresponding weights are used for calculating the value of local binary pattern. As for Figure 6.6, the calculation of local binary pattern is as follows:

CT density of center pixel = 100
CT density of 8 pixels = [200, 30, 50, 250, 150, 10, 200, 20]
Binarization result = [1, 0, 1, 0, 1, 0, 0, 1]
Value of local binary pattern = $128 \times 1 + 64 \times 0 + 32 \times 1 + 16 \times 0 + 8 \times 1 + 4 \times 0 + 2 \times 0 + 1 \times 1 = 169$

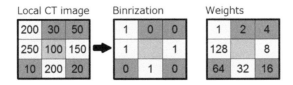

Figure 6.6   Representative example of the calculation of local binary pattern.

Formally, the calculation of local binary pattern is represented as follows:

$$LBP(x, R, P) = \sum_{i=0}^{P-1} 2^i \times s(d_i)$$
$$d_i = I(n(x, R, i)) - I(x),$$

where x is the center pixel in which the value of local binary pattern is calculated, R is the distance between the center pixel and the surrounding pixels, P is the number of the surrounding pixels, $n(x, R, i)$ is the ith surrounding pixel around the center pixel x, $I(u)$ is the CT density of pixel u, and $s(v)$ is an indicator function, where $s(v)$ is 1 if $v \geq 0$ and 0 otherwise. In the current study, rotation invariant and uniform pattern were used for calculating local binary pattern.

By use of local binary pattern, the local CT images are represented by values of local binary pattern because edge, corner, and spot can be assigned to different values of local binary pattern. By collecting the values of local binary pattern and calculating the histogram of its values, the local structure of lung nodules can be captured. One previous study [15] showed that a histogram of local binary pattern was useful for CADx of lung nodule. In local binary pattern, the number of histogram bins is dependent on the number of surrounding pixels. For example, when the number of surrounding pixels is 8, the number of histogram bins is 11 in the rotation-invariant and uniform pattern. By changing the number of surrounding pixels and the distance between the center pixel and surrounding pixels, the local structure on a different scale can be evaluated by using local binary pattern.

6.2.1.2.5 Combined Use of Local Binary Pattern and CT Density. Previously, classification of emphysema subtypes was performed using both local binary pattern and CT density [49]. In the current study, the combined use of these two types of feature extraction was also evaluated for classification of lung nodules. As in the previous study [49], a 2D histogram of local binary pattern and CT density was used.

6.2.1.2.6 Feature Vector and Machine Learning. By the feature extraction step described in the previous subsections, the CT images of lung nodule were represented by feature vectors x. For example, x is {nodule size, patient age, patient sex} in the feature vector of radiological and clinical findings. For each of the 73 lung nodules, $\{x, y\}$ is collected, where y represents the type of lung nodule; if $y = 0$, then the lung nodule is benign; otherwise, it is lung cancer. As shown, the labels of the 73 lung nodules in LUNGx can be obtained from the LUNGx website.

After collecting the data $\{x, y\}$ of the 73 lung nodules, the data $\{x, y\}$ were fed to the algorithms of machine learning. A support vector machine and a random forest were used as algorithms of machine learning in CADx. For the support vector machine, C was used for controlling the support vector machine with a linear kernel. There were several hyperparameters for controlling the random forest. In the current study, the effect of the following three hyperparameters of the random

TABLE 6.1   Hyperparameters of Feature Extraction

Feature	Hyperparameter	Hyperparameter Choice/Range
Radiological and clinical findings	No hyperparameter	
Histogram of CT density	B_c	5, 10, 15, 20, 25, 30, 35, or 40
Histogram of local binary pattern	LBP_R	1, 2, 3, 4, 5, 6, 7, 8, or 9
	LBP_P	8, 16, 24, 32, 40, 48, 56, 64, 72, or 80

forest were evaluated: number of tree, maximum number of features for tree, and depth of tree.

6.2.1.2.7 Hyperparameters. The following hyperparameters were used for controlling the conventional type of CADx:

- For radiological and clinical findings, there is no hyperparameter.
- The histogram of CT density has one hyperparameter: number of histogram bins, B_c.
- The histogram of local binary pattern has two hyperparameters. Hereafter, the distance between the center pixel and surrounding pixels and the number of surrounding pixels are denoted by LBP_R and LBP_P, respectively.
- For the support vector machine, there is one hyperparameter: C.
- For the random forest, there are three hyperparameters: number of tree (RF_n), maximum number of features for tree (RF_f), and depth of tree (RF_d).

Tables 6.1 and 6.2 summarize the hyperparameters that affected the performance of the conventional type of CADx. For the combined use of local binary pattern and CT density, there are three hyperparameters, and its histogram bins are determined by LBP_P and B_c.

6.2.1.3 CADx with DCNN

The outline of CADx with DCNN is shown in Figure 6.7. To perform nodule classification without feature extraction, 2D-DCNN derived from VGG16 [50] was used in CADx with DCNN. As shown in Figures 6.5 and 6.7, there were two major differences between the conventional type of CADx and CADx with DCNN: (1) steps of feature extraction and machine learning were removed from the conventional type of CADx, and (2) DCNN was added in CADx with DCNN. For implementing 2D-DCNN, python-3.5 (http://www.python.org), keras (http://keras.io), and Tensorflow (http://www.tensorflow.org) were used. Geforce GTX 980 or 1080 was used as a graphics processing unit.

TABLE 6.2   Hyperparameters of Machine Learning

Algorithm	Hyperparameter	Hyperparameter Choice/Range
Support vector machine	C	$2^{-6}-2^{12}$
Random forest	RF_n	100, 300, or 500
	RF_f	10%, 30%, 50%, 70%, or 90% of original feature vector
	RF_d	1, 2, 3, 4, 5, 6, 7, or 8

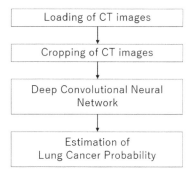

Figure 6.7 Diagram of CADx with DCNN.

6.2.1.3.1 Image Preprocessing. The CT images of LUNGx were loaded, and its voxel size was converted to $1 \times 1 \times 1$ mm. As in the conventional type of CADx, the CT images, including the lung nodule, were cropped. In CADx with DCNN, three 2D images of three orthogonal planes (axial, coronal, and sagittal images) were extracted from the CT images. The three orthogonal planes were set on the center of the 3D images, and the three 64×64 2D images of three orthogonal planes were extracted. When the 2D images were extracted, the size of 2D images was converted to 112×112. Three representative 2D images of three orthogonal planes are shown in Figure 6.8. As a result of this image processing, each lung nodule was represented as three 2D images with size = 112×112, and a pair of these three 2D images and corresponding label were referred to as a batch. Before feeding batches to DCNN, the range of pixel value in the 2D images of each patch was changed from [–1,000, 1,000] to [–1, 1] by using the transformation $t = s/1,000$, where s is the pixel value before the transformation and t is the pixel value after the transformation.

6.2.1.3.2 Input Data and Architecture of DCNN. For each of the 73 lung nodules, a batch (a pair of three 2D images and label) was obtained. Based on the notation in the conventional type of CADx, $\{x, y\}$ represents a batch in the CADx with DCNN, where x is three 2D images and y is the label of x. After collecting $\{x, y\}$ of the 73 lung nodules, the batches $\{x, y\}$ were fed to 2D-DCNN.

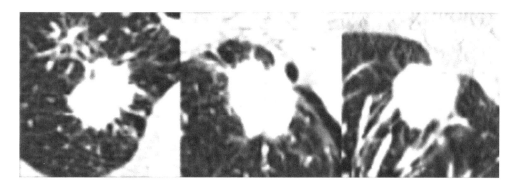

Figure 6.8 Three 2D images of three orthogonal planes obtained from lung cancer (LUNGx).

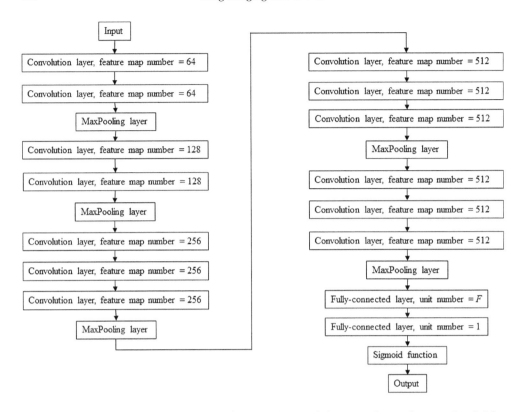

Figure 6.9 Architecture of VGG16. The kernel size of the convolution layer is (3, 3). The activation function is omitted in this figure, except for the sigmoid function.

The architecture of 2D-DCNN in CADx with DCNN was derived from VGG16 [50]. For the enhancement of robustness, transfer learning was used in CADx with DCNN using VGG16. The following modification was applied to the architecture of VGG16 in the current study. Figure 6.9 shows a schematic illustration of the modified VGG16. First, fully connected (FC) layers of VGG16 were removed, and the last layer of VGG16 after removing the FC layers was connected to a new FC layer (the number of unit in this new FC layer is denoted by F). Then an FC layer with 1 unit, whose output is converted to the probability of lung cancer, was added as the prefinal layer of 2D-DCNN. Dropout was applied between the two FC layers, and the strength of dropout was denoted by D ($D = 0$ indicated no dropout, and $D = 1$ indicated full dropout and no connection between the two FC layers). Rectified linear units (ReLU) were used as an activation function of the FC layer with F units. To convert the output of the final FC layer to the probability of lung cancer, sigmoid function was used. For transfer learning, learnable parameters of VGG16 pretrained with IMAGENET [51] were used, and these learnable parameters of VGG16 were fine-tuned using stochastic gradient descent (SGD). The learning rate of SGD is represented as R. The fine-tuning of parameters was not performed in several layers of VGG16, and V represents the number of layers where parameters was not fine-tuned. When training 2D-DCNN, data augmentation was performed.

TABLE 6.3   Hyperparameters of CADx with DCNN

Hyperparameter	Hyperparameter Choice/Range
Number of batches (B)	100
Number of epochs (E)	10, 15, 20, or 25
Learning rate (R)	6×10^{-7}, 7×10^{-7}, 8×10^{-7}, 9×10^{-7}, or 1×10^{-6}
Number of layers where parameters were not fine-tuned (V)	7, 11, or 15
Number of units in the FC layer (F)	96, 128, 160, 192, 224, or 256
Strength of dropout between the two FC layers (D)	0.2, 0.3, 0.4, 0.5, or 0.6

6.2.1.3.3 Hyperparameters.   The following hyperparameters were used for CADx with DCNN:

- B was the number of batches in training DCNN.
- E was the number of epochs in training DCNN.
- R was the learning rate of SGD.
- V was the number of layers where learnable parameters were not fine-tuned.
- F was the number of units in the FC layer.
- D was the strength of dropout between the two FC layers.

Table 6.3 summarizes the hyperparameters which affected performance of CADx with DCNN.

6.2.1.4 Hyperparameter Optimization and Evaluation of CADx

The hyperparameter of the conventional type of CADx was dependent on the type of feature extraction and the algorithms of machine learning. At most, the conventional type of CADx had the six adjustable hyperparameters. On the other hand, the number of adjustable hyperparameters of CADx with DCNN was constant, and CADx with DCNN had the five adjustable hyperparameters. These hyperparameters were optimized by use of a random search [52].

In both the conventional type of CADx and CADx with DCNN, cross validation was performed for evaluating the CADx performance, and cross-validated accuracy was used for a performance metric. Accuracy was calculated using the following equation:

$$\text{accuracy} = \frac{TP + TN}{TP + TN + FP + FN},$$

where *TP*, *TN*, *FP*, and *FN* are true positives, true negatives, false positives, and false negatives, respectively. For the conventional type of CADx, leave-one-out cross validation was performed. On the other hand, because of computational cost, 3-fold cross validation was performed for CADx with DCNN. For the CADx system where the best accuracy was obtained, the area under the curve was calculated.

6.2.2 False-Positive Reduction for CADe of Lung Nodules

CADe of lung nodules judges the existence of lung nodules in chest CT images. Because the CADe system produces several nonnodule candidates, systems of false-positive reduction are frequently used that classify nodule candidates generated by the CADe system and discard nonnodule candidates. In this section, a false-positive reduction system was developed. For this purpose, LUNA16 data set [41, 42] was used in the current study. Because the LUNA16 data set was large, the false-positive reduction system utilized 3D-DCNN. As in CADx, neither nodule segmentation nor feature extraction was used in the false-positive reduction system.

6.2.2.1 LUNA16 Data Set

The purpose for using LUNA16 [41, 42] was twofold: to develop a nodule detection and a false-positive reduction system. The LUNA16 data set was derived from the LIDC-IDRI data set [43]. The organizers of LUNA16 excluded CT scans with a slice thickness greater than 2.5 mm from LIDC-IDRI. As a result, 888 CT scans are included in LUNA16. Based on annotation results of LIDC-IDRI, organizers of LUNA16 determined the ground truth of lung nodules, and the definition of lung nodule of LUNA16 consisted of the following two points: (1) the nodule size was larger than 3 mm, and (2) the nodule was accepted by at least three of four radiologists in the annotation results of LIDC-IDRI. To provide training data on the false-positive reduction system, candidates_V2.csv is available on the LUNA16 website (https://luna16.grand-challenge.org/). In candidates_V2.csv, more than half a million candidate locations and 1,558 locations of true lung nodules are stored. In the current study, candidates_V2.csv was used for developing the false-positive reduction system.

6.2.2.2 Outline of the False-Positive Reduction System with DCNN

Roughly, the outline of the false-positive reduction system with 3D-DCNN was similar to that of CADx with 2D-DCNN shown in Figure 6.7. The major differences between the false-positive reduction system with 3D-DCNN and CADx with 2D-DCNN were as follows: (1) the dimension of input data to DCNN (3D vs 2D) and (2) the use of transfer learning. For implementation of 3D-DCNN, python-3.5, keras (https://keras.io/), and Tensorflow (https://www.tensorflow.org/) were also used. Geforce GTX 1080 Ti was used as the graphics processing unit.

6.2.2.3 Image Preprocessing

The CT images of LUNA16 were loaded, and its voxel size was converted to $1 \times 1 \times 1$ mm. Based on the candidate locations stored in candidates_V2.csv, the CT images were cropped from the chest CT images with the volume of interest. The size of the volume of interest was set to $32 \times 32 \times 32$ mm ($32 \times 32 \times 32$ voxels). The cropped $32 \times 32 \times 32$ images were used as inputs to the false-positive reduction systems. In small portions of the candidate locations, it was not possible to locate the $32 \times 32 \times 32$ volume of interest because several candidate locations were at the marginal zone of chest CT images. Such candidate locations were ignored in the current study.

6.2.2.4 Input Data and Architecture of DCNN

After the preprocessing, 753,599 3D images (size $32 \times 32 \times 32$) were obtained, including 1,558 nodules and 752,041 nonnodules. For each of these 3D images, its corresponding label was obtained from candidates_V2.csv. By using the notation of $\{x, y\}$ used in CADx, x represents the $32 \times 32 \times 32$ 3D images and y represents label of x; if $y = 0$, then x does not contain lung nodules, and if $y = 1$, then x contains lung nodules.

Because the input data to DCNN were 3D, 3D-DCNN was used in the false-positive reduction system. The architecture of 3D-DCNN in the false-positive reduction system is shown in Figure 6.10. Except for the 3D inputs and the padding of convolution layers, the architecture of 3D-DCNN was similar to VGG16 [50] of 2D-DCNN used in CADx with DCNN. It consists of five blocks of convolution and max pooling layers, which are followed by two FC layers. In the five blocks, ReLU was used as the activation function between the convolution and max pooling layers. Between the two FC layers, ReLU was used. To convert the output of the last FC layer to the probability of a nodule, the sigmoid function was used. Dropout was also used in 3D-DCNN. The kernel size of each convolution layer is (3, 3, 3). The number of feature maps in the first convolution layer was denoted by F_C, the number of the unit in the prefinal FC layer was denoted by F, and the strength of dropout was denoted by D. Learnable parameters of 3D-DCNN were trained using Adam. The learning rate of Adam was represented as R. When training

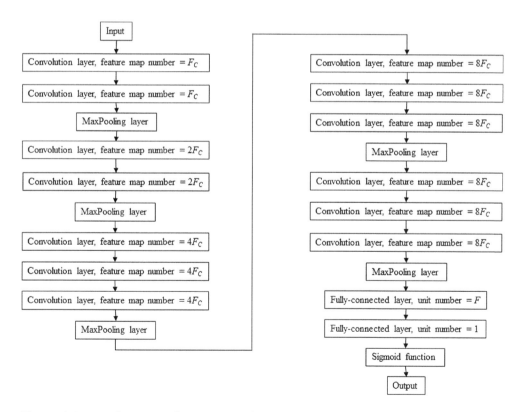

Figure 6.10 Architecture of 3D-DCNN. The kernel size of the convolution layer is (3, 3, 3). The activation function was omitted in this figure, except for the sigmoid function.

TABLE 6.4　Hyperparameters of 3D-DCNN

Hyperparameter	Hyperparameter Choice/Range
Number of batches (B)	50 or 100
Number of epochs (E)	10, 15, 20, 25, or 30
Learning rate (R)	0.0002–0.00002
Number of feature maps in the first convolution layer (F_C)	8 or 16
Number of units in the FC layer (F)	16–128
Strength of dropout (D)	0.2, 0.4, or 0.6
Ratio between nodule and nonnodule in the training data (RT)	0.5, 0.2, or 0.1

3D-DCNN, data augmentation for 3D images was performed. In addition, the ratio between nodule and nonnodule in the training data (RT) was modified during data augmentation because the LUNA16 data set was extremely unbalanced. Because pretrained parameters of 3D-DCNN were not widely available, transfer learning was not used.

6.2.2.5 Hyperparameters

The following hyperparameters were used for 3D-DCNN, and Table 6.4 summarizes the hyperparameters of 3D-DCNN:

- B was the number of batches in training DCNN.
- E was the number of epochs in training DCNN.
- R was the learning rate of Adam.
- F_C was the number of feature maps in the first convolution layer.
- F was the number of units in the FC layer.
- D was the strength of dropout.
- RT was the ratio between nodule and nonnodule in the training data.

6.2.2.6 Hyperparameter Optimization and Evaluation of False-Positive Reduction

Patient-based splitting of training data and testing data was performed, and 682,318 and 71,281 3D images (size 32 × 32 × 32) were used for training of 3D-DCNN and evaluating its performance, respectively. These two sets of data were nonoverlapping, and candidates obtained from one patient were not divided into training data and testing data. Because of computational cost, cross validation was not performed. The number of adjustable hyperparameters of 3D-DCNN was seven, and these hyperparameters were optimized empirically.

Because the data of false-positive reduction were extremely unbalanced, accuracy is not suitable for the performance metric. Therefore, the average precision of testing data was used for the performance metric. Average precision represents the area under the curve of precision and recall, and precision and recall are calculated using the following equations:

$$\text{precision} = \frac{TP}{TP + FP}$$

$$\text{recall} = \frac{TP}{TP + FN}$$

6.3 Results

6.3.1 Results of CADx

6.3.1.1 Results of the Conventional Type of CADx

For the conventional type of CADx, the top three results of cross-validated accuracy are summarized in Tables 6.5–6.8 and Figure 6.11. As shown in the Tables 6.5–6.8, the best accuracy was obtained in the CADx using a 2D histogram of local binary pattern and CT density; the best accuracy was 80.8%.

For the CADx using a 2D histogram of local binary pattern and CT density, the area under the curve ranged from 0.756 to 0.818; the best area under the curve (0.818) was obtained in the following hyperparameters: $B_C = 20$, $LBP_R = 9$, $LBP_P = 56$, $RF_n = 300$, $RF_f = 50\%$, and $RF_d = 7$.

TABLE 6.5   Top Three Results of CADx Using Radiological and Clinical Findings in Leave-One-Out Cross Validation

Rank	Algorithm of Machine Learning	Hyperparameters	Accuracy (%)
1	RF	$RF_n = 100$, $RF_f = 10\%$, $RF_d = 5$	60.3
2	RF	$RF_n = 100$, $RF_f = 10\%$, $RF_d = 7$	58.9
3	RF	$RF_n = 100$, $RF_f = 10\%$, $RF_d = 4$	58.9

Abbreviation: RF, random forest.

TABLE 6.6   Top Three Results of CADx Using Histogram of CT Density in Leave-One-Out Cross Validation

Rank	Algorithm of Machine Learning	Hyperparameters	Accuracy (%)
1	SVM	$B_c = 5$, $C = 256$	64.4
2	SVM	$B_c = 35$, $C = 256$	64.4
3	RF	$B_c = 5$, $RF_n = 500$, $RF_f = 70\%$, $RF_d = 5$	61.6

Abbreviations: SVM, support vector machine; RF, random forest.

TABLE 6.7   Top Three Results of CADx Using Histogram of Local Binary Pattern in Leave-One-Out Cross Validation

Rank	Algorithm of Machine Learning	Hyperparameters	Accuracy (%)
1	RF	$LBP_R = 5$, $LBP_P = 32$, $RF_n = 500$, $RF_f = 10\%$, $RF_d = 5$	68.5
2	RF	$LBP_R = 4$, $LBP_P = 24$, $RF_n = 500$, $RF_f = 50\%$, $RF_d = 8$	68.5
3	SVM	$LBP_R = 6$, $LBP_P = 40$, $C = 64$	65.8

Abbreviations: SVM, support vector machine; RF, random forest.

TABLE 6.8   Top Three Results of CADx Using 2D Histogram of Local Binary Pattern and CT Density in Leave-One-Out Cross Validation

Rank	Algorithm of Machine Learning	Hyperparameters	Accuracy (%)
1	RF	$B_C = 20, LBP_R = 9, LBP_P = 80, RF_n = 300, RF_f = 30\%, RF_d = 8$	80.8
2	RF	$B_C = 20, LBP_R = 9, LBP_P = 56, RF_n = 300, RF_f = 50\%, RF_d = 7$	79.5
3	RF	$B_C = 5, LBP_R = 7, LBP_P = 56, RF_n = 300, RF_f = 30\%, RF_d = 5$	79.5

Abbreviation: RF, random forest.

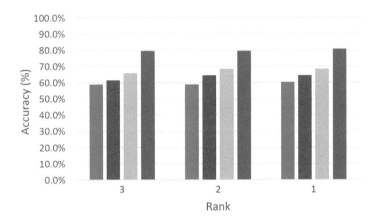

Figure 6.11   Top three results of CADx accuracy of the conventional type of CADx in leave-one-out cross validation. Blue, red, green, and purple bars represent results of radiological and clinical findings, histogram of CT density, histogram of local binary pattern, and 2D histogram of local binary pattern and CT density, respectively.

6.3.1.2 Results of CADx with DCNN

Table 6.9 summarizes the top three results of cross-validated accuracy of CADx with DCNN in 3-fold cross validation. The best accuracy was 68.7% in CADx with DCNN. While different types of cross validation were used between the conventional type of CADx and CADx with DCNN, the cross-validated accuracy of CADx with DCNN was worse than that of CADx using 2D histogram of local binary pattern and CT density (68.7% vs. 80.8%).

TABLE 6.9   Top Three Results of CADx With DCNN in Threefold Cross Validation

Rank	Hyperparameters	Accuracy (%)
1	$E = 10, R = 8 \times 10^{-7}, V = 15, F = 128, D = 0.3$	68.7
2	$E = 10, R = 9 \times 10^{-7}, V = 15, F = 256, D = 0.2$	65.9
3	$E = 25, R = 1 \times 10^{-6}, V = 15, F = 192, D = 0.3$	65.8

TABLE 6.10   Confusion Matrix When False Positives Were One per Patient

	Prediction of Nodule	Prediction of Nonnodule
Actual nodule	116	26
Actual nonnodule	87	71,052

TABLE 6.11   Confusion Matrix When False Positives Were Two per Patient

	Prediction of Nodule	Prediction of Nonnodule
Actual nodule	125	17
Actual nonnodule	176	70,963

6.3.2 Results of False-Positive Reduction

By optimizing hyperparameters empirically, the following hyperparameters were used in 3D-DCNN: $B = 50$, $E = 20$, $R = 0.00002$, $F_C = 16$, $F = 16$, $D = 0.3$, and $RT = 0.5$. Its average precision was 0.801. Tables 6.10 and 6.11 show the confusion matrices when the number of false positives per patient were one and two, respectively; Among 142 lung nodules in the test sets, 116 and 125 lung nodules were correctly classified as lung nodules by the false-positive reduction system.

6.4 Discussion

In this chapter, public data sets were used for the development and evaluation of CAD of lung nodules because it is relatively easy for readers of this chapter to obtain these public data sets and try to develop their own CAD of lung nodules.

In the current study, two types of CAD systems were built for evaluation of lung nodules: the CADx system for estimating lung cancer probability and the false-positive reduction system of CADe for distinguishing between nodules and non-nodules. The CADx system and the false-positive reduction system of the current study were built using the LUNGx data set and the LUNA16 data set, respectively. Except for the nodule size obtained by radiologists, the results of nodule segmentation were not utilized in the current study. Nevertheless, the accuracy and area under the curve of CADx using 2D histogram of local binary pattern and CT density were 80.8% and 0.818, respectively. Explicit feature extraction was not performed in CADx with DCNN or the false-positive reduction system, and acceptable performance was obtained in the false-positive reduction system.

The number of data in LUNA16 was much larger than that in LUNGx (753,599 in LUNA16 and 73 in LUNGx). On the other hand, LUNA16 was extremely imbalanced, and LUNGx was balanced; LUNA16 included 1,558 nodules and 752,041 non-nodules, and LUNGx included 36 lung cancers and 37 benign lung nodules. Because of these characteristics of the two data sets, a different method was adopted for each.

6.4.1 CADx

Previously, an observer study was performed using the 73 lung nodules of LUNGx Challenge, and the observer study included six radiologists [40]. Results of the observer study show that the area under the curve of the six radiologists ranged from 0.70 to 0.85. While the CADx system of the current study was evaluated mainly by accuracy, the best value of the area under the curve was 0.818 in the conventional type of CADx system (CADx using 2D histogram of local binary pattern and CT density). According to the results of the observer study and the current study, at least in the LUNGx data set, it is expected that the diagnostic accuracy of the CADx system in the current study might be comparable to that of radiologists. However, because the number of lung nodules was not large in LUNGx, the CADx system might overfit LUNGx data set.

In LUNGx data set, many CADx systems were evaluated previously. Although the CADx results of the current study were based on the ground truth provided by LUNGx Challenge, the results cannot be compared to the results of other participants in the LUNGx Challenge; other participants used the LUNGx data set only for testing their systems, and the CADx systems of other participants were trained on different independent training data. One previous study showed that an efficient CADx system was built by using the LUNGx data set and support vector machine [20]. Because the previous study used surrogate ground truth obtained from radiologists for constructing their CADx system, it was difficult to compare the diagnostic accuracy of the CADx systems between the current study and the previous study.

The conventional type of CADx was built using the three types of feature extraction: radiological and clinical findings, histogram of CT density, and histogram of local binary pattern. While CADx using CT density and/or local binary pattern did not utilize results of nodule segmentation, the performance of CADx using 2D histogram of local binary pattern and CT density might be comparable to that of radiologists. This result shows that even if nodule segmentation was not performed, 2D histogram of local binary pattern and CT density could provide useful information for classifying lung nodules between lung cancer and benign lung nodules. This validates the hypothesis that CADx could be performed reliably without nodule segmentation.

Although results of recent studies suggest that deep learning (DCNN) is superior to the conventional machine learning algorithm, deep learning requires a large number of training data. To compare the performance of CADx in the small data set, both the conventional type of CADx and CADx with DCNN were built by use of LUNGx data set in the current study. The results of CADx show that performance of the conventional type of CADx was superior to CADx with DCNN, although cross validation in the conventional type of CADx was different from that in CADx with DCNN. The author speculates that the performance difference was caused by the computational cost of DCNN and the number of training data in LUNGx. Even if a graphics processing unit were used, the computational cost of CADx with DCNN would be much larger than that of the conventional type of CADx. As a result, the computational cost of CADx with DCNN hindered the optimization of hyperparameters of CADx with DCNN. In addition, the small number of training data decreased the generalizability of DCNN. Considering the trade-off between computational cost and performance, the author suggests that the conventional type of CADx (feature extraction based on handcrafted algorithms and machine learning) should be tried when the number of training data is small. Generally, it is more difficult to collect training data for medical image analysis than for other fields of image analysis. Combined use of handcrafted algorithms and machine learning may be useful more frequently in medical image analysis than in other fields of image analysis.

6.4.2 False-Positive Reduction

To compare 2D-DCNN used in CADx with 3D-DCNN used in the false-positive reduction system, the VGG16-like network of 3D-DCNN was used in the false-positive reduction system of the current study. The performance of false-positive reduction with 3D-DCNN was acceptable, although that of CADx with 2D-DCNN was not. As shown, because deep learning requires a large number of training data, the number of training data of the LUNGx data set was too small to train 2D-DCNN fully. On the other hand, 3D-DCNN could be trained successfully by use of the LUNA16 data set, and the average precision of the false-positive reduction system was acceptable. These results of 2D-DCNN and 3D-DCNN validate that if a large number of training data is available, DCNN is useful for CAD of lung nodules. It is also validated that neither nodule segmentation nor feature extraction is necessary for CAD with DCNN if training data are plentiful.

Because the LUNA16 data set was extremely imbalanced, data augmentation was used for modifying the ratio between nodules and nonnodules in the training data. Although the author tested the 3D-DCNN training without modification of the ratio between nodules and nonnodules, it was difficult to train 3D-DCNN without the modification of the nodule ratio.

Although the author tested the combined use of handcrafted algorithms, machine learning, and adjustment of class weights for imbalanced data in a false-positive reduction system, the performance was much worse than that of 3D-DCNN. Therefore, the author shows only the results of 3D-DCNN in this chapter.

6.4.3 Limitations

There were several limitations in the current study. First, the author did not evaluate the CADx systems using other data sets. Therefore, the robustness of the CADx systems was not apparent in the current study. It might be possible that the CADx systems strongly overfit the LUNGx data set. Second, optimization of the false-positive reduction system was not fully performed. For comparison between 2D-DCNN using a small data set (LUNGx) and 3D-DCNN using a large data set (LUNA16), the network architecture of 3D-DCNN (VGG16-like) was restricted. Because there were more than half a million nodule data in LUNA16, a more complex and efficient network structure could be used in 3D-DCNN. According to the LUNA16 website, descriptions of several systems of CADe and false-positive reduction systems are available. Visit the LUNA16 website for an efficient network structure of 3D-DCNN that is useful for false-positive reduction. Third, the current study did not investigate the number of training data for efficient training of DCNN. Although the current study shows that 73 lung nodules of LUNGx was not a large enough number to train the VGG16-like network of 2D-DCNN, the author did not evaluate precisely the effect of the number of lung nodule on the diagnostic ability of CAD of lung nodules.

6.4.4 Conclusion

At least in LUNGx data set, the conventional type of CADx was superior to CADx with 2D-DCNN and might be comparable to radiologists. The performance of false-positive reduction was acceptable by use of VGG16-like 3D-DCNN, the LUNA16 data set, and correction of imbalanced data.

Acknowledgments

This study was supported by JSPS KAKENHI (grant no. JP16K19883). The author thanks Sumiaki Matsumoto for his mentoring.

References

1. Siegel RL, Miller KD, Jemal A. Cancer statistics, 2016. *CA Cancer J Clin.* 2016;66(1):7–30.
2. Naidich DP, Marshall CH, Gribbin C, Arams RS, McCauley DI. Low-dose CT of the lungs: preliminary observations. *Radiology.* 1990;175(3):729–731.
3. Kernstine KH, Reckamp KL. *Lung Cancer: A Multidisciplinary Approach to Diagnosis and Management.* New York, Demos Medical; 2011.
4. National Lung Screening Trial Research Team. Reduced lung-cancer mortality with low-dose computed tomographic screening. *N Engl J Med.* 2011;365(5):395–409.
5. Zurawska JH, Jen R, Lam S, Coxson HO, Leipsic J, Sin DD. What to do when a smoker's CT scan is "normal"? Implications for lung cancer screening. *Chest.* 2012;141(5):1147–1152.
6. Lung CT Screening Reporting and Data System (Lung-RADS). Available at: https://www.acr.org/Quality-Safety/Resources/LungRADS. Accessed: January 20, 2018.
7. Cao P, Liu X, Yang J, et al. A multi-kernel based framework for heterogeneous feature selection and over-sampling for computer-aided detection of pulmonary nodules. *Pattern Recognit.* 2017;64:327–346.
8. Suzuki K. A review of computer-aided diagnosis in thoracic and colonic imaging. *Quant. Imaging Med. Surg.* 2012;2(3):163–176.
9. Kawagishi M, Chen B, Furukawa D, et al. A study of computer-aided diagnosis for pulmonary nodule: comparison between classification accuracies using calculated image features and imaging findings annotated by radiologists. *Int J Comput Assist Radiol Surg.* 2017;12(5):767–776.

10. Litjens G, Kooi T, Bejnordi BE, et al. A survey on deep learning in medical image analysis. *Med Image Anal*. 2017 Dec;42:60–88.

11. Lee SLA, Kouzani AZ, Hu EJ. Automated detection of lung nodules in computed tomography images: a review. *Mach Vis Appl*. 2012;23(1):151–163.

12. Teramoto A, Fujita H, Yamamuro O, Tamaki T. Automated detection of pulmonary nodules in PET/CT images: ensemble false-positive reduction using a convolutional neural network technique. *Med Phys*. 2016;43(6):2821–2827.

13. Valente IR, Cortez PC, Neto EC, Soares JM, de Albuquerque VH, Tavares JM. Automatic 3D pulmonary nodule detection in CT images: a survey. *Comput Methods Programs Biomed*. 2016;124:91–107.

14. Schubert T, Eggensperger K, Gkogkidis A, Hutter F, Ball T, Burgard W. Automatic bone parameter estimation for skeleton tracking in optical motion capture. *Proc. IEEE International Conference on Robotics and Automation (ICRA)*. 2016:5548–5554.

15. Arai K, Herdiyeni Y, Okumura H. Comparison of 2D and 3D local binary pattern in lung cancer diagnosis. *Int J Adv Comput Sci Appl*. 2012;3(4):89–95.

16. Aberle DR, Abtin F, Brown K. Computed tomography screening for lung cancer: has it finally arrived? Implications of the National Lung Screening Trial. *J Clin Oncol*. 2013;31(8):1002–1008.

17. Hua KL, Hsu CH, Hidayati SC, Cheng WH, Chen YJ. Computer-aided classification of lung nodules on computed tomography images via deep learning technique. *OncoTargets Ther*. 2015;8:2015–2022.

18. Suzuki K. Computer-aided detection of lung cancer. In *Image-Based Computer-Assisted Radiation Therapy*. Singapore: Springer Singapore; 2017:9–40.

19. Benzakoun J, Bommart S, Coste J, et al. Computer-aided diagnosis (CAD) of sub-solid nodules: evaluation of a commercial CAD system. *Eur J Radiol*. 2016;85(10):1728–1734.

20. Nishio M, Nagashima C. Computer-aided diagnosis for lung cancer: usefulness of nodule heterogeneity. *Acad Radiol*. 2017;24(3):328–336.

21. Doi K. Computer-aided diagnosis in medical imaging: historical review, current status and future potential. *Comput Med Imaging Graph*. 2007;31(4–5):198–211.

22. de Carvalho Filho AO, Silva AC, Cardoso de Paiva A, Nunes RA, Gattass M. Computer-Aided Diagnosis of Lung Nodules in Computed Tomography by Using Phylogenetic Diversity, Genetic Algorithm, and SVM. *J Digit Imaging*. 2017 Dec;30(6):812–822.

23. Way TW, Hadjiiski LM, Sahiner B, et al. Computer-aided diagnosis of pulmonary nodules on CT scans: segmentation and classification using 3D active contours. *Med Phys* 2006;33:2323–2337.

24. El-Baz A, Beache GM, Gimel'farb G, et al. Computer-aided diagnosis systems for lung cancer: challenges and methodologies. *Int J Biomed Imaging*. 2013;2013:942353.

25. Shin HC, Roth HR, Gao M, et al. Deep convolutional neural networks for computer-aided detection: CNN architectures, dataset characteristics and transfer learning. *IEEE Trans Med Imaging* 2016;35(5):1285–1298.

26. Nomura Y, Higaki T, Fujita M, et al. Effects of iterative reconstruction algorithms on computer-assisted detection (CAD) software for lung nodules in ultra-low-dose CT for lung cancer screening. *Acad Radiol*. 2017;24(2):124–130.

27. Roth HR, Lu L, Liu J, et al. Improving Computer-Aided Detection Using Convolutional Neural Networks and Random View Aggregation. *IEEE Trans Med Imaging*. 2016 May;35(5):1170–81.

28. Anirudh R, Thiagarajan JJ, Bremer T, Kim H. Lung nodule detection using 3D convolutional neural networks trained on weakly labeled data. Proc. SPIE 9785, Medical Imaging 2016: Computer-Aided Diagnosis, 978532.

29. Chen H, Xu Y, Ma Y, Ma B. Neural network ensemble-based computer-aided diagnosis for differentiation of lung nodules on CT images. *Acad Radiol*. 2010; 17(5):595–602.

30. Lin D, Vasilakos AV, Tang Y, Yao Y. Neural networks for computer-aided diagnosis in medicine: a review. *Neurocomputing*. 2016;216:700–708.

31. Nibali A, He Z, Wollersheim D. Pulmonary nodule classification with deep residual networks. *Int J Comput Assist Radiol Surg*. 2017;12(10):1799–1808.

32. Matsumoto S, Kundel HL, Gee JC, Gefter WB, Hatabu H. Pulmonary nodule detection in CT images with quantized convergence index filter. *Med Image Anal*. 2006; 19(3):343–352.

33. Ciompi F, Chung K, van Riel SJ, et al. Towards automatic pulmonary nodule management in lung cancer screening with deep learning. *Sci Rep*. 2017;7:46479.

34. Hussein S, Gillies R, Cao K, Song Q, Bagci U. TumorNet: lung nodule characterization using multi-view convolutional neural network with Gaussian process. Proc. IEEE 14th International Symposium on Biomedical Imaging (ISBI 2017).

35. Liang M, Tang W, Xu DM, et al. Low-dose CT screening for lung cancer: computer-aided detection of missed lung cancers. *Radiology* 2016;281(1):279–288.

36. Gulshan V, Peng L, Coram M, et al. Development and validation of a deep learning algorithm for detection of diabetic retinopathy in retinal fundus photographs. *JAMA*. 2016;316(22):2402–2410.

37. Esteva A, Kuprel B, Novoa RA, et al. Dermatologist-level classification of skin cancer with deep neural networks. *Nature*. 2017;542(7639):115–118.

38. Clark K, Vendt B, Smith K, et al. The Cancer Imaging Archive (TCIA): maintaining and operating a public information repository. *J Digit Imaging*. 2013;26(6):1045–1057.

39. Armato SG 3rd, Hadjiiski L, Tourassi GD, et al. LUNGx Challenge for computerized lung nodule classification: reflections and lessons learned. *J Med Imaging*. 2015;2(2):020103.

40. Armato SG 3rd, Drukker K, Li F, et al. LUNGx Challenge for computerized lung nodule classification. *J Med Imaging*. 2016;3(4):044506.

41. Lung nodule analysis 2016. Available at: https://luna16.grand-challenge.org. Accessed: January 20, 2018.

42. Setio AAA, Traverso A, de Bel T, et al. Validation, comparison, and combination of algorithms for automatic detection of pulmonary nodules in computed tomography images: the LUNA16 challenge. *Med Image Anal*. 2016;42:1–13.

43. Armato SG 3rd, McLennan G, Bidaut L, et al. The Lung Image Database Consortium (LIDC) and Image Database Resource Initiative (IDRI): a completed reference database of lung nodules on CT scans. *Med Phys*. 2011;38(2):915–931.

44. Chang C-C, Lin C-J. LIBSVM: a library for support vector machines. *ACM Trans Intell Syst Technol*. 2011;2(3):1–27.

45. Breiman L. Random forests. *Mach Learn*. 2001;45(1):5–32.

46. Kamiya A, Murayama S, Kamiya H, Yamashiro T, Oshiro Y, Tanaka N. Kurtosis and skewness assessments of solid lung nodule density histograms: differentiating malignant from benign nodules on CT. *Jpn J Radiol*. 2014;32(1):14–21.

47. Ojala T, Pietikainen M, Maenpaa T. Multiresolution gray-scale and rotation invariant texture classification with local binary patterns. *IEEE Trans Pattern Anal Mach Intell*. 2002;24(7):971–987.

48. Ojala T, Pietikainen M, Harwood D. A comparative study of texture measures with classification based on featured distributions. *Pattern Recognit.* 1996;29(1):51–59.
49. Sørensen L, Shaker SB, de Bruijne M. Quantitative analysis of pulmonary emphysema using local binary patterns. *IEEE Trans Med Imaging.* 2010:29(2):559–569.
50. Simonyan K, Zisserman A. Very deep convolutional networks for large-scale image recognition. *arXiv.* 1409.1556.
51. Russakovsky O, Deng J, Su H, et al. ImageNet Large Scale Visual Recognition Challenge. *Int. J. Comput. Vis.* 2015;115(3):211–252.
52. Bergstra J, Bengio Y. Random search for hyper-parameter optimization. *J Mach Learn Res.* 2012;13:281–305.

7

Automated Lung Cancer Detection From PET/CT Images Using Texture and Fractal Descriptors

K. Punithavathy, Sumathi Poobal, and M. M. Ramya

Contents

7.1 Introduction

Cancer is the second leading cause of death universally; close to one in six deaths is due to cancer [1]. Lung cancer is the principal cause of cancer-associated deaths around the world, characterized by low survival rates and aggressiveness [2–4]. Up to the last decade, lung cancer was not common in India, but an alarming increase in the number of incidents has occurred in recent years [4, 5]. From 58% to 73% of people diagnosed in the initial stage have a survival of 5 years, whereas only 2%–13% of lung cancer cases diagnosed at the terminal stage live past 5 years [6–8]. Early detection and adequate treatment helps in better long-term survival of up to 73%.

Medical imaging involves the application of techniques and processes to create images of the various parts of the body for diagnosis and treatment. Several medical imaging methods are available in medical diagnostics, such as X-ray–based methods of medical imaging, imaging techniques without the use of ionizing radiation, and molecular imaging techniques. X-ray–based medical imaging methods include conventional X-ray, computed tomography (CT) and mammography. Magnetic resonance imaging (MRI) and ultrasound imaging operate without ionizing radiation. Molecular imaging techniques, such as positron emission tomography (PET), use radioactive substances to view the body parts at cellular and molecular levels. To correlate the biological processes with anatomical information, molecular imaging techniques are integrated with CT and MRI scanners. PET/CT combines PET and CT scanners into a single device to acquire sequential images from both devices in the same session that are combined into a single superimposed image. Thus, functional imaging acquired by PET can be more accurately correlated with anatomic imaging acquired by CT scan. PET/CT is a supreme imaging technique in lung cancer diagnosis, staging, and treatment planning, as it provides morphological and anatomical information [9–13]. A major drawback in PET/CT is the false-positive (FP) result due to inflammation or infection [14, 15]. Also in PET/CT, the CT scans performed at minimal energy settings to reduce the radiation effects result in poor image quality, hence affecting diagnostic accuracy [16]. There has been a steady rise in the number of imaging studies and the volume of images collected from these studies. This burdens the medical expert in interpretation and may result in error-prone diagnosis. Also, there are a limited number of radiologists available. Therefore, computer-aided diagnosis (CAD) systems are highly essential to assist radiologists in lung cancer diagnosis with increased speed, accuracy, minimal diagnostic errors, and less time [17].

CAD plays a major complementary role in medical diagnosis [18]. CAD systems are developed with computer algorithms that are based on the knowledge of image interpretation by medical experts. Image processing techniques and artificial intelligence (AI) are applied in CAD to detect abnormalities, and a suitable classifier is used for classification [19]. Several researchers have made significant contributions in developing CAD systems to diagnose various cancers from medical images [20, 21]. Output from CAD systems has been used as a second opinion by the radiologists in interpretation and decision making. Many commercial systems are available for lung cancer detection on chest radiographs and CT scans. To improve the accuracy of lung cancer diagnosis, CAD systems have been developed using texture analysis (TA) of PET/CT images [22]. Such CAD systems comprise the essential stages: (1) preprocessing, (2) segmentation to focus on the region of interest (ROI), (3) feature extraction and detection of abnormalities, and (4) classification.

The quality of medical images is degraded by the artifacts due to noise and variations in contrast. PET/CT images are affected by artifacts that are caused by metallic implants, respiratory motion, and use of contrast [23–25]. An extensive review has been carried out on the application of traditional preprocessing techniques, such as median filtering, Wiener filtering, and Gaussian filtering, on CT images to reduce the noise present in lung CT images [26]. Traditional contrast enhancement techniques, such as histogram equalization (HE) and contrast-limited adaptive histogram equalization (CLAHE), have been widely used to improve the contrast of medical images. However, medical image enhancement using these traditional techniques is not automatic and tends to produce overenhancement in non-ROIs [27]. In detecting suspicious regions from medical images, a prime focus is on enhancing the ROIs. Hence, fuzzy-based image enhancement techniques are preferred in lung cancer diagnosis [27].

Image intensity is considered to be an important image feature, but it is not a contributive image attribute in lung cancer detection, as there is no significant variation in intensity at the boundary of normal and cancerous regions. TA is used to describe and quantify the roughness, smoothness, silkiness, or bumpiness in terms of the spatial variation in pixel intensities. TA is found highly useful in various applications, including remote sensing and medical image processing. Much meaningful image information is available in medical images with image textures. Any abnormalities present in the medical images change the appearance of the texture of the regions. Hence, TA plays a key role in discriminating between normal and abnormal regions in medical images. Fourteen texture features proposed by Haralick et al. [28] are found beneficial in image classification. Few researchers have analyzed the first- and second-order statistical texture features to detect lung cancer from chest radiographs and from CT images [29–37]. Statistical second-order texture features extracted from PET/CT images have been utilized to detect the presence of lung cancer [38]. However, texture features might be insufficient to identify and classify smaller lymph nodes.

Medical images are characterized by irregular complex tissue structures that cannot be quantified by traditional Euclidean geometry. Hence, fractal geometry has been used widely to analyze these medical images [39, 40]. The fractal dimension (FD) is used to indicate the amount of surface roughness, and it has noninteger values. Several approaches are used to estimate FD, such as box counting (BC) and differential box counting (DBC) methods, and fractal analysis has been carried out for segmenting various natural texture images, classification of breast mammograms, and retinal images [41–43]. Fractal analysis has been found significant to find the aggressiveness of the lung cancer from CT images [44] and from PET/CT images [45].

Classification algorithms play an important role in CAD systems in detecting the malicious regions from medical images. CAD systems developed by several researchers to detect lung cancer have been analyzed and reviewed critically, and it was observed that several CAD systems produced promising results in sensitivity and specificity. However, the level of automation was not satisfactory due to the manual operations involved in segmentation. Also, the ability to detect various types of nodules, the number of FPs, and validation of these systems have not shown significant improvement. Hence, these CAD systems can be improved in the future for a high level of automation and a reduced number of FPs [46]. A CAD system using a back-propagation neural network classifier with optimal network parameters has been implemented to test chest X-ray images and produced 80% accuracy for lung cancer classification [47]. An artificial neural network (ANN)–based lung cancer detection system has been established and utilized first-order texture features extracted from CT images [48, 49]. A CAD system was designed for early lung cancer detection in which the first-order statistical texture features and color information were fed as input to ANN for classification [50].

A fully automated lung cancer detection system was attempted by a few researchers. A CAD system for lung cancer detection with various classifiers was reviewed extensively [51]. Machine learning (ML) techniques, such as ANN and support vector machine (SVM), have been examined to classify lung CT images. Significant texture features yielded a better accuracy of 98.4% using ANN compared to 93.2% by SVM [52]. Classification using the Hopfield neural network achieved 98% accuracy in detecting lung cancer [53]. An ANN of a two-level CAD system was implemented and tested for automatic lung cancer detection from chest radiographic images [54]. Critical analysis was carried out in selecting optimal network parameters, such as number of hidden neurons in the neural network classifier, to produce better accuracy [55]. A CAD system based on ANN was designed and developed for lung cancer detection from PET/CT images. This CAD system fixed the optimal network parameters after many trials and utilized significant texture and fractal features for lung cancer classification. Performance of the classifier with many training algorithms was compared, and it was found that the Levenberg-Marquardt (LM) back-propagation algorithm produced an improved classification accuracy of 92.5% [56]. Recent studies have demonstrated that SVM has been found as a popular ML tool in the classification of medical images. SVM makes use of set of points (support vectors) to identify and establish the boundary. Several researchers developed a CAD system with an SVM classifier for automatic lung cancer detection and classification using the extracted texture features from CT images [57–60]. A new computerized system was developed using the SVM classifier to improve the diagnostic accuracy and was tested on texture features of PET/CT images [61–65].

This present study focuses on establishing a CAD system to perform automatic lung cancer detection using texture and fractal features from lung PET/CT images.

7.2 Materials and Methods

7.2.1 Image Data Set

This method involved a retrospective study of 18F-FDG PET/CT images from 82 patients. Patients underwent PET/CT scan after administering an intravenous injection. CT images were initially acquired, and PET images were acquired using attenuation-corrected CT data with GE Discovery 16. Fused PET/CT images of dimension 256×256 were considered for this study. Images taken during the period 2015–2016 were collected from Anderson Diagnostics and Labs, Chennai, India. Two expert nuclear medicine physicians interpreted the results obtained by this method and compared them with the ground truths. Detailed information of the data collected for this study is listed in Table 7.1.

A few sample normal lung PET/CT images are shown in Figure 7.1, and a few lung cancer PET/CT images in various stages are shown in Figure 7.2.

In Figure 7.2, image A1 has a lesion in the left lung measuring 31×35 mm with a maximum standardized uptake value (SUV_{max}) of 15 and in stage II. Image A2 is

TABLE 7.1   Patient Data

Patient count (male/female/total)	50/32/82
Patient age (minimum/maximum/median)	27/71/53
Benign/malignant image count	34/48
Malignant (stages II/III/IV)	12/21/15

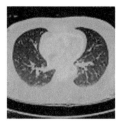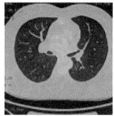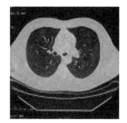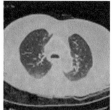

Figure 7.1   Normal lung PET/CT images.

stage III lung cancer image having a lesion in the left lung of size 35×28 mm with SUV_{max} of 6. Image A3 is a stage IV lung cancer image with a lesion in the right lung measuring 37×43 mm with SUV_{max} of 16. Image A4 is an 80% contrast-reduced stage IV lung cancer image with a lesion in the right lung of 60×39 mm and SUV_{max} of 10. In image A4, the contrast is intentionally reduced to illustrate a degraded image due to poor contrast when images are captured at a low radiation dose in minimizing the radiation effects. Contrast reduction at various levels, such as 20%, 40%, 60%, and 80%, has been experimented with and investigated in the main phases of this method.

7.2.2 Methodology

The objective of this chapter is to develop a CAD system to detect lung cancer using texture and fractal features from lung PET/CT images. The overall flow diagram of this method is depicted in Figure 7.3. The CAD system includes the following major steps: preprocessing, feature extraction, and classification. In the preprocessing step, filtering techniques and fuzzy-image enhancement were applied on RGB PET/CT images to denoise and improve the contrast. Meaningful image features, such as texture and fractal, were extracted from the enhanced images. Finally, supervised classification methods were applied to classify the images as normal or cancerous.

7.2.2.1 Denoising Techniques
Many real-time images, including medical images, suffer from noise and poor contrast. Medical images are affected by artifacts that are caused by factors such as data acquisition errors and the inability of the reconstruction algorithm to represent the

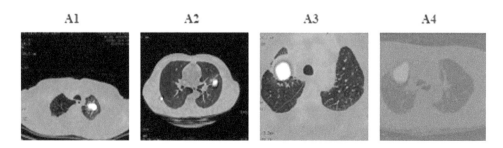

Figure 7.2   Lung cancer PET/CT images in various stages.

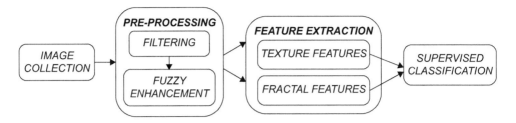

Figure 7.3 Overall flow diagram of the developed CAD system for lung cancer.

anatomy. Quality of medical images is affected by these artifacts, and this in turn affects the accuracy of medical image diagnosis. Hence, image processing techniques are applied on medical images to remove the noise present and to improve image quality. PET/CT images contain artifacts due to metallic implants, respiratory motion, and application of contrast [23–25]. These artifacts lead to the possibility of FP results due to more uptake of radioactive tracer. However, the knowledge and use of appropriate algorithms reduce these artifacts and thereby improve the quality of medical images.

7.2.2.1.1 Traditional Filtering Techniques. Traditional filters used for noise removal are classified as spatial domain and frequency domain methods. Spatial domain filters work directly on the pixels of an image to perform noise removal. In the frequency domain method, an image is transformed to another domain; denoising is done there, and inverse transformation is applied to get the improved image. Various spatial domain filters include mean, median, Gaussian, and Wiener filtering techniques. The choice of filters for denoising medical images depends on the type of noise present in them. The Wiener filter performs better in case of Gaussian, Poisson, and speckle noise. For impulse noise, the median filter outperforms all other filters.

The quality of lung PET/CT images is affected by the presence of additive Gaussian noise. The Wiener filter performs better in the removal of additive noise with edges and fine details of images preserved [38, 56]. Hence, Wiener filtering was used in this study to denoise the additive noise present in lung PET/CT images. It uses the prior statistical knowledge of signal and noise. The Wiener filter estimates the local mean and standard deviation by using a neighborhood with size m by n. The operation involves inverse filtering and noise smoothing. This proves to be optimal in reducing the overall mean square error (MSE). Operation of the Wiener filter is better understood in the frequency domain, and the transfer function is chosen to minimize MSE. The transfer function of Wiener filter is given as

$$W(u, v) = \frac{H*(u,v)}{|H(u,v)|^2 + \frac{S_\eta(u,v)}{S_f(u,v)}} \tag{1}$$

where $H(u,v)$ is the Fourier transform of the point spread function and $S_f(u,v)$ and $S_\eta(u,v)$ are the power spectral density of image and noise, respectively. Commonly used traditional filters were tried on lung PET/CT images, and their performance was compared with performance metrics, such as MSE and peak signal-to-noise ratio (PSNR). The Wiener filter produces the best reconstruction in terms of least MSE by reducing the effect of additive noise.

7.2.2.2 Contrast Enhancement

Contrast defines the difference in the intensity between the adjacent regions in an image, and it is an important image feature to detect any abnormalities. Hence, it is essential to go for noise removal and enhance the contrast of medical images before further processing for diagnosis or analysis. The main goal of image enhancement is to increase image quality so that interpretation from the enhanced features can be improved. Extensive research has been carried out in developing many techniques for medical image enhancement.

7.2.2.2.1 Traditional Enhancement Techniques.   HE methods enhance image contrast by using the image histogram. CLAHE is the most widely used traditional HE method in contrast enhancement. These techniques tend to improve the contrast of medical images by modifying the gray-level histogram. Even though they sharpen the boundaries, they result in overenhancement and the loss of important local information, which may lead to poor diagnosis. To overcome these drawbacks, fuzzy-image enhancement has been utilized in this study. Fuzzy rule–based enhancement improves enhancement by making the high-intensity regions brighter and low-intensity regions more dark [45, 56].

7.2.2.2.2 Fuzzy-Image Enhancement.   Medical images represent tissue characteristics as the spatial relationship between anatomical structures. Abnormality present in any medical images can be detected by the deviation in the spatial relationship between anatomical structures. Lung PET/CT images exhibit fuzziness, as they contain fewer sharp edges than other medical images. Hence, fuzzy enhancement is chosen to enhance the contrast of lung PET/CT images. Fuzzy-image enhancement techniques are nonlinear and knowledge based to process the ambiguous data. The general structure of the fuzzy-image processing technique is shown in Figure 7.4.

Fuzzy-image processing includes three steps: fuzzification (Φ), fuzzy membership function (Γ), and defuzzification (ψ). A fuzzy enhanced image is described as

$$I_1(i, j) = \psi\left(\Gamma\left(\Phi\left(I(i,j)\right)\right)\right) \tag{2}$$

In fuzzification, crisp pixels of the input image $I(i, j)$ are mapped to the fuzzy plane. A suitable fuzzy membership function is used to map the fuzzy values to new values. New membership values are remapped into the gray-level values to obtain a fuzzy enhanced image. Normalization was used in fuzzification and expressed as

$$\mu(i,j) = \left(I(i, j)\right)/255 \tag{3}$$

The objective of this method is to focus on the detection of lung cancer and with an understanding that the cancerous regions have more uptakes of radioactive materials, thus exhibiting high intensity. To enhance the contrast of the cancerous regions

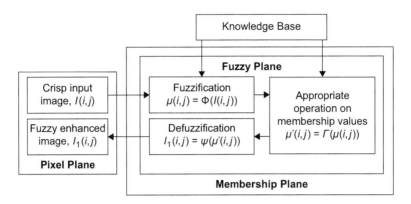

Figure 7.4   Fuzzy-image processing—general structure.

and suppress the contrast of other non-ROIs in lung PET/CT images, four times the cubic function was selected as a membership function. The membership modified image is mathematically expressed as

$$\mu'(i,j) = \begin{cases} 4 * \mu(i,j)^3 & \text{if } \mu(i,j) \leq 0.5 \\ 1 - 4 * \left[1 - \left(\mu(i,j)\right)\right]^3 & \text{if } \mu(i,j) > 0.5 \end{cases} \quad (4)$$

The defuzzification method utilized a threshold T selected from the histogram of modified membership image, $\mu'(i,j)$ and a gain factor G to enhance the cancerous regions. Non-ROIs, such as the background and regions surrounding the lung, were reduced in contrast and brightness. The optimum value of T and G were fixed after many experimental trials to achieve the desired enhancement and to eliminate under- and overenhancement.

The fuzzy enhanced image is denoted by $I_1(i,j)$ and described by

$$I_1(i,j) = \begin{cases} 0 & \text{if } \mu'(i,j) \leq 0 \\ 255 * G * \mu'(i,j) & \text{if } 0 < \mu'(i,j) < T \\ 255 & \text{if } \mu'(i,j) \geq T \end{cases} \quad (5)$$

The contrast-to-noise ratio (CNR) is used as a performance metric to evaluate the performance of enhancement algorithms.

7.2.2.3 Feature Extraction
7.2.2.3.1 TA.
Traditional intensity-based thresholding techniques may not contribute much to accurate segmentation and lung cancer detection. TA plays a vital role in medical diagnosis, as various regions in medical images have unique texture information. TA methods are found useful in studying and discriminating distinct

as well as subtle textures in multimodality medical images, such as those of PET/CT [66]. The texture of an image represents the structural arrangement of various objects in an image. Feature extraction is the preliminary stage of image TA. Results attained from this stage are used for segmentation and classification. Texture features described by mathematical expressions are computed from the spatial distribution of pixels. Structural, statistical, and transform-based methods are used to extract the texture features from an image. Structural approaches are used to represent texture by primitives. The structural approach is advantageous in providing a good symbolic description of the image; however, this approach is more useful for synthesis than for image analysis.

Statistical methods derive a set of statistics from the spatial distribution of pixels. They compute the local features of each pixel in an image to investigate the spatial distribution of gray values. Statistical features include first- and second-order statistical methods. In first-order statistical TA, texture features are extracted from the histogram of image intensity. First-order statistical texture features are mean, variance, coarseness, skewness, kurtosis, energy, and entropy. The first-order statistical approach is simple and uses standard descriptors, such as mean and variance, to characterize image textures. However, this approach does not consider correlations between pixel neighborhoods, and it measures the frequency of a particular gray level only at a random image location. Hence, the second-order statistical texture approach is preferred in medical diagnosis.

In second-order statistical TA, texture features are extracted based on the probability of finding a pair of gray levels at a specified distance and orientation over the entire image. Gray level co-occurrence matrix (GLCM) is a matrix obtained by finding the probability of occurrence of a pair of gray-level values and is used to extract second-order statistical texture features. Two image textures can be discriminated based on the difference in the second-order statistics of the textures. Figure 7.5 depicts the co-occurrence matrix directions for the extraction of texture features. This method analyzed the texture features of Haralick et al. [28] by using a co-occurrence matrix pattern in the horizontal direction with unit distance.

Table 7.2 lists the Haralick texture features and their mathematical expressions that were analyzed in the study.

The information provided by a few texture features may have a significant correlation or of be less significance. A feature selection strategy is therefore used to eliminate redundant or irrelevant information.

7.2.2.3.2 Fractal Analysis. Fractal geometry has been found as a useful area of mathematics in quantifying complex, irregular biological structures that cannot be

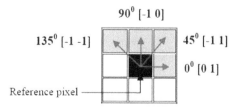

Figure 7.5 Co-occurrence matrix directions for extracting texture features.

TABLE 7.2   Haralick Second-Order Statistical Texture Features

Texture Featurewide	Formula
Autocorrelation	$tf_1 = \sum_{i=1}^{N_g} \sum_{j=1}^{N_g} (ij)p(i,j)$
Contrast	$tf_2 = \sum_{i=1}^{N_g} \sum_{j=1}^{N_g} (i-j)^2 p(i,j)$
Dissimilarity	$tf_3 = \sum_{i=1}^{N_g} \sum_{j=1}^{N_g} |i-j| p(i,j)$
Energy	$tf_4 = \sum_{i=1}^{N_g} \sum_{j=1}^{N_g} p(i,j)^2$
Entropy	$tf_5 = -\sum_{i=1}^{N_g} \sum_{j=1}^{N_g} p(i,j)\log\big(p(i,j)\big)$
Homogeneity	$tf_6 = \sum_{i=1}^{N_g} \sum_{j=1}^{N_g} \frac{1}{1+(i+j)^2} p(i,j)$
Maximum probability	$tf_7 = \max_{i,j} p(i,j)$
Sum average	$tf_8 = \sum_{i=2}^{2N_g} i\, p_{x+y}(i)$
Sum entropy	$tf_9 = \sum_{i=2}^{2N_g} p_{x+y}(i)\log\big\{p_{x+y}(i)\big\}$
Sum variance	$tf_{10} = \sum_{i=2}^{2N_g} \big(i-\mu_{x+y}\big)^2 i\, p_{x+y}(i)$
Difference variance	$tf_{11} = \sum_{i=0}^{N_g-1} \big(i-\mu_{x-y}\big)^2 p_{x-y}(i)$
Difference entropy	$tf_{12} = -\sum_{i=0}^{N_g-1} p_{x-y}(i)\log\big\{p_{x-y}(i)\big\}$
Information measures of correlation 1	$tf_{13} = \dfrac{HXY - HXY1}{\max(HX, HY)}$
Information measures of correlation 2	$tf_{14} = \big(1-\exp\big(-2(HXY2 - HXY)\big)\big)^{1/2}$

Notation:

$p(i,j)$ is the (i,j)th entry in normalized GLCM $= \dfrac{P(i,j)}{R}$

N_g is number of distinct gray levels in quantized image

TABLE 7.2   Haralick Second-Order Statistical Texture Features (*Continued*)

Texture Featurewide	Formula

$$p_x(i) = \sum_{j=1}^{N_g} p(i,j); \ p_y(j) = \sum_{i=1}^{N_g} p(i,j)$$

$\mu_x, \mu_y, \sigma_x, \sigma_y$ are the means and standard deviations of p_x and p_y, respectively

$$p_{x+y}(i) = \sum_{i=1}^{N_g} \sum_{j=1}^{N_g} p(i,j); \ i+j = k; k = 2, \ 3 \ldots 2N_g$$

$$p_{x-y}(i) = \sum_{i=1}^{N_g} \sum_{j=1}^{N_g} p(i,j); |i-j| = k; \ k = 0, \ 1 \ldots N_g - 1$$

$$HX = -\sum_{i=1}^{N_g} p_x(i)\log\{p_x(i)\}; \ HY = -\sum_{i=1}^{N_g} p_y(i)\log\{p_y(i)\}$$

$$HXY = -\sum_{i=1}^{N_g} p(i,j)\log\{p(i,j)\}$$

$$HXY1 = -\sum_{i=1}^{N_g} \sum_{j=1}^{N_g} p(i,j)\log\{p_x(i)p_y(j)\}$$

$$HXY2 = -\sum_{i=1}^{N_g} \sum_{j=1}^{N_g} p_x(i)p_y(j)\log\{p_x(i)p_y(j)\}$$

described by Euclidean geometry [67]. The fractal approach characterizes a textured region by a single measure of noninteger dimension, known as FD, and is useful in many applications other than statistical approaches. FD describes the amount of irregularity or surface texture. A number of techniques are available to estimate the FD of objects, and BC approach is the most commonly used method to estimate the FD of a binary image. The FD of an image can be estimated for its full image, termed as global FD, or for a local region specified by a neighborhood of pixels, known as local FD. In medical image analysis, to discriminate between normal and cancerous regions, local FD is more preferred than global FD. Various factors, such as the tissue characteristics of an image, local neighborhood size, and box width, determine the value of FD. The value of FD changes as the size of the local neighborhood varies [42]. Fractal analysis on digital images has been carried out with various neighborhood sizes, such as 5×5 and 17×17, using the DBC technique [41–43]. This method utilized the DBC technique to estimate the local FD of grayscale images [38]. In the DBC approach, an $M \times M$ image is considered as a three-dimensional spatial space with (x, y) as spatial coordinates of the pixels and the third axis (z) representing the gray-level value of pixels. Grids of size $s \times s$ are used to cover the (x, y) space, where $M/2 \geq s \geq 2$, scale factor $r = s/M$, and s is an integer. Each grid contains a column of boxes with dimension $s \times s \times s$ for an image of size 256×256 with 256 gray levels. The number of boxes needed to cover grid (i, j) is calculated as

$$n_r(i,j) = l - k + 1 \tag{6}$$

where l is the box number with highest intensity and k is the box number whose intensity is minimum. Taking all grids into account, the total number of boxes required to cover the entire image is expressed as

$$N(r) = \sum_{i,j} n_r(i, j) \tag{7}$$

This $N(r)$ is counted for different values of r, and the log-log plot between $N(r)$ and $(1/r)$ was done. The slope of the plot gives an estimate of the FD of an image and is given by

$$FD = \log(N(r))/\log(1/r) \tag{8}$$

Highly complex, irregular fractal structures exhibit greater FD values [44]. Fractal objects having various textures and spatial arrangements may result in the same FD value because of the combined differences in roughness, coarseness, and directionality. Mandelbrot and Pignoni [67] introduced lacunarity as a complementary parameter to differentiate fractal objects yielding similar FD. Lacunarity analyzes the distribution of holes in an object to measure the amount of nonuniformity in an image. Lacunarity [44] is computed by

$$\text{Lacunarity} = \left(\text{Variance}/\text{Mean}^2\right) - 1 \tag{9}$$

Six fractal features, $f_1 - f_6$, have been identified and derived [41] for natural image texture segmentation. Five fractal features, $f_1 - f_5$, derived from the original image, high- and low-gray-valued images, and horizontal and vertical smoothened images, were found significant in classifying mammograms. However, f_6 was insignificant in the classification of medical images. Hence, the original image is averaged over 4 pixels in the neighborhood, and the estimated FD is taken as a new sixth fractal feature [43, 45] in classifying medical images. This method investigated these six fractal features on fuzzy enhanced images in lung cancer diagnosis.

The high- and low-gray-valued images I_2 and I_3 are obtained from the fuzzy enhanced image $I_1(i, j)$ using thresholds L_1 and L_2, respectively, and defined as

$$I_2(i, j) = \begin{cases} I_1(i, j) - L_1; & \text{if } I_1(i, j) > L_1 \\ 0 & \text{otherwise} \end{cases} \tag{10}$$

$$I_3(i, j) = \begin{cases} 255 - L_2; & \text{if } I_1(i, j) > (255 - L_2) \\ I_1(i, j) & \text{otherwise} \end{cases} \tag{11}$$

where $L_1 = \min + \dfrac{\text{avg}}{2}$, $L_2 = \max - \dfrac{\text{avg}}{2}$, and min, max, and avg are minimum, maximum, and average pixel intensity values of image $I_1(i, j)$, respectively.

Horizontal and vertical smoothened images denoted by I_4 and I_5 are defined as

$$I_4(i,j) = \frac{1}{5} \sum_{k=1}^{5} I_1(i, j+k) \tag{12}$$

$$I_5(i,j) = \frac{1}{5} \sum_{k=1}^{5} I_1(i+k, j) \tag{13}$$

The averaged image I_6 over a neighborhood of 4 pixels is given by

$$I_6(i,j) = \frac{1}{4} \sum_{i=i}^{i+1} \sum_{j=j}^{i+1} I_1(i,j) \tag{14}$$

Lung segmentation is a crucial step in automatic lung cancer detection and is more challenging. Conventional methods in lung segmentation may fail to identify the nodules attached to the pleura and the chest wall. To automate the process of lung cancer detection and to identify the lesions that are attached to the other structures of the lung, a unique segmentation method was employed in this method. Images $I_1 - I_6$ were segmented to subimages of size 128×128 pixels with 50% overlapping in four directions. The total number of subimages obtained is given by the formula

$$N_S = \left(\frac{2 \times \text{Row or column dimension of the input image}}{\text{Row or column dimension of the subimage}} - 1 \right)^2 \tag{15}$$

The segmented images of $I_1 - I_6$ are denoted as I_{pN}, where $p = 1, 2 \ldots 6$ and $N = 1, 2 \ldots N_S$.

Segmented images I_{pN} were fractally transformed using equation 16 and are given as

$$f_{pN}(i,j) = FD\{I_{pN}(i+l, j+k); -W \le l, k \le W\}; p=1, 2\ldots6; N=1, 2\ldots N_S \tag{16}$$

The fractal analysis was carried out on lung PET/CT images with various neighborhood sizes defined by $(2W + 1) \times (2W + 1)$ and optimized based on the results obtained from an experimental study [45]. FD_{avg} and lacunarity were computed from $f_{pN}(i,j)$ to obtain the fractal features $ff_1 - ff_{12}$. Fractal thresholds $T_1(p)$ and $T_2(p)$ were selected from the estimated FD_{avg} and lacunarity of the fractal subimages f_{pN} and are given in equation 17:

$$T_1(p) = \text{Max}\left(FD_{avg}\left(f_{pN} \right) \right); \quad T_2(p) = \text{Min}\left(\text{Lacunarity}\left(f_{pN} \right) \right) \tag{17}$$

Fractal subimages with high FD_{avg} and low lacunarity were identified, and cancerous regions were extracted based on the conditions given in equation 18:

FD of pixels in identified $f_{pN} > T_1(p)$; lacunarity of pixels in identified $f_{pN} < T_2(p)$

$$\tag{18}$$

7.2.2.3.3 Morphology.   Morphological operators are used to extract the edges of the cancerous regions accurately by filling the small gaps found in the extracted edges of the cancerous regions. Morphological dilation with a disk-shaped structuring element was utilized in this study, as it matches well with the shape of the lung [45]. Mathematical morphology is a powerful tool in extracting the shape features of an image that are useful in the description and representation of the region shape.

7.2.2.3.4 Feature Selection.   The texture and fractal analysis extracts features that describe important image properties. Combined texture and fractal features were utilized in this method to improve the diagnostic accuracy of lung cancer detection. However, some of the extracted features may have greater significance, and some features may be insignificant and hence not contributive in lung cancer detection and classification. Significant features are selected based on the study of the range of texture and fractal values of normal and cancerous regions [45, 56]. A reduced feature set improves the performance of the automated classification system [66]. Significant features are fed as inputs to the supervised classifier for automatic classification of lung PET/CT images as normal or cancerous ones.

7.2.2.4 Classification

7.2.2.4.1 Data Set Preparation.   A data set was prepared with the extracted features (three texture and 10 fractal features) from various regions of the lung PET/CT images. Samples were taken from various locations of the images: 50% of the samples from normal regions and 25% of the samples from cancerous regions and from the boundaries of each cancerous region. A total of 1,072 samples were collected and used in classification; 70% of the data were used for training the classifier, and 30% of the data were used for testing the performance of the classifiers.

7.2.2.4.2 ML Techniques.   A huge amount of data have been obtained due to the remarkable advancements in image acquisition devices and the volume of images per single study. This makes it highly challenging and more interesting in medical image analysis. This tremendous, rapid growth in diagnostic medical imaging and modalities needs extensive and wearying efforts by medical expert. This may liable to human error and may have interobserver variations in interpretation. ML and AI techniques have made remarkable progress recently and have played a vital role in medical image analysis, CAD, and image segmentation. ML and AI techniques help medical experts make speedy, automatic diagnosis with improved accuracy. There are two types of ML techniques: supervised learning and unsupervised learning. Supervised ML uses a known set of input and output (target) to make predictions, whereas in unsupervised ML, predictions are made from data sets of input without target values. To train a supervised learning model, an appropriate algorithm is chosen, and then inputs are passed to obtain the response. The supervised learning algorithm develops a model based on the training and makes predictions for new test data that are not used in training. The most commonly used supervised classifiers include decision trees, discriminant analysis, k-nearest neighbors, the Naive Bayes classifier, neural networks, and SVM. The extracted features for a number of observations are taken as a matrix and fed as input to the classifier.

7.2.2.4.3 Decision Trees.   A decision tree uses branching methodology to demonstrate all probable outcomes of a decision. It is a popular ML algorithm and graphical representation that makes decisions based on certain conditions. In a decision tree, the internal node, branch, and leaf node represent the test on the feature, the outcome of the test, and the class label, respectively. The classification rules are represented through the path from the root to the leaf node. These ML algorithms make decisions under uncertainty. Optimal decisions can be arrived at by traversing through forward and backward calculation paths. Decision trees consider only one feature at a time and are not suitable for actual data in the decision space. A decision tree with a higher number of decisions results in reduced accuracy. This method analyzed the three decision tree models: a simple decision tree with a maximum of four splits, a medium tree with a maximum of 20 splits, and a complex tree with a maximum of 100 splits. A medium tree with 20 splits with the Gini diversity index as the split criterion helped make a coarse distinction between the two classes (normal and cancerous) of lung PET/CT images.

7.2.2.4.4 Discriminant Analysis.   Discriminant analysis (DA) is a kind of supervised ML algorithm used in statistics and pattern recognition. Linear DA assigns objects to different classes based on the constructed discriminant equations. It predicts the class of a new set of inputs by maximizing the distance between the mean of each class and minimizing the spreading within the class itself. Linear DA is the preferred classification algorithm to classify linear data with more than two classes. A quadratic DA classifier is used to classify two or more classes by a quadratic surface. As the data set generated from the texture and the fractal features of lung PET/CT images are not linearly separable, DA techniques are not suitable for classifying lung cancer images. To have a complete analysis and to compare various ML techniques, DA has been applied in this method and tested for its performance.

7.2.2.4.5 k-Nearest Neighbor.   The k-nearest neighbor (k-NN) is the most widely used nonparametric, lazy ML technique in classification. It is a simple algorithm in which the entire training data set and all possible cases are stored. A new case is being assigned to a class, and prediction is made by its k-nearest neighbors, measured by a similarity. Similarity is measured by a distance function, such as Euclidean, Manhattan, Minkowski for continuous variables, and the Hamming distance for categorical variables. The performance and behavior of the algorithm depend on the value of k, and its selection depends on the data. Proper selection of k is a challenging one in k-NN modeling. This method was tried with various odd values of

k ranging from 1 to 13 (square root of the training samples/2) and analyzed the performance. A Euclidean distance metric was used to establish the nearest neighbors. The value of k that results in better accuracy and minimum training error is considered the optimal value. Accurate classification is achieved with $k = 1$; however, it overfits the boundaries. Higher values of k reduced the error rate, and a minima was reached. After the minima, the error increases with increasing values of k. In this study, $k = 11$ produced better accuracy and minimal training error and hence was fixed as the optimal value.

7.2.2.4.6 Naive Bayes Classifier.   The Naive Bayes (NB) classifier is the most popular supervised learning method based on the grouping of similarities. It uses Bayes' theorem of probability to predict each class, and the class with the highest probability is considered the most likely class. The NB classifier predicts based on the *naive* assumption that all the features are mutually independent, i.e. there is no way to know anything about other variables when given an additional variable. The NB algorithm is useful for a moderate to large training data set with several features. The NB classifier is suitable for document classification, subjective analysis content, e-mail spam filtering, and disease prediction.

7.2.2.4.7 ANNs.   ANNs represent a promising area that has been successfully applied in the medical field for cancer detection, biochemical analysis, and the identification of pathological conditions [47–50, 53, 54, 63]. An ANN mimics the human brain to process the information, structured with series of layers and a number of artificial neurons (nodes) in each layer. ANNs contain 3 layers, namely input hidden and output layers. Each neuron in the hidden layer is fully connected to the every neuron in the input and output layers. Initially, ANN is trained with a known set of input and outputs. The training is performed using back-propagation or gradient-descent learning algorithms. Back-propagation learning algorithms are most widely used in which the error (i.e., the difference between the actual and the predicted output) is calculated and back propagated to the previous layers to adjust the weights and biases so that the MSE is minimum. Learning happens in ANN with iterative adjustment of its weights and bias to produce desired output. Careful selection of ANN parameters determines the performance of the network. Experimental trials were conducted on number of hidden neurons, learning rate, and momentum to fix optimal network parameters [55, 56].

The number of hidden neurons plays a major role in achieving the desired network performance. The upper bound for the number of hidden neurons was computed by using equation 19:

$$N_h = \frac{N_{ts}}{\alpha(N_i + N_o)} \tag{19}$$

where N_i and N_o represent the number of input and output neurons, respectively; N_{ts} is the number of training samples and parameter; and α is a range from 2 to 10; $\alpha = 2$

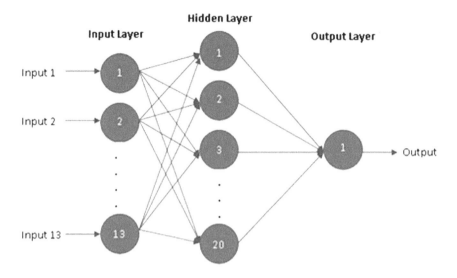

Figure 7.6   ANN architecture with optimal neurons.

was used, as it produced better performance without overfitting. The mean value of the input and output neurons was considered as the lower bound of hidden neurons. Many trials with various hidden neurons ranging from 10 to 25 (obtained from lower and upper bounds) were conducted, and an optimum of 20 hidden neurons was used based on the minimum MSE achieved. The LM back-propagation algorithm was found to be a better learning algorithm with a learning rate of 0.3 and momentum of 0.9 in classifying lung PET/CT images [56].

The architecture of the utilized ANN is shown in Figure 7.6. ANN is structured with 13 input neurons corresponding to three texture and 10 fractal features, a hidden layer with 20 neurons, and an output neuron to classify the lung PET/CT image as normal or cancerous.

7.2.2.4.8 SVM.   SVM was invented by V. N. Vapnik in 1998 and has become a popular tool in pattern recognition, face detection, text characterization, and various applications. SVM has become more popular and powerful in the field of medical diagnosis [57, 59–62]. SVM is a supervised ML algorithm for classification in which the data set teaches SVM about the classes. Learned SVM tends to classify the new data into various classes by finding a hyperplane to separate various classes. Figure 7.7 illustrates the SVM.

Consider the problem of classifying lung cancer images with the extracted features and their classes. A trained SVM model must predict whether the given image is a normal one or shows lung cancer. To find the hyperplane in separating various classes, a weight vector (*w*) and a bias (*b*) are used. The function of the hyperplane can be expressed as

$$w^T x + b = 0 \qquad (20)$$

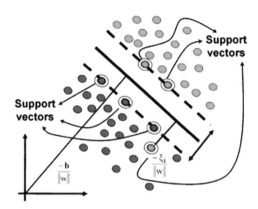

Figure 7.7   Demonstration of the SVM.

The data points are termed normal or cancerous based on the value of the hyperplane function and described as

$$\text{Normal if } w^T x + b < 0;$$
$$\text{Cancerous if } w^T x + b > 0 \qquad (21)$$

The maximum margin classification rule is followed in choosing the hyperplane. The distance between the closest data points for each class to the hyperplane is considered the margin. The closest data points are known as the support vectors. SVMs are categorized as linear and nonlinear: linear for solving linear problems and nonlinear kernels, such as the radial basis function (RBF) kernel, for nonlinear problems. The selection and use of appropriate SVM kernels depend on the data and the application. With an objective of detecting and classifying lung cancer, the training data are very complex and not linearly separable. Hence, the linear kernel is not helpful, and SVM with nonlinear kernels is considered a suitable model in the classification of lung PET/CT images. SVM yields greater efficiency and no overfitting of the data in high-dimensional space. Automatic detection of cancerous regions was performed by using the texture and fractal thresholds. Detected cancerous regions were then superimposed on the RGB lung PET/CT images. Experimental results achieved from this method were validated by two expert nuclear physicians.

7.2.2.5 Performance Measures
The performance measures utilized in image preprocessing are PSNR and CNR and given by equations 22 and 23:

$$\text{PSNR (dB)} = 10 \log_{10} \frac{\max^2}{\frac{1}{mn} \sum_{i=0}^{m-1} \sum_{j=0}^{n-1} \left[I(i,j) - I_F(i,j) \right]^2} \qquad (22)$$

where $I(i, j)$ is the original image and $I_F(i, j)$ is the filtered image and

$$CNR = \frac{\mu_f - \mu_n}{\sigma_n} \tag{23}$$

where μ_f is the mean of the original image and μ_n and σ_n are the mean and standard deviation of the difference image, respectively, between the original and enhanced images. MSE, sensitivity, specificity, and accuracy are the performance measures to evaluate the performance of the classifier and given in equations 24–27:

$$MSE = \frac{1}{N} \sum_{i=1}^{N} e_i^2 = \frac{1}{N} \sum_{i=1}^{N} \left(target_i - actual_i \right)^2 \tag{24}$$

$$Sensitivity = \frac{TP}{TP + FN} \tag{25}$$

$$Specificity = \frac{TN}{FP + TN} \tag{26}$$

$$Accuracy = \frac{TP + TN}{Total\ number\ of\ samples} \tag{27}$$

where TP = true positive, FN = false negative, FP = false positive, and TN = true negative. A perfect classifier has sensitivity and specificity of 100%.

7.3 Results

This method analyzed lung PET/CT images retrospectively to detect and classify lung cancer using texture and fractal feature descriptors. MATLAB R2013a was used to implement this method and tested on lung PET/CT images of size 256×256.

To remove the noise due to image artifacts and enhance the contrast of the lung PET/CT images, Wiener filtering and fuzzy-image enhancement were applied. RGB lung PET/CT images were converted into grayscale images and then denoised using Wiener filtering. Traditional contrast enhancement techniques produce overenhancement in non-ROIs, leading to poor diagnosis. Hence, fuzzy enhancement was carried out to enhance the lung PET/CT images. A gain factor and a threshold were used to enhance highly textured cancerous regions and non-ROIs, such as background, and regions surrounding the lung were reduced in contrast and brightness. It was observed from the histogram of the modified image that the cancerous region's intensity was above 0.9. Hence, T was fixed at 0.9 for better enhancement. Thus, the pixels ranging from 0 to 0.89 were suppressed in contrast, and pixels with values equal to or greater than 0.9 were enhanced in contrast. To minimize overenhancement in non-ROIs, a gain factor, G, was introduced in defuzzification. Trials were conducted with various values of G ranging from 0.3 to 0.9. The results illustrated that very low values of G resulted in underenhancement, whereas high values of G produced overenhancement and thus did not contribute to lung cancer detection. Hence, an optimal gain factor of 0.6 was arrived at based on experimental results.

The images might be degraded in quality when they are acquired at a low radiation dose to minimize the effects of radiation. This degraded image could affect the diagnosis. Lung PET/CT images with intentionally reduced contrast levels at 20%, 40%, 60%, and 80% were tested by the fuzzy enhancement method used in this study. It was found that fuzzy enhancement resulted in an improved enhancement for images with 80% contrast reduced. Hence, fuzzy-image enhancement could benefit in improving the contrast of poor-quality images and thereby improve medical image interpretation. Figure 7.8 shows preprocessed images using Wiener filtering and fuzzy enhancement for a normal lung, lung cancer images in stages II–IV, and contrast-reduced stage IV lung PET/CT images.

Wiener filtering has been found efficient in removing the additive noise present in input images and preserving the fine details. Fuzzy enhancement helped to achieve the desired enhancement.

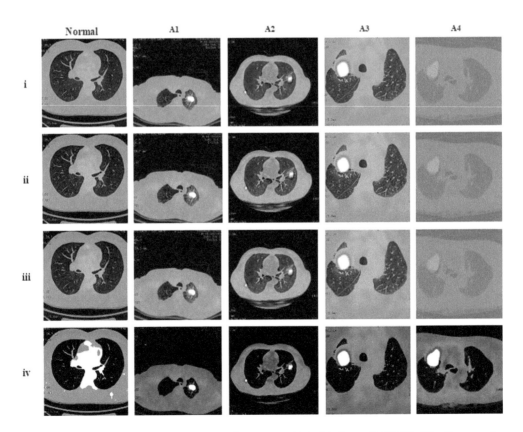

Figure 7.8 Original and preprocessed images: (i) RGB lung PET/CT. (ii) Gray scale. (iii) Wiener filtered image. (iv) Fuzzy enhanced image.

TABLE 7.3   Comparison of Performance Measures of Preprocessing Techniques

Preprocessing Technique	Normal	A1	A2	A3	A4
		PSNR (dB)			
Wiener filtering	36.60	43.01	39.73	39.78	51.76
Median filtering	35.39	39.64	38.03	38.39	50.57
Gaussian filtering	33.80	38.00	36.18	36.39	41.63
		CNR (dB)			
Fuzzy enhancement	8.28	7.03	4.42	12.55	6.02
CLAHE	68.16	26.23	22.04	27.94	23.90

A comparison of the performance of the preprocessing techniques is provided in Table 7.3.

It is observed from Table 7.3 that Wiener filter outperformed median and Gaussian filters in terms of PSNR values. Fuzzy enhancement outperformed the CLAHE technique by improving the contrast of cancerous regions, thereby improving the accurate detection of lung cancer.

Fuzzy enhanced images were subjected to TA to extract meaningful texture information. Fuzzy enhanced images were divided into nonoverlapping smaller subimages of size 5 × 5 to calculate GLCMs and to extract texture features. Second-order statistical texture features listed in Table 7.2 were extracted for normal and abnormal images. A floating graph was plotted for the range of values of 14 texture features for normal and abnormal images and is shown in Figure 7.9.

Texture features that show nonoverlap in their values between normal and abnormal were selected as significant features. It is clear from the graph in Figure 7.9 that only three texture features show nonoverlapping values and hence are considered significant texture features. They are tf_1 (autocorrelation), tf_8 (sum average), and tf_{10}

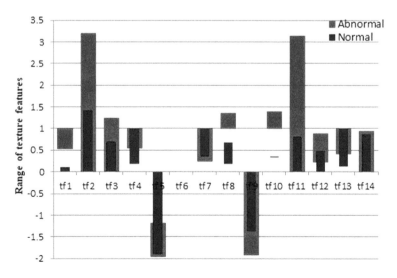

Figure 7.9   Floating graph to demonstrate the selection of significant texture features.

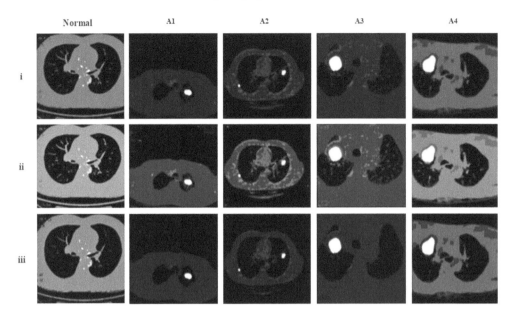

Figure 7.10 Significant texture features: (i) Autocorrelation. (ii) Sum average. (iii) Sum variance.

(sum variance). Figure 7.10 shows the significant texture features for a normal image, three abnormal images, and a contrast-reduced abnormal image.

Fractal analysis was carried out to improve the accuracy of lung cancer diagnosis. The fuzzy enhanced images were considered for the fractal analysis. The initial study of fractal analysis started with dividing the enhanced images into smaller subimages of size 128×128 to estimate the local FD. Estimation of local FD is preferred over global FD in analyzing the texture of medical images by fractal geometry to distinguish normal and cancerous regions. Neighborhood size plays a vital role in estimating the FD, and the value of FD changes as the neighborhood size changes. The effect of neighborhood size in estimating FD was analyzed for lung PET/CT images ranging from 3×3 to 15×15. A neighborhood size of 5×5 was fixed, as the features of the cancerous regions were well identified, whereas the size beyond 5×5 resulted in blurring of the image features due to oversmoothing. Images $I_1 - I_6$, obtained using equations 5 and 10–14, were fractally transformed using equation 16; FD_{avg} and lacunarity were computed for these six images. Hence, a total of 12 fractal features, ff_1–ff_{12}, were estimated for normal as well as abnormal images. Fractal features $ff_1 - ff_6$ correspond to FD_{avg}, and $ff_7 - ff_{12}$ correspond to lacunarity. It was observed that abnormal regions in lung PET/CT images exhibited high FD_{avg} and low lacunarity. The range of fractal feature values for normal and abnormal images was tabulated and plotted as a floating graph. Significant fractal features were selected based on the nonoverlapping values and hence considered for a further stage of classification. Figure 7.11 depicts the plot of the fractal features as a floating chart.

It is evident from Figure 7.11 that ff_3 and ff_9 estimated from the modified image I_3 showed overlap in values between normal and abnormal images. Hence, these

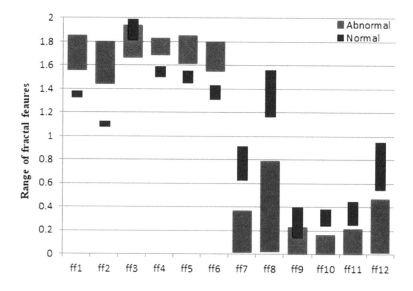

Figure 7.11 Floating graph to demonstrate the selection of significant fractal features.

features were not contributive in discriminating between normal and abnormal images and not considered for further steps in lung cancer detection. Figure 7.12 shows the fractally transformed images for a normal image, abnormal images, and a contrast-reduced abnormal image from which the significant fractal features FD_{avg} and lacunarity were extracted.

Extracted significant texture and fractal features were combined, and a total of 13 features were used in classification; 1,072 observations for these 13 combined features were taken from various regions of normal and abnormal images. These observations were arranged as a matrix and fed as input to the supervised classifier. Supervised classification using ANN with a number of training algorithms was implemented in lung cancer detection from PET/CT images, and it was observed that the LM algorithm produced better classification accuracy [56]. Fourteen supervised classifiers, including decision trees, DA, k-NN, the NB classifier, ANN with the LM training algorithm, and SVM with various kernels, were tried, and their comparative performance was analyzed for finding the best classifier in classifying lung cancer from lung PET/CT images. The performance measures, such as sensitivity, specificity, and accuracy, obtained for all 14 classifiers are listed in Table 7.4.

A confusion matrix table is used to describe the performance of a classifier on test data. Confusion matrixes produced by all 14 classifiers were used to construct a comparison plot to analyze their performance. Figure 7.13 shows the comparison plot demonstrating TP, TN, FP, (type I error), and FN (type II error) obtained with the testing data set for the 14 classifiers. A better classifier could result in improved accuracy by reducing both type I and type II errors. A perfect classifier must have 100% of all three performance measures (sensitivity, specificity, and accuracy).

It is seen from Figure 7.13 that almost all the 14 supervised classifiers produced comparable sensitivity by reducing the number of FNs (type II error), except for

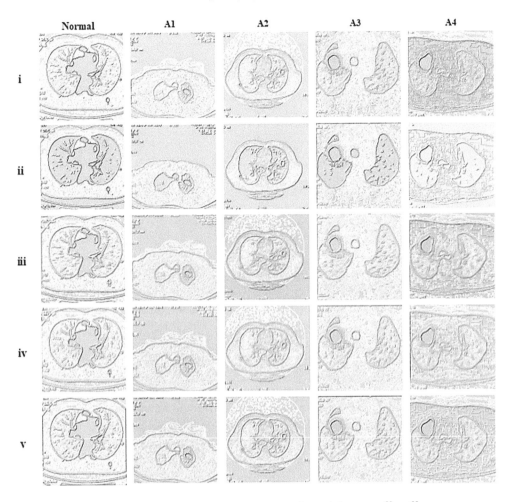

Figure 7.12 Fractally transformed images to extract fractal features $ff_1 - ff_{12}$.

linear DA, quadratic DA, and linear SVM. However, many classifiers have not produced better specificity and have failed to reduce the number of FPs (type I error), which reduced the classification accuracy. The classifiers linear DA, quadratic DA, quadratic SVM, and SVM with RBF kernel of width $\sigma = 0.1$ produced specificities ranging from 60% to 80%. SVM with polynomial kernel of order 2 produced 0% specificity. SVM with polynomial kernel of order 3 produced low specificity of 34.28%. A few classifiers, that is, k-NN (with $k = 11$), the NB classifier, ANN with the LM algorithm, and SVM with RBF kernel of widths $\sigma = 0.5$ and $\sigma = 1$, yielded high specificity. It is seen from the comparison plot of 14 supervised classifiers analyzed in this method that SVM with RBF kernel of $\sigma = 1$ yielded better sensitivity and specificity with a minimum number of FPs and FNs. Figure 7.14 shows the plot of sensitivity, specificity, and accuracy for all 14 classifiers analyzed in this method. It is deduced from Table 7.4 and Figures 7.13 and 7.14 that SVM with RBF kernel $\sigma = 1.0$ (classifier N) outperformed all classifiers in specificity and accuracy.

TABLE 7.4 Comparison of Performance Measures of Various Classifiers Analyzed in This Method

Classifier Code	Classifier Name	Sensitivity (%)	Specificity (%)	Accuracy (%)
A	Decision trees (medium) Maximum splits = 20	98.61	94.28	97.19
B	DA (linear)	83.67	60.33	73.10
C	DA (quadratic)	73.50	80.54	75.90
D	k-NN ($k = 11$)	98.61	96.19	97.81
E	NB classifier	98.61	91.42	96.26
F	ANN with LM algorithm	92.60	92.30	92.50
G	SVM (linear kernel)	81.65	87.08	83.80
H	SVM (quadratic kernel)	96.40	76.23	87.30
I	SVM (polynomial, order 1)	95.74	84.70	90.76
J	SVM (polynomial, order 2)	100.00	0	67.29
K	SVM (polynomial, order 3)	100.00	34.28	78.50
L	SVM (RBF kernel $\sigma = 0.1$)	95.57	80.00	88.52
M	SVM (RBF kernel $\sigma = 0.5$)	97.44	90.08	94.12
N	SVM (RBF kernel $\sigma = 1.0$)	98.61	97.14	98.13

Texture and fractal thresholds were used to extract the cancerous regions, and morphological dilation, followed by thinning, was used to extract the edges of the cancerous regions accurately. Extracted cancerous regions were then superimposed onto the lung RGB PET/CT image. The results produced by the CAD system were validated by expert nuclear physicians. Figure 7.15 shows the final results of the developed CAD system in lung cancer detection and the ground-truth images.

The results of the developed CAD system for lung cancer detection were appreciable, as the system clearly identifies and detects cancerous regions accurately. The performance metrics attained in this method substantiate that the segmented results show similarity with ground truths and demonstrate the robustness of this method.

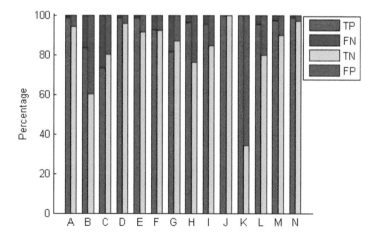

Figure 7.13 Comparison plot of performance of the 14 classifiers.

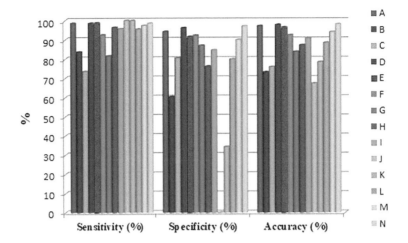

Figure 7.14 Performance comparison of the various classifiers.

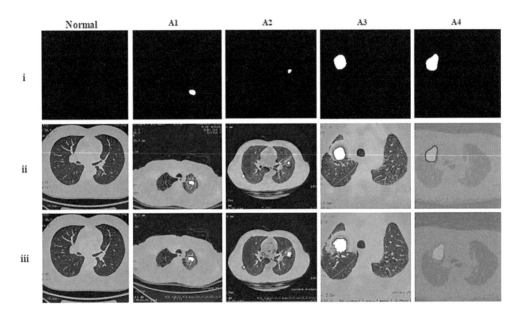

Figure 7.15 Visual comparison of results of CAD system. (i) Detected cancerous regions. (ii) Lung PET/CT images marked with cancerous regions. (iii) Ground-truth images.

7.4 Discussion

The diagnostic accuracy of various established CAD systems using various imaging modalities in lung cancer detection was analyzed and compared with this method of lung cancer detection using texture and fractal features from PET/CT images. The observations are listed in Table 7.5.

Many CAD systems utilized the texture features in detecting lung cancer from CT images, and little research has been carried out from PET/CT images. Supervised

TABLE 7.5 Comparison of Existing and Developed CAD Systems in Lung Cancer Detection

Contributors	Features	Classifier	Database	Classification Accuracy (%)
Al-Fehoum et al. [29]	Statistical texture features	Supervised classifier	CT images	97.33
Udeshani et al. [31]	Statistical texture features	ANN	Chest X-ray images	88
Ahmad et al. [33]	Statistical texture features	ANN	Chest radiographs	98
Ganeshan et al. [34]	Statistical texture features	Not specified	CT images	95
Hossain et al. [35]	Statistical texture features	SVM	CT images	83.7
Xiuhua et al. [36]	Statistical texture features	SVM	CT images	81.5
Kuruvilla et al. [49]	Statistical texture features	ANN	Lung CT images	93.3
Almas et al. [50]	Statistical texture features	ANN	Chest radiographs	80
Parveen et al. [57]	Statistical texture features	SVM with RBF kernel	Lung CT images	90.5
Pham et al. [58]	Statistical texture features	SVM	CT images	70
Shukla et al. [59]	Statistical texture features	SVM with RBF kernel	Lung CT	92.5
Sui et al. [60]	Statistical texture features	SVM	Low-dose CT lung images	92.94
Gao et al. [61]	Statistical texture features	SVM with RBF kernel	Lung PET/CT images	86
Zhao et al. [65]	Statistical texture features	SVM	PET/CT	95.6
Al-Kadi et al. [44]	Fractal features: FD_{avg}, lacunarity	Not specified	Contrast-enhanced CT images	83.5
Irianto et al. [47]	Complete images	ANN	X ray	80
Taher et al. [53]	Intensity features	Hopfield neural network	Sputum color images	98
Penedo et al. [54]	Curvature peak space	ANN	Chest radiographs	89
Guo et al. [62]	Multiple image features (SUV mean, heterogeneity, CT textures)	SVM	Lung PET/CT images	NA
Gutte et al. [63]	Diagnostic features	ANN	Lung PET/CT images	92
Wang et al. [64]	Texture and diagnostic features (SUV)	CNN	PET/CT images	86
Developed CAD system by this method	Texture and fractal features	SVM	PET/CT images	98.13

classifiers, such as ANN and SVM, were mostly used. CAD systems have been developed to detect lung cancer from chest radiographic images [31, 33, 50, 53]. All these CAD systems classify lung cancer based on the extracted first- and second-order statistical texture features. Median filtering and HE were employed in preprocessing of CT images, and lung segmentation was performed using region-based techniques. This developed CAD system utilized six first-order and four second-order statistical texture features in classification of lung cancer by ANN. This method produced an accuracy of 88% [31]. A CAD system was established for lung cancer detection from chest radiographic images with five extracted first-order texture features. Region-based segmentation was used to segment lung regions, and classification was done by using k-means. With a fewer number of features extracted and unsupervised classification, the accuracy yielded was 80% [50]. The CAD system developed by Ahmad et al. [33] utilized six first-order and 11 second-order statistical texture features in lung cancer classification by ANN. Linear DA and principal components analysis were used for feature selection and dimensionality reduction. This resulted in an improved accuracy of 98%. Hence, it is observed that the selection of significant features resulted in an improved accuracy for chest radiographic images.

Many researchers have carried out TA and utilized supervised classifiers in lung cancer detection from CT images [29, 34–36, 44, 49, 57–60]. The CAD system developed by Pham et al. [58] implemented TA and synthesis to extract four first-order and 20 second-order texture features. This method of texture synthesis and estimating optimal levels of noise addition to enhance texture characteristics of lymph nodes on CT does not contribute to improved accuracy. The accuracy obtained was 70% with the SVM classifier [58]. Automatic lung cancer detection implemented by Xiuhua et al. [36] extracted 14 texture features using a curvelet transform. The classification accuracy was 81.5% with the SVM classifier. A CAD system has been established to detect lung cancer from contrast-enhanced CT images. This method used two fractal features, FD_{avg} and lacunarity, and identified the images as aggressive with the fractal threshold and achieved an accuracy of 83.5% [44]. An accuracy of 83.7% was achieved in a CAD system with 14 second-order texture features extracted. Thresholding and region-based methods were used for lung segmentation [29, 35]. A chi-square–based classification outperformed the SVM classifier [35]. Histogram and morphological features were extracted, and an accuracy of 97.33% was achieved [29]. A lung cancer classification method was developed from CT images and used first-order texture features for classification. Morphological operations were used to segment the lungs and ANN with the gradient-descent algorithm with a variable learning rate, and momentum was used to classify lung images. This method achieved an accuracy of 93.3% [49]. A CAD system was established to classify CT lung images using extracted first-order texture features and yielded an accuracy of 95% [34]. Some CAD systems have utilized region-based and watershed algorithms to segment the lungs [57, 59, 60]. First- and second-order texture features were extracted, and the SVM classifier was used. Comparable accuracy was achieved by all these methods: 90.5% [57], 92.5% [59], and 92.94% [60].

A few researchers have attempted to implement a CAD system for lung cancer detection from PET/CT images [61–65]. These methods utilized thresholding for lung segmentation and extracted the first- and second-order texture features. Supervised classifiers, such as ANN and SVM, were used for lung cancer classification. Methods developed by Gao et al. [61] and Wang et al. [64] have resulted in an accuracy of 86%, whereas the methods by Guo et al. [62] and Zhao et al. [65] produced comparable accuracy of 92% and 95.6%, respectively. Even though all these methods yielded a better accuracy, texture features might not be suitable for classifying small lymph nodes [64]. However, employing suitable preprocessing techniques and utilizing fractal texture features could result in improved accuracy. This method utilized Wiener filtering to eliminate additive noise and fuzzy-image enhancement to improve the contrast of PET/CT images. Texture and fractal features were extracted, and the SVM classifier was used in classification. It is clearly evident from Table 7.5 that the developed CAD system using this method for lung cancer detection from PET/CT images using the SVM classifier with RBF kernel $\sigma = 1$ achieved an enriched accuracy of 98.13%.

7.5 Conclusion

The development of an automated lung cancer detection method using texture and fractal descriptors was aimed for in this chapter. Fuzzy-image enhancement offered improved contrast for regions of high texture and was found useful in lung cancer detection. Texture features based on a statistical approach and fractal analysis were found highly useful for detecting and classifying distinct and subtle textures in dual-modality medical images. Significant features were selected from the extracted feature set based on their relevance and contribution in lung cancer detection. This reduced the dimensionality and improved the classification accuracy. This method utilized three texture features and 10 fractal features to detect lung cancer from PET/CT images. From the experimental results, it can be deduced that the combined texture and fractal features were found significant in lung cancer detection.

The data set obtained with these features were linearly nonseparable. The RBF kernel used in the SVM classifier mapped the linearly nonseparable features well into linearly separable ones. The bell-shaped characteristics centered at each support vector, and an appropriate width of the bell-shaped surface worked well in classifying lung cancer. The SVM classifier with RBF kernel width $\sigma = 1$ yielded better classification accuracy than the other classifiers. It is also observed that the classification accuracy produced by k-NN and decision trees is comparable to the results produced by SVM. However, the specificity produced by SVM is higher than that of k-NN and decision tress, thus yielding better classification accuracy. Hence, this chapter concludes that the SVM classifier with RBF kernel width $\sigma = 1$ is the better classifier for lung cancer diagnosis compared to other classifiers analyzed in this method and yielded an accuracy of 98.13%.

Acknowledgment

The authors would like to express their sincere thanks to the nuclear radiologists at Anderson Diagnostics and Labs, Chennai, India, for providing the image data set, precious time, meaningful input, and critical validation of the output. Authors also thank the management of the Hindustan Institute of Technology and Science for their motivation and encouragement to carry out the research work.

References

1. World Health Organization. Cancer. http://www.who.int/mediacentre/factsheets/fs297/en.

2. Malik PS, Raina V. Lung cancer: prevalent trends and emerging concepts. *Indian J Med Res.* 2015;141:5–7.

3. Noronha V, Pinninti R, Patil VM, Joshi A, Prabhash K. Lung cancer in the Indian subcontinent. *S Asian J Cancer.* 2016;5(3):95–103.

4. Ali I, Wani WA, Saleem K. Cancer scenario in India with future perspectives. *Cancer Ther.* 2011;8:56–70.

5. Gwalani P. Lung cancer catches Indians early. July 10, 2014. Accessed December 13, 2016 from https://timesofindia.indiatimes.com.

6. Parikh PM, Ranade AA, Govind B, et al. Lung cancer in India: current status and promising strategies. *S Asian J Cancer.* 2016;5(3):93–95.

7. Behera D, Balamugesh T. Lung cancer in India. *Indian J Chest Dis Allied Sci.* 2004;46(4):269–282.

8. Beadsmoore CJ, Screaton NJ. Classification, staging and prognosis of lung cancer. *Eur J Radiol.* 2003;45(1):8–17.

9. Tsukamoto E, Ochi S. PET/CT today: system and its impact on cancer diagnosis. *Ann Nucl Med.* 2006;20(4):255–267.

10. Joshi SC, Pant I, Khan FA, Shukla AN, Gokula K. Role of integrated PET/CT fusion in lung carcinoma. *Int J Health Sci.* 2008;2(2008):97–101.

11. Ambrosini V, Nicolini S, Caroli P, et al. PET/CT imaging in different types of lung cancer: an overview. *Eur J Radiol.* 2012;81(5):988–1001.

12. Hernández D. The role of PET/CT imaging in lung cancer. *J Cancer Ther.* 2015;6:690–700.

13. Wang HQ, Zhao L, Zhao J, Wang Q. Analysis on early detection of lung cancer by PET/CT scan. *Asia Pac J Cancer Prev.* 2015;16(6):2215–2217.

14. Griffeth LK. Use of PET/CT scanning in cancer patients: technical and practical considerations. *Baylor Univ Med Proc.* 2005;18(4):321–330.

15. Hochhegger B, Alves GRT, Irion KL, et al. PET/CT imaging in lung cancer: indications and findings. *J Bras Pneumol.* 2015;41(3):264–274.

16. http://eradiology.bidmc.harvard.edu/LearningLab/gastro.

17. Van Ginneken B, Schaefer-Prokop CM, Prokop M. Computer-aided diagnosis: how to move from the laboratory to the clinic. *Radiology.* 2011;261(3):719–732.

18. Doi K. Computer-aided diagnosis in medical imaging: historical review, current status and future potential. *Comput Med Imaging Graph.* 2007;31(4):198–211.

19. Castellino RA. Computer aided detection (CAD): an overview. *Cancer Imaging.* 2005; 5(1):17–19.

20. Tang J, Agaian S, Thompson I. Guest editorial: computer-aided detection or diagnosis (CAD) systems. *IEEE Syst J.* 2014;8(3):907–909.

21. Lee H, Chen YP. Image based computer aided diagnosis system for cancer detection. *Expert Syst Appl.* 2015;42(12):5356–5365.

22. Hatt M, Tixier F, Pierce L, et al. Characterization of PET/CT images using texture analysis: the past, the present … any future? *Eur J Nucl Med Mol Imaging.* 2017;44(1):151–165.

23. Blodgett TM, Mehta AS, Mehta AS, et al. PET/CT artifacts. *Clin Imaging.* 2011;35:49–63.

24. Sureshbabu W, Mawlawi O. PET/CT imaging artifacts. *J Nucl Med Technol.* 2005;33(3):156–161.

25. Pettinato C, Nanni C, Farsad M, et al. Artefacts of PET/CT images. *Biomed Imaging Intervent J.* 2006; 2(4):e60.

26. Mahersia H, Zaroug M, Gabralla L. Lung cancer detection on CT scan images: a review on the analysis techniques. *Int J Adv Res Artif Intell.* 2015;4(4):38–45.

27. Preethi SJ, Rajeswari K. Membership function modification for image enhancement using fuzzy logic. *Int J Emerg Trends Technol Comput Sci.* 2013;2(2):114–118.

28. Haralick RM, Shanmugam K. Textural features for image classification. *IEEE Trans Syst Man Cybern.* 1973;3(6):610–621.

29. Al-Fehoum AS, Jaber EB, Al-Jarrah MA. Automated detection of lung cancer using statistical and morphological image processing techniques. *J Biomed Graphics Comput.* 2014;4(2):33–42.

30. Xie G, Cao T, Yan C. Wu Z. Texture features extraction of chest HRCT images based on granular computing. *J Multimedia.* 2010;5(6):639–647.

31. Udeshani KAG, Meegama RGN, Fernando TGI. Statistical feature-based neural network approach for the detection of lung cancer in chest x-ray images. *Int J Image Process.* 2011;5(4):425–434.

32. Cox GS, Hoare FJ, de Jager G. Experiments in lung cancer nodule detection using texture analysis and neural network classifiers. *In Third South African Workshop on Pattern Recognition, Pretoria*; 1992;31:136–142.

33. Ahmad MS, Naweed MS, Nisa M. Application of texture analysis in the assessment of chest radiographs. *Int J Video Image Process Netw Secur.* 2009;9(9):32–36.

34. Ganeshan B, Abaleke S, Young RCD Chatwin CR, Miles KA. Texture analysis of non-small cell lung cancer on unenhanced computed tomography: initial evidence for a relationship with tumour glucose metabolism and stage. *Cancer Imaging.* 2010; 10(1):137–143.

35. Hossain MRI, Ahmed I, Kabir MH. Automatic lung cancer detection using GLCM features. In: Jawahar C, Shan S (Eds.), *Computer Vision - ACCV 2014 Workshops. Lecture Notes in Computer Science, 9010*, Springer, Cham, 2015:109–121.

36. Xiuhua G, Tao S, Haifeng W, et al. Support vector machine prediction model of early-stage lung cancer based on curvelet transform to extract texture features of CT image. *World Acad Sci Eng Technol, Int J of Biomed Biolog Eng.* 2010;4(11):539–543.

37. Zayed N, Elnemr HA. Statistical analysis of Haralick texture features to discriminate lung abnormalities. *J Biomed Imaging.* 2015;2015:1–8.

38. Punithavathy K, Ramya MM, Poobal S. Analysis of statistical texture features for automatic lung cancer detection in PET/CT images. Paper presented at the International Conference on Robotics, Automation, Control, and Embedded Systems (RACE), Chennai, India; February 18–20, 2015.

39. Lopes R, Betrouni N. Fractal and multifractal analysis: a review. *Med Image Anal.* 2009;13(4):634–649.

40. Chen CC, DaPonte JS, Fox MD. Fractal feature analysis and classification in medical imaging. *IEEE Trans Med Imaging.* 1989;8(2):133–142.

41. Chaudhuri BB, Sarkar N. Texture segmentation using fractal dimension. *IEEE Trans Pattern Anal Mach Intell.* 1995;17(1):72–77.

42. Pant T. The Role of Fractal Dimension, Lacunarity and Multifractal Dimension for Texture Analysis in SAR Image—A Comparison Based Analysis. In: Lobiyal DK, Mohapatra DP, Nagar A, Sahoo MN (Eds.), *Proceedings of the International Conference on Signal, Networks, Computing, and Systems. Lecture Notes in Electrical Engineering,* 395. Springer, New Delhi, 2017; 127–136.

43. Sankar D, Thomas T. Classification of mammograms into normal, benign and malignant based on fractal features. *Int J Image Graphics Signal Process.* 2016;8(3):36–44.

44. Al-Kadi OS, Watson D. Texture analysis of aggressive and nonaggressive lung tumor CE CT images. *IEEE Trans Biomed Eng.* 2008;55(7):1822–1830.
45. Punithavathy K, Soundararajan R, Poobal S, Ramya MM. Fractal based lung cancer detection from fuzzy enhanced PET/CT images. *Int J Pure Appl Math.* 2017; 117(7):427–444.
46. Firmino M, Morais AH, Mendoça RM, et al. Computer-aided detection system for lung cancer in computed tomography scans: review and future prospects. *Biomed Eng Online.* 2014;13(1):41.
47. Irianto BG, Mak'ruf MR, Titisari D. Identification of lung cancer using a back propagation neural network. *Indonesian J Electr Eng Comput Sci.* 2015;16(1):91–97.
48. Hussain MA, Ansari TM, Gawas PS, Chowdhury NN. Lung cancer detection using artificial neural network and fuzzy clustering *Int J Adv Res Comput Commun Eng.* 2015;4(3):360–363.
49. Kuruvilla J, Gunavathi K. Lung cancer classification using neural networks for CT images. *Comput Methods Programs Biomed.* 2014;113(1):202–209.
50. Almas P, Bariu KS. Detection and classification of lung cancer using artificial neural network. *Int J Adv Comput Eng Commun Technol.* 2012;1(1):62–67.
51. Chauhan D, Jaiswal V. Development of computational tool for lung cancer prediction using data mining. *Int J Comput Appl Technol Res.* 2016;5(7):417–421.
52. Kohad R, Ahire V. Application of machine learning techniques for the diagnosis of lung cancer with ANT colony optimization. *Int J Comput Appl.* 2015;113(18):34–41.
53. Taher F, Werghi N, Al-Ahmad H, Sammouda R. Lung cancer detection by using artificial neural network and fuzzy clustering methods. *Am J Biomed Eng.* 2012;2(3):136–142.
54. Penedo MG, Carreira MJ, Mosquera A, Cabello D. Computer-aided diagnosis: a neural-network-based approach to lung nodule detection. *IEEE Trans Med Imaging.* 1998;17(6):872–880.
55. Karsoliya S. Approximating number of hidden layer neurons in multiple hidden layer BPNN architecture. *Int J Eng Trends Technol.* 2012;3(6):714–717.
56. Punithavathy K, Poobal S, Ramya MM. Artificial neural network based lung cancer detection for PET/CT images. *Indian J Sci Technol.* 2018;10(42):1–13.
57. Parveen SS, Kavitha C. Classification of lung cancer nodules using SVM kernels. *Int J Comput Appl.* 2014;95(25):25-28.
58. Pham TD, Watanabe Y, Higuchi M, Suzuki H. Texture analysis and synthesis of malignant and benign mediastinal lymph nodes in patients with lung cancer on computed tomography. *Sci Rep.* 2017;7:43209.
59. Shukla N, Narayane A, Nigade A, Yadav K, Mhaske H. Lung cancer detection and classification using support vector machine. *Int J Eng Comput Sci.* 2015;4(11):14983–14986.
60. Sui Y, Wei Y, Zhao D. Computer-aided lung nodule recognition by SVM classifier based on combination of random undersampling and SMOTE. *Comput Math Methods Med.* 2015; 2015:1-13.
61. Gao X, Chu C, Li Y, et al. The method and efficacy of support vector machine classifiers based on texture features and multi-resolution histogram from 18 F-FDG PET-CT images for the evaluation of mediastinal lymph nodes in patients with lung cancer. *Eur J Radiol.* 2015;84(2):312–317.
62. Guo N, Yen RF, El Fakhri G, Li Q. SVM based lung cancer diagnosis using multiple image features in PET/CT. Paper presented at the Nuclear Science Symposium and Medical Imaging Conference (NSS/MIC), San Diego, CA, USA; Oct 31, 2015:1–4.

63. Gutte H, Jakobsson D, Olofsson F, et al. Automated interpretation of PET/CT images in patients with lung cancer. *Nucl Med Commun.* 2007;28(2):79–84.

64. Wang H, Zhou Z, Li Y, et al. Comparison of machine learning methods for classifying mediastinal lymph node metastasis of non-small cell lung cancer from 18F-FDG PET/CT images. *EJNMMI Res.* 2017;7(1):11.

65. Zhao J, Ji G, Qiang Y, et al. A new method of detecting pulmonary nodules with PET/CT based on an improved watershed algorithm. *PloS One.* 2015;10(4):e0123694.

66. Nailon WH. Texture analysis methods for medical image characterisation. In: Mao Y (Ed.), *Biomedical Imaging.* Intech Publishing, Croatia, 2010: 75–100.

67. Mandelbrot BB. *The Fractal Geometry of Nature.* New York, NY: W. H. Freeman; 1982.

8

Lung Cancer Risk of a Population Exposed to Airborne Particles: The Contribution of Different Activities and Microenvironments

L. Stabile and G. Buonanno

Contents

8.1 Introduction

Airborne particles, also known as aerosols, represent solid and liquid particles from a few nanometers to tens of micrometers in diameter transported by a carrying gas (i.e., air) [1–3]. Due to their different origins, sizes, shapes, and chemical compositions, airborne particles represent a complex thermodynamic mixture [4].

In the past decades, increasing interest was paid by the scientific community to the exposure to airborne particles and the related health effects. Indeed, a number of papers were recently published to highlight the respiratory and cardiovascular outcomes due to the short- or long-term exposure to different particle sizes and origins [5–13]. Results of these studies highlight a greater effect of submicron particles with respect to larger ones, likely due to their greater capacity to enter the lungs: such recognized health effects acted as a boost for new exposure assessment studies investigating particle metrics (e.g., submicron particles) still not considered by actual air quality standards [14–20].

In addition to respiratory and cardiovascular outcomes, airborne particles were recently classified by the International Agency for Research on Cancer, which is part of the World Health Organization, as carcinogenic to humans (group 1) based on sufficient evidence that exposure is associated with an increased risk of lung cancer [21, 22]. Such a carcinogenic effect of airborne particles is strictly related to the amount of carcinogenic compounds carried by the particles [23] and the efficiency of those particles in crossing the respiratory systems and depositing in the deepest regions of the lungs [24]. The relationship between exposure and risk still represents a main challenge for scientists; indeed, it could allow estimating a priori the risk of a typical population when their exposure scenario is known.

This chapter aims to provide a comparison in terms of particle-related lung cancer risk among different exposure scenarios: to this end, a lung cancer risk model considering the effect of both sub- and supermicron particles [25] was adopted. Before discussing the research carried out by the authors in different scientific papers, a short informative section is provided to give the reader more background.

8.1.1 Dimensional Classification of Airborne Particles

The International Organization for Standardization [26] has defined an aerosol as "a metastable suspension of solid or liquid particles in a gas." The term "metastable" was due to the dynamic behavior of such particles, which can be suddenly affected by thermodynamic processes, leading to the formation of new particles through nucleation phenomena, the coagulation of previous existing particles, the enlargement of particles due to condensation phenomena, and the removal of particles due to sedimentation, diffusion, and impaction [4]. Particle size ranges from a few nanometers (in theory slightly larger than molecules) up to 100 μm, even if particles larger than 10 μm are not interesting from a health risk assessment point of view. Since particle shape can strongly differ from being spherical, particle diameter, as usually mentioned, refers to an equivalent diameter, that is, the diameter of a sphere having the same properties of that under investigation. Typically, the aerodynamic diameter is used to measure and classify particles: it is defined as the diameter of an idealized sphere with unit density having a settling velocity identical to that of the particle in question [27].

On the basis of aerodynamic diameter, PM_{10}, $PM_{2.5}$, and PM_1 are defined as the mass concentrations of particles that pass through a size-selective inlet with a 50% cutoff efficiency at 10-, 2.5-, and 1-μm aerodynamic diameter, respectively. $PM_{2.5}$ are also known as "fine particles," whereas the $PM_{2.5-10}$ fraction (evaluated as the difference between PM_{10} and $PM_{2.5}$ concentrations) is commonly termed "coarse particles."

The previously mentioned mass particle concentration fractions are affected mostly by supermicron particles, which have a higher mass than submicrometric ones. Nonetheless, the number of such supermicron particles is quite negligible

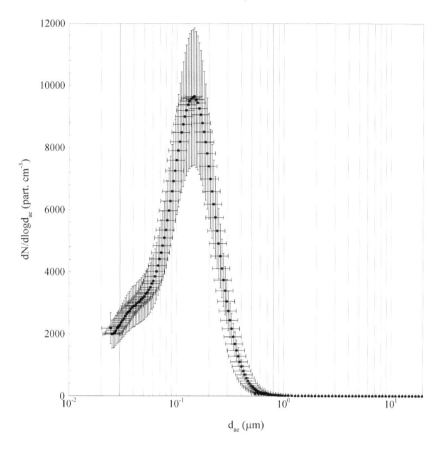

Figure 8.1 Example of particle number distribution measured at a rural site in central Italy (figure reproduced from Buonanno et al. [28] with permission).

with respect to the submicron ones. As an example, in Figure 8.1, a particle number distribution measured by Buonanno et al. [28] at a rural sampling site in central Italy was reported. The number distribution is dominated by particles smaller than 1 μm, such as ultrafine particles (UFPs) and nanoparticles (defined as particles smaller than 100 and 50 nm, respectively), whose mass contribution is almost negligible. Indeed, submicron particles are commonly expressed not in terms of mass concentrations but rather in terms of number or surface area concentrations.

Moreover, particle size can be roughly considered a marker of the origin: the emission of submicron particles (and then particle number, surface area, and PM_1 concentrations) is due mainly to combustion activities (e.g., vehicular traffic, biomass, and cigarettes [29–35]), whereas supermicron particles (and in particular the coarse fraction) are strongly affected by mechanical processes (e.g., resuspension and erosion, [15, 19, 36–39]). Summarizing, then, the dimensional classification of the airborne particles indirectly refers to the most representative particle metrics and to particle origin.

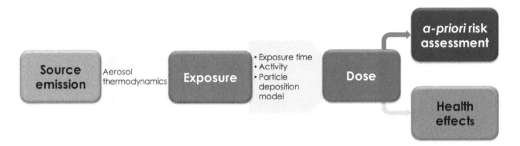

Figure 8.2   Exposure chain of airborne particles.

8.1.2 From Particle Emission to Dose Received by a Population

To evaluate the possible health effects due to the inhalation of airborne particles, toxicological and epidemiological studies are trying to determine dose–response relationships for different diseases [40–44]. Such relationships could be also used for a priori risk assessments of the population for different exposure scenarios. Therefore, the evaluation of dose is a key aspect since it represents the connecting point between exposure and the possible outcomes, as shown in the exposure chain reported in the Figure 8.2. In particular, the figure highlights the chain of physicochemical events from particle emission to their related health effects and risks for human populations. Indeed, the particles emitted by sources typically undergo sudden thermodynamic processes leading to possible variations in terms of size, chemical composition, and concentrations. Thus, the aerosols inhaled by people at a certain spatial and temporal distance from the emitting source can be significantly different from those freshly emitted: as an example, people walking on curbs in an urban area are exposed to particle concentrations much lower than those measured at the vehicle tailpipe section due to the dilution effect typically affecting particles emitted in outdoor environments [45, 46]. This represents a key point to be considered by air quality experts and regulatory authorities; in fact, the regulations released over the years aiming to reduce source emissions could be ineffective in terms of protecting human health. Indeed, to reduce the possible health effects, the dose of inhaled and deposited particles should be reduced; therefore, the actual exposure to particles in the different microenvironments in which people reside should be taken into consideration.

The dose received by people can be only estimated on the basis of particle deposition models and time activity patterns, whereas the exposure of the population can actually be measured. The dose of particles (δ) received by people in the alveolar and tracheobronchial regions of the lungs when performing a certain activity in a specific microenvironment can be calculated as the product of the particle concentration in the people exposed, the deposition efficiency in the alveolar and tracheobronchial regions, and the volume of air inhaled by people, as expressed by the equation 1:

$$\delta_{Alv+TB} = \sum_i C(D_i) \cdot DF(D_i, \text{activity})_{Alv+TB} \cdot T \cdot IR_{\text{activity}} \tag{1}$$

Here, C represents the particle concentration of the ith particle size (D) expressed in terms of number, surface area, or mass; DF represents the deposition fraction in the alveolar and tracheobronchial regions (estimated through different particle deposition models available in the scientific literature as a function of the particle size and the human activity [24, 47, 48]); T is the exposure time at that concentration; and IR is the inhalation rate of the exposed population, which is a function of the activity performed, gender, and age [24]. Summarizing, then, the evaluation of the dose is strictly related to the exposure assessment [49] and thus to the spatial scale adopted to measure such exposure. With regard to the exposure assessment of the population, Cattaneo et al. [50] documented five different spatial scales: (1) "city scale," the broadest and most common scale used to characterize air quality across several city blocks using remote measurements; (2) "outdoor scale," which is representative of particle exposure outside buildings, where the population typically live or work; (3) "indoor scale," which reflects indoor-based exposure in buildings; (4) "individual scale," where the sampling location is within 3 m of the person; and (5) "personal scale," using handheld instruments carried as personal monitors able to sample aerosols from the "breathing zone" of the person. To date, most of the epidemiological studies analyzing the exposure-outcome relationships are based only on measurements performed at the city scale [13, 51], that is, the data typically provided by the regulatory authorities in a city. The limit values of airborne particles in outdoor environments (and thus in urban areas) are currently defined in terms of PM_{10} and $PM_{2.5}$ [52, 53]. To map outdoor air quality in terms of PM_{10} and $PM_{2.5}$, current European legislation [52] suggests a limited number of fixed sampling points as representative of the exposure of the entire urban population living within this area; however, this approach does not take into account personal exposure factors, factors related to mode of transport, traffic and meteorological factors, or variations in particle concentrations due to meteorological conditions and source emission properties, which can strongly affect the real exposure of the population. This is an oversimplified approach due to the spatial variability of particulate matter in cities [19, 20, 54]; moreover, the method is even less valid for UFPs, which are recognized as having greater spatial variability than PM_{10} [30, 55]. Since several studies have demonstrated that airborne particle monitoring through fixed stations provides inadequate evaluations and is not related to the exposure of the entire population, measurements as close as to the exposed population are required. Therefore, measurements in each microenvironment where the investigated persons spend time are needed, or, even better, individual/personal monitoring could be used to evaluate the actual exposure to airborne particles of people living or working in or crossing several urban microenvironments [18, 56, 57]. Such personal monitoring should also include the UFPs, which are currently not considered in the normative guidelines [58]. The exposure characterization at indoor/outdoor scales or at individual/personal scales could solve a further main limitation of the current air quality standards, namely, the lack of standards for exposure in indoor environments, which represent the environments where the population spend a longer time fraction of the day.

Summarizing, then, on the basis of the previously mentioned spatial scales, two main exposure assessment approaches can be used: the indirect and the direct exposure assessment approach. The indirect approach is characterized by the measurement of particle concentrations in different microenvironments in which a population resides at indoor and outdoor scales through stand-alone instruments. On the other hand, the direct approach is based on measurements at the individual/personal scales by means of handheld monitors; such monitors are typically characterized by inferior meteorological performance with respect to stand-alone laboratory instruments but allow following the person under investigation during the day in each microenvironment in which one resides.

8.1.3 Lung Cancer Risk Model

The toxicity of aerosols is clearly related to the compounds carried by the particles; some of these compounds are listed by the International Agency for Research on Cancer as group 1 carcinogens (i.e., characterized by an evident carcinogenetic effect on humans), and a causal relationship was established between exposure to these agents and human cancer. Among these, polycyclic aromatic hydrocarbons (PAHs) and some heavy metals could be considered major contributors to human exposure through the respiratory tract. PAHs are organic compounds with two or more fused aromatic rings formed during incomplete combustion. In general, the carcinogenic properties of PAHs increase with the number of aromatic rings [59]. The PAHs emitted by combustion sources are present in the gaseous phase (semivolatile) and are associated with particles (particle bound). Baek et al. [60] found that two- and three-ring PAHs were mainly in the gas phase, while four-ringed PAHs were in both the gas phase and the particle phase and five- and six-ringed PAHs were mainly attached to particles. Benzo[a]pyrene (BaP) is the most extensively studied PAH and is the usual marker for carcinogenic levels of PAHs in epidemiology and environmental studies. The World Health Organization International Program on Chemical Safety [61] represents a source of information on the relative carcinogenic potency of PAHs, and the European Union developed an extensive body of legislation establishing health-based standards for PAHs and heavy metals in the air. In particular, the annual mean concentration of BaP, as a representative for PAHs (1 ng m^{-3}), As (6 ng m^{-3}), Cd (5 ng m^{-3}), and Ni (20 ng m^{-3}), was established by Directive 2004/107/EC [62]. The corresponding estimated lifetime lung cancer risk due to PAHs is 8.7 cases per 100,000 people with chronic inhalational exposure to 1 ng m^{-3} of BaP over a lifetime of 70 years. Based on this information, the U.K. government's Expert Panel on Air Quality Standards recommended a U.K. standard for BaP of 0.25 ng m^{-3} [63], and when proposing an action plan to reduce environmental health risks in Sweden, the Swedish Governmental Commission on Environmental Health [64] proposed a value of 0.1 ng m^{-3} as the long-term average limit for BaP. This level corresponds to a theoretical lifetime cancer risk of 1×10^{-5} [65].

On the basis of the findings summarized in the previous section, the evaluation of risk associated with real exposure is particularly complex because (1) data on fixed sampling points are not representative of real outdoor exposure because of the high particle concentration decay with respect to distance from the source, (2) outdoor exposure represents only a fraction of personal integrated exposure since individuals also move through multiple indoor microenvironments, (3) no air quality standards considering other particle metrics (number and surface area) are defined [66], and (4) existing risk models for chemicals use mass as the dosimetry to assess the health effect. Consequently, health effects induced by UFPs are usually not considered, and they are strongly underestimated when assessing exposure to particulate matter. More recently, Sze-To et al. [25] proposed a new model to assess the lung cancer risk associated with both sub- and supermicron particles. Indeed, they realized that classical lung cancer risk model based only on particle mass as dosimetry underestimated by a large amount the actual lung cancer data provided by epidemiological studies. Therefore, they calculate the contribution of submicron particles, expressed as particle surface area metrics, to the lung cancer risk and introduced a coefficient to correlate the particle surface area–based cancer potency of the chemical in the form of particulate matter to the mass-based cancer potency of the chemical. The lung cancer risk equation developed by Sze-To et al. [25] allows one to evaluate the total excess lifetime cancer risk (ELCR), which represents the additional or extra risk of developing cancer due to exposure to a toxic substance incurred over the lifetime of an individual, conventionally assumed to be 70 years:

$$\mathrm{ELCR} = \frac{1}{BW}\left(\sum_{i}^{n} SF_i \cdot \frac{m_i}{\mathrm{PM}_{10}}\right) \cdot \left[c_f \cdot \delta_{alv+TB} + \delta_{PM10}\right] \tag{2}$$

where BW is the average body weight of the population (70 kg); SF_i is the inhalation slope factor used to describe the lifetime cancer potency of the ith pollutant (i.e., the percent increase in the risk of getting cancer associated with exposure to a unit concentration of a chemical every day for a lifetime, here assumed equal to 70 years); m_i is the mass concentration of the ith pollutant present on the PM_{10} mass; c_f is the previously mentioned conversion coefficient (6.6×10^{-13} mg nm^{-2}), obtained by Sze-To et al. [25], representing the equivalent toxicity of the particle surface area metric expressed as particle mass; and δ_{Alv+TB} and δ_{PM10} represent the doses received by the investigated population in terms of alveolar- and tracheobronchial-deposited surface area and PM_{10}, respectively. The SFs of the carcinogenic chemicals were provided by the Office of Environmental Health Hazard Assessment [67]: in particular, SF values for PAHs (expressed as BaP), As, Cd, and Ni are equal to 3.9, 15.1, 6.3, and 0.91 kg day mg^{-1}, respectively. The term $\sum_{i}^{n} SF_i \cdot \frac{m_i}{PM_{10}}$ represents the SF of the mixture of the n carcinogenic pollutants on PM_{10} and are hereafter reported as SF_m.

The lung cancer risk model proposed by Sze-To et al. [25] represents a useful tool for engineers and air quality experts due to its feasibility; indeed, it was applied in some research aiming to provide an estimate of the lung cancer risk of a population exposed to different sources and/or residing in different microenvironments [17, 34, 35, 68–71]. Those using such model should be aware that it presents limitations due to the simplifying hypotheses typically adopted in its application. In particular, the main simplification is due to the chemical composition of the aerosol, which is considered uniform within the entire particle size range; this is usually not true since UFPs and coarse particles could present different formation processes [72]. Including size-dependent particle chemistry in the model would require chemical composition data characteristics of each size range for all the sources investigated, which are not currently provided by the scientific literature. A further aspect to be considered in the risk model uncertainty is the conversion coefficient c_f: it represents the equivalent toxicity of the particle surface area metric expressed as particle mass and, at first, was considered to not depend on aerosol typology and size by Sze-To et al. [25]. Therefore, this hypothesis merits an in-depth analysis involving both aerosol experts and toxicologists aiming to assess the toxicity of the two particle metrics for different aerosols. Summarizing, then, on the basis of such limitations, the model can be used primarily to give an estimate of the order of magnitude of the risk. In the next section, such a model was applied to different exposure scenarios. The first case study represents the application of the lung cancer risk model to doses received by the Italian population; in particular, the population investigated was nonsmoking and not exposed to particles emitted by indoor biomass-burning systems. The dose data were evaluated on the basis of an indirect approach through measurements performed at outdoor and indoor scales in other previous studies. The second case study deals with the dose and risk contribution of the exposure to indoor biomass-burning systems; in particular, open and closed fireplaces as well as pellet stoves were investigated.

8.2 Case Studies

8.2.1 Italian Nonsmoking Population

The primary objective of the research was to characterize the major contributors to lung cancer risk for the Italian population on the basis of the risk assessment scheme described in section 8.1.3. To this end, the daily exposure of people of different age-groups to PAHs, regulated heavy metals (As, Cd, and Ni), and airborne particles were considered; moreover, the time activity patterns reported in the Italian Human Activity Pattern Survey were adopted to estimate the dose and risk of a typical nonsmoking population. The investigated population was not exposed to biomass-burning phenomena typical of residential heating through fireplaces and stoves; such an exposure scenario was studied separately and reported in section 8.2.2.

8.2.1.1 Methodology
ELCR was evaluated through equation 2 described in section 8.1.3; here, to take into account the variability of the exposure during an individual's lifetime, the curve of ELCR as a function of age was reconstructed, modifying equation 2 for the ith pollutant and for an individual at age τ as

$$\mathrm{ELCR}_i(\tau) = c_f \frac{SF_i}{70} \int_\tau^0 \frac{m_i}{PM_{10}}(t) \frac{\delta_{Alv+TB}(t)}{BW(t)} dt + \frac{SF_i}{70} \int_\tau^0 \frac{m_i}{M_{10}}(t) \frac{\delta_{PM_{10}}(t)}{BW(t)} dt \qquad (3)$$

where the number 70 is due to the fact that the slope factor is evaluated on a conventional life duration equal to 70 years and t and τ are expressed in years.

    PAHs and heavy metal concentrations in the air were obtained from national environmental protection agencies. Indeed, annual concentrations measured by local environmental protection agencies in the urban areas of Turin and Milan, as well as in Apulian and Sicilian cities, were considered for northern and southern

Italy, respectively. With regard to cooking activities, the frequency distributions of BaP/PM$_{10}$, As/PM$_{10}$, Cd/PM$_{10}$, and Ni/PM$_{10}$ mass ratios were obtained using the values measured by See and Balasubramanian [73].

The estimate of daily surface area and mass deposition of airborne particles was performed through an indirect exposure assessment using the statistical analysis procedure reported in Buonanno et al. [74]: (1) matching the locations (microenvironments) where each exposed person spends time, (2) verifying particle number size distributions to which people are exposed in each microenvironment, (3) determining inhalation rates as a function of age and specific activity levels of the exposed population, and (4) estimating the fraction of inhaled particles that are deposited. With regard to the evaluation of Italian daily time activity patterns, data were obtained from Bastone et al. [75, 76] and Soggiu et al. [77, 78] for northern and southern Italy, respectively. Inhalation rates as a function of the different activities and age-groups were obtained from U.S. Environmental Protection Agency (EPA) [79] and Adams [80], whereas the average body weight of the Italian population was provided by the World Health Organization [81], Zoppi et al. [82], and Masali [83].

Data on the exposure to particles in each microenvironment where the Italian population was exposed were obtained from our previous studies conducted in Cassino, a typical, busy town located in south-central Italy and summarized in Buonanno et al. [74]. In particular, particle size distributions used to evaluate the daily particle dose were fitted through a lognormal distribution, and these data were used to perform a Monte Carlo simulation to generate both particle number distributions and daily time activity patterns. In particular, (1) for each activity, a sample of 100 particle number distributions was generated according to a random distribution between the minimum and maximum values for the corresponding microenvironment; (2) for each age-group, a sample of 10^6 daily time activity pattern combinations were generated following a Gaussian distribution; and (3) a random sample of 10^6 combinations of the generated particle size number distributions, as well as the daily time activity patterns, was obtained. On the basis of the 10^6 different generated combinations, the daily surface area and mass-deposited doses for each age-group were estimated.

8.2.1.2 Results

8.2.1.2.1 Dose. Table 8.1 reports the average daily alveolar and tracheobronchial particle number and surface area deposited doses as a function of age-group, gender, and location (northern and southern Italy). The daily alveolar particle number (and surface area) deposited for males from all age-groups ranged from 1.39×10^{11} particles (2.28×10^{15} nm^2) in northern Italy to 1.51×10^{11} particles (2.51×10^{15} nm^2) in southern Italy. The corresponding values for females ranged from 1.44×10^{11} particles (2.64×10^{15} nm^2) in northern Italy to 1.51×10^{11} particles (2.56×10^{15} nm^2) in southern Italy. Such values are larger than those estimated for the tracheobronchial region due to the higher deposition fractions in the alveolar regions [24]. In fact, the daily tracheobronchial doses in terms of particle number (surface area) received by the Italian population considering all the age-groups, ages, and locations were in the range 3.44×10^{10} to 1.07×10^{11} particles (4.96×10^{14} – 1.75×10^{15} nm^2).

TABLE 8.1 Daily Doses in Terms of Particle Number and Surface Area Received by the Italian Population as a Function of Age, Gender, and Location (Data Reported as Average ± Standard Deviation) (Table Adapted From Buonanno et al. [74])

Age-Groups	Alveolar Number (Particles)	Alveolar Surface Area (nm^2)	Tracheobronchial Number (Particles)	Tracheobronchial Surface Area (nm^2)
		Females, Northern Italy		
<1	—	—	—	—
1–5	$5.26 \pm 0.24 \times 10^{10}$	$1.21 \pm 0.10 \times 10^{15}$	$3.73 \pm 0.34 \times 10^{10}$	$5.05 \pm 0.39 \times 10^{14}$
6–10	$6.90 \pm 0.36 \times 10^{10}$	$1.40 \pm 0.13 \times 10^{15}$	$3.44 \pm 0.18 \times 10^{10}$	$4.96 \pm 0.41 \times 10^{14}$
11–18	$9.75 \pm 0.66 \times 10^{10}$	$1.80 \pm 0.16 \times 10^{15}$	$4.31 \pm 0.25 \times 10^{10}$	$6.99 \pm 0.64 \times 10^{14}$
19–40	$2.03 \pm 0.45 \times 10^{11}$	$3.16 \pm 0.87 \times 10^{15}$	$8.93 \pm 1.80 \times 10^{10}$	$1.26 \pm 0.35 \times 10^{15}$
41–65	$2.45 \pm 0.57 \times 10^{11}$	$4.10 \pm 1.30 \times 10^{15}$	$1.07 \pm 0.24 \times 10^{11}$	$1.65 \pm 0.52 \times 10^{15}$
>65	$1.95 \pm 0.57 \times 10^{11}$	$4.17 \pm 1.40 \times 10^{15}$	$9.20 \pm 2.60 \times 10^{10}$	$1.75 \pm 0.58 \times 10^{15}$
		Males, Northern Italy		
<1	—	—	—	—
1–5	$5.36 \pm 0.29 \times 10^{10}$	$1.30 \pm 0.13 \times 10^{15}$	$3.96 \pm 0.39 \times 10^{10}$	$5.41 \pm 0.47 \times 10^{14}$
6–10	$7.15 \pm 0.44 \times 10^{10}$	$1.41 \pm 0.13 \times 10^{15}$	$3.57 \pm 0.21 \times 10^{10}$	$5.07 \pm 0.45 \times 10^{14}$
11–18	$8.83 \pm 0.49 \times 10^{10}$	$1.51 \pm 0.11 \times 10^{15}$	$3.74 \pm 0.15 \times 10^{10}$	$5.41 \pm 0.40 \times 10^{14}$
19–40	$2.13 \pm 0.50 \times 10^{11}$	$3.05 \pm 0.79 \times 10^{15}$	$8.16 \pm 1.70 \times 10^{10}$	$1.03 \pm 0.26 \times 10^{15}$
41–65	$2.24 \pm 0.49 \times 10^{11}$	$3.29 \pm 0.79 \times 10^{15}$	$8.60 \pm 1.70 \times 10^{10}$	$1.12 \pm 0.27 \times 10^{15}$
>65	$1.82 \pm 0.43 \times 10^{11}$	$3.15 \pm 1.00 \times 10^{15}$	$7.28 \pm 1.60 \times 10^{10}$	$1.09 \pm 0.35 \times 10^{15}$
		Females, Southern Italy		
<1	$1.17 \pm 0.02 \times 10^{11}$	$8.13 \pm 0.15 \times 10^{14}$	$4.60 \pm 0.17 \times 10^{10}$	$7.50 \pm 0.38 \times 10^{14}$
1–5	$8.31 \pm 0.33 \times 10^{10}$	$2.08 \pm 0.12 \times 10^{15}$	$4.46 \pm 0.16 \times 10^{10}$	$7.67 \pm 0.37 \times 10^{14}$
6–10	$9.17 \pm 0.36 \times 10^{10}$	$2.02 \pm 0.15 \times 10^{15}$	$4.27 \pm 0.15 \times 10^{10}$	$7.11 \pm 0.46 \times 10^{14}$
11–18	$1.10 \pm 0.04 \times 10^{11}$	$2.24 \pm 0.12 \times 10^{15}$	$4.85 \pm 0.14 \times 10^{10}$	$8.72 \pm 0.47 \times 10^{14}$
19–40	$1.99 \pm 0.07 \times 10^{11}$	$2.95 \pm 0.36 \times 10^{15}$	$8.40 \pm 0.28 \times 10^{10}$	$1.14 \pm 0.04 \times 10^{15}$
41–65	$2.26 \pm 0.08 \times 10^{11}$	$3.96 \pm 0.57 \times 10^{15}$	$9.87 \pm 0.41 \times 10^{10}$	$1.58 \pm 0.09 \times 10^{15}$
>65	$1.77 \pm 0.03 \times 10^{11}$	$3.85 \pm 0.56 \times 10^{15}$	$8.17 \pm 0.17 \times 10^{10}$	$1.60 \pm 0.05 \times 10^{15}$
		Males, Southern Italy		
<1	$8.95 \pm 0.33 \times 10^{10}$	$7.21 \pm 0.41 \times 10^{14}$	$4.14 \pm 0.19 \times 10^{10}$	$5.20 \pm 0.42 \times 10^{14}$
1–5	$5.58 \pm 0.25 \times 10^{10}$	$1.42 \pm 0.13 \times 10^{15}$	$4.32 \pm 0.26 \times 10^{10}$	$5.96 \pm 0.43 \times 10^{14}$
6–10	$6.91 \pm 0.29 \times 10^{10}$	$1.42 \pm 0.12 \times 10^{15}$	$3.50 \pm 0.14 \times 10^{10}$	$5.14 \pm 0.41 \times 10^{14}$
11–18	$1.42 \pm 0.05 \times 10^{11}$	$2.28 \pm 0.11 \times 10^{15}$	$5.47 \pm 0.15 \times 10^{10}$	$7.97 \pm 0.40 \times 10^{14}$
19–40	$2.25 \pm 0.08 \times 10^{11}$	$3.47 \pm 0.59 \times 10^{15}$	$8.40 \pm 0.26 \times 10^{10}$	$1.14 \pm 0.41 \times 10^{15}$
41–65	$2.47 \pm 0.13 \times 10^{11}$	$4.20 \pm 0.98 \times 10^{15}$	$9.39 \pm 0.46 \times 10^{10}$	$1.41 \pm 0.10 \times 10^{15}$
>65	$2.26 \pm 0.12 \times 10^{11}$	$4.05 \pm 0.89 \times 10^{15}$	$8.46 \pm 0.43 \times 10^{10}$	$1.48 \pm 0.11 \times 10^{15}$

Slightly higher dose values were estimated for people living in southern Italy (compared to northern Italy) and for females (compared to males). However, these differences are lower than the corresponding standard deviations and therefore have to be considered not significant. With regard to the age effect, the doses were recognized to increase from younger (1–18 years old) to older (19–65 years old) age-groups and to decrease for people >65 years old. The age effect is related mostly to the level of particle concentration in the different microenvironments where people spend their time. In fact, when compared to adults (41–65 years old), the percentage difference in alveolar (tracheobronchial) number deposition for children (6–10 years old) and the elderly (>65 years old) was equal to 74% (57%) and 17% (14%), respectively.

To identify the main contributors to the previously mentioned daily dose value, Figure 8.3 reports the time contribution for each activity as well as the average

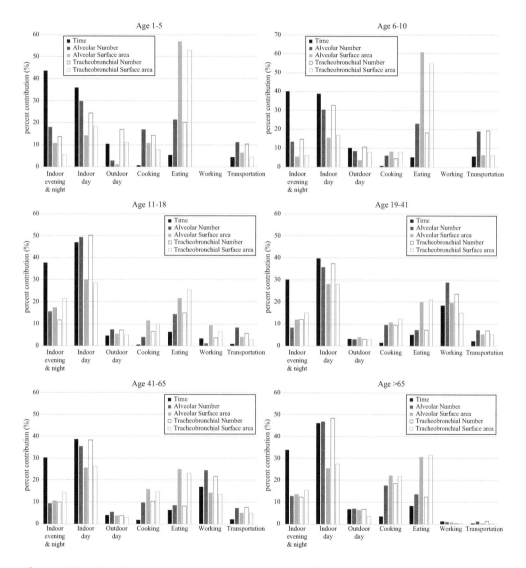

Figure 8.3 Contributions to daily activity patterns and average daily alveolar and tracheobronchial particle number and surface area deposited of the different human activities carried out by the age-groups investigated. Activities were grouped into seven main activities (figure adapted from Buonanno et al. [74]).

TABLE 8.2   Classification of Activities Performed by Citizens in the Seven Main Microenvironments

Microenvironment	Activities
Transportation	Trip and use of time not specified, round-trip to work
Working	Nonindustrial workplaces, profitable work, main and secondary jobs, work-connected activities, studying, school, institute or university, voluntary job and meetings, voluntary work in an organization
Eating	Eating and drinking (including home and restaurant)
Cooking	Cooking
Outdoor, day	Gardening and animal care, construction and restoration, sport and outdoor activities, physical workout, productive exercise, sports-connected activities
Indoor, day	Personal care; other personal care; studying, not specified; studying in free time; activities for home and family, not specified; housework, clothes care and folding; purchasing goods and services; home maintenance; baby care; helping adult family members; helping other family members; active activities; social activities and entertainment; social life; entertainment and culture; inactivity; hobbies and computer science; art and hobbies; computing; playing; media; reading; watching TV, DVD, or videos; listening to the radio or a recording
Indoor, evening and night	Sleeping

daily alveolar and tracheobronchial particle number and surface area doses for each activity. The activities are grouped into seven main activities/microenvironments (summarized in Table 8.2). The microenvironment that mainly contributed to the daily doses (80%–95%) received by all the age-groups under investigation is the indoor one (where sleeping, indoor day, cooking, eating, and working activities take place), whereas low contributions were recognized for outdoor and transportation microenvironments. The huge effect of the indoor microenvironment is due to both the high time fraction spent therein and the high concentrations experienced during some indoor activities. In particular, even if the time duration of cooking and eating activities is negligible, their contributions to the surface area daily doses were found to be even larger than 50%. The high exposures experienced during such activities are related to the high particle emission factors of cooking activities [31, 84, 85] and the reduced air exchange rate typical of naturally ventilated buildings, which are not able to properly dilute the emitted particles [86, 87]. The percent contribution of cooking and eating activities was found to be larger for the population younger than 5 years and older than 65 years (i.e., the population spending most of their time at home and having all their meals at home).

8.2.1.2.2 Risk.   Table 8.3 reports ELCR for an entire lifetime obtained on the basis of the exposure to B[a]P, As, Cd, and Ni for both northern and southern Italy. Data show that Italian females had higher ELCR values for both northern and southern Italy with respect to Italian males ($p < 0.01$). The level of risk associated with particle mass

TABLE 8.3 ELCR for the Italian Population: Contributions of Ultrafine Particles (UFPs, Expressed in Terms of Particle Surface Area, S) and Supermicron Particles (PM$_{10}$, Expressed in Terms of Particle Mass, M) (Table Reproduced from Buonanno et al. [68] with Permission)

		Males (North)	Females (North)	Males (South)	Females (South)
B[a]P	UFPs (S)	$1.08 \times 10^{-3} \pm 3.1 \times 10^{-6}$	$1.97 \times 10^{-3} \pm 3.1 \times 10^{-6}$	$1.25 \times 10^{-3} \pm 3.1 \times 10^{-6}$	$1.57 \times 10^{-3} \pm 3.2 \times 10^{-6}$
	PM$_{10}$ (M)	$0.80 \times 10^{-5} \pm 4.1 \times 10^{-7}$	$0.87 \times 10^{-5} \pm 4.5 \times 10^{-7}$	$0.34 \times 10^{-5} \pm 1.9 \times 10^{-7}$	$0.37 \times 10^{-5} \pm 2.2 \times 10^{-7}$
As	UFPs (S)	$9.84 \times 10^{-3} \pm 3.6 \times 10^{-6}$	$1.36 \times 10^{-2} \pm 4.5 \times 10^{-6}$	$8.15 \times 10^{-3} \pm 3.2 \times 10^{-6}$	$1.03 \times 10^{-2} \pm 3.4 \times 10^{-6}$
	PM$_{10}$ (M)	$3.5 \times 10^{-5} \pm 2.3 \times 10^{-6}$	$3.8 \times 10^{-5} \pm 2.5 \times 10^{-6}$	$8.7 \times 10^{-5} \pm 5.2 \times 10^{-6}$	$9.6 \times 10^{-5} \pm 5.5 \times 10^{-6}$
Cd	UFPs (S)	$1.14 \times 10^{-3} \pm 2.1 \times 10^{-7}$	$1.60 \times 10^{-3} \pm 4.1 \times 10^{-7}$	$1.10 \times 10^{-3} \pm 2.6 \times 10^{-6}$	$1.41 \times 10^{-3} \pm 3.1 \times 10^{-6}$
	PM$_{10}$ (M)	$0.39 \times 10^{-5} \pm 2.9 \times 10^{-7}$	$0.42 \times 10^{-5} \pm 3.1 \times 10^{-7}$	$3.9 \times 10^{-5} \pm 2.8 \times 10^{-6}$	$4.3 \times 10^{-5} \pm 3.0 \times 10^{-6}$
Ni	UFPs (S)	$4.53 \times 10^{-3} \pm 1.1 \times 10^{-6}$	$6.17 \times 10^{-3} \pm 1.3 \times 10^{-6}$	$5.50 \times 10^{-3} \pm 3.2 \times 10^{-6}$	$6.90 \times 10^{-3} \pm 3.2 \times 10^{-6}$
	PM$_{10}$ (M)	$1.5 \times 10^{-5} \pm 1.1 \times 10^{-6}$	$1.6 \times 10^{-5} \pm 1.1 \times 10^{-6}$	$1.7 \times 10^{-5} \pm 1.2 \times 10^{-6}$	$1.9 \times 10^{-5} \pm 1.1 \times 10^{-6}$
Total	UFPs (S)	1.66×10^{-2}	2.33×10^{-2}	1.60×10^{-2}	2.02×10^{-2}
	PM$_{10}$ (M)	6.19×10^{-5}	6.69×10^{-5}	1.46×10^{-4}	1.62×10^{-4}

(supermicron particles, PM_{10}) was negligible in comparison to surface area (UFPs) even if it was still higher than the maximum acceptable level of 10^{-5}–10^{-6} suggested by the World Health Organization and the EPA. The data clearly highlight that the widespread use of mass as a dosimetry in the risk assessment of exposure to particulate matter fails to consider the elevated risk of hazardous agents in the form of UFPs. In fact, the contribution of UFPs to ELCR for males and females living in northern and southern of Italy was equal to 1.66×10^{-2}/1.60×10^{-2} and 2.33×10^{-2}/2.02×10^{-2}, respectively. These values are two to three orders of magnitude higher than those for PM_{10}, as also reported by Sze-To et al. [25] in their case study on the exposure to cooking emissions in Hong Kong. These estimates suggest that a significant fraction of the lung cancer risk related to airborne particles can be attributed to UFPs. Concerning the contribution of the different compounds, the main contribution to ELCR was due to the amount of heavy metal deposited onto airborne particles: in particular, the average contributions of B[a]P, As, Cd, and Ni to the overall ELCR were equal to 8%, 55%, 7%, and 30%, respectively.

To compare these results to the official data on cancer in Italy, the data collected by the National Cancer Registry for 2014 were analyzed: such data revealed that the overall ELCR for the Italian population (including the smoking population) was equal to 1.1×10^{-1} and 2.7×10^{-2} for males and females, respectively [88]. Thus, the ELCR data here determined for the nonsmoking Italian population were equal to 15% and 81% of the official national ELCR values for males and females, respectively. While these data are based on the entire Italian population, including smokers, ex-smokers, and nonsmokers, the ELCRs reported here are for nonsmokers and smoke-free microenvironments. Even if smoking is by far the most important preventable cause of lung cancer in the world, it is already known that factors other than smoking (such as inhaling ambient particulate matter) play an important role in causing lung cancer in Italy [89]; therefore, the incidence of lung cancer related to air quality in the microenvironments resided in is hereinafter reported.

The overall lung cancer mortality rate (I) for the entire Italian population, including smokers, ex-smokers, and nonsmokers, was estimated by Forastiere et al. [89] as

$$I = I_0 \cdot f_n + I_0 \cdot RR_s \cdot f_s + I_0 \cdot RR_e \cdot f_e \tag{4}$$

where I_0 is the lung cancer mortality rate not attributable to smoking (background rate); f_n, f_s, and f_e are the fractions of nonsmokers, smokers, and ex-smokers, respectively; and RR_s and RR_e represent the rate ratios for smokers and ex-smokers compared to nonsmokers. Based on the actual fraction of Italian smokers (0.26 for males and 0.16 for females) and ex-smokers (0.31 for males and 0.16 for females), the excess life cancer risk for nonsmokers is 2.58×10^{-2} for males and 1.77×10^{-2} for females. Therefore, ELCR values determined for nonsmoking Italian population calculated here (1.63×10^{-2} and for males and 2.18×10^{-2} for females) are quite similar to those proposed by Forastiere et al. [89]; that is, the contribution of airborne particle inhalation to ELCR for the overall nonsmoking population represents the main cause of lung cancer risk apart from smoking. Hence, a significant percentage of lung cancer risk for nonsmoking females could be prevented by improving indoor air quality, particularly during cooking activities.

Figure 8.4 presents the contribution to average ELCR for different activities carried out by the Italian population. The average contributions of indoor microenvironments to ELCR in northern and southern Italy were equal to 97.9%/98.5% and 98.4%/98.8% for males and females, respectively. Among the indoor microenvironments, homes were the major contributors to ELCR. For northern and southern Italy, we found that the average contribution from home microenvironments was equal to 74.9%/76.3% and 76.3%/80.6% for males and females, respectively. The contribution was greater for females compared to males and for southern compared to northern Italy, which is likely due to the previously mentioned high doses received during cooking activities. Also, in terms of ELCR, the average contribution of cooking and eating activities to ELCR for males/females was equal to 34.0%/40.6% and 34.2%/30.4%, respectively. Therefore, despite similar contributions received during eating activities, males and females showed very different values during cooking activities. This difference is better highlighted in Figure 8.4b, where the number of lung cancer cases per 100,000 persons is reported for the seven activities/microenvironments. On average, females present 322 more cases with respect to males due to cooking activities. Given the Italian lifestyle, this is certainly a significant and influential parameter in the evaluation of lung cancer risk from airborne particles. The lowest direct contribution was from transportation, even if it cannot be considered negligible.

The total ELCR over an entire lifetime (70 years) did not account for the variability of exposure during an individual lifetime. To this end, the ELCR slope as function of age (and then lifestyle) was evaluated according equation 3. ELCR cumulative trends as a function of age were estimated for UFPs ($ELCR_{UFP}$) in relation to both PAH content and total heavy metal (As, Cd, and Ni) content and are reported in Figure 8.5. The contribution of PM_{10} to ELCR was ignored since it can be considered negligible (Table 8.3). Clearly, ELCR increases with age, even if a different growth rate is used for the different stages of life. In particular, $ELCR_{UFP}$ shows a decreasing slope in the range 0–18 years and a constant (or increasing) slope for people older than 18. The different slopes in these two age ranges are due to the different dose rates ($\delta_S(t)$) and body weight ($BW(t)$) functions such that during childhood and adolescence, the increase in body weight $BW(t)$ is faster than $\delta_S(t)$, while during adulthood, the increase in dose rate is larger than the increase in body weight. Moreover, $ELCR_{UFP}$ trends, considering both PAHs and heavy metals, highlight the effect of the different lifestyles that are characteristic of males and females. In particular, considering people living in northern Italy, the influence of gender is negligible for people under age 18 because during childhood and adolescence, northern people have similar lifestyles and are therefore exposed to similar doses. On the other hand, the effect of lifestyle is clearly recognizable during adulthood, with ELCR for females increasing at a higher rate

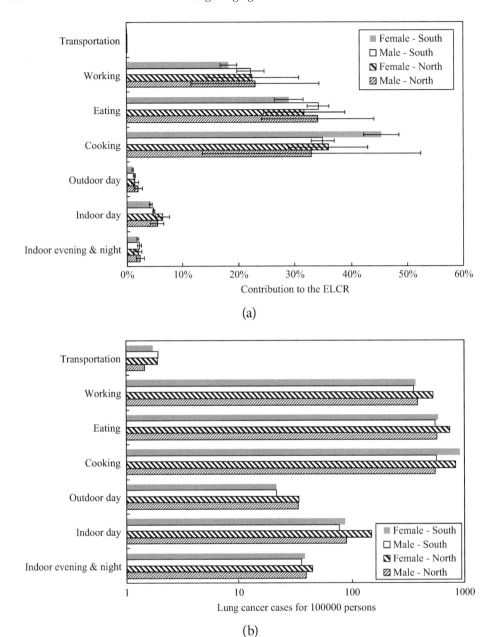

(a)

(b)

Figure 8.4   "Contribution to the average ELCR of different activities (a) for the 7 activities/ microenvironments and number of lung cancer cases for 100 000 persons (b) for the 7 activities/ microenvironments" (figure reproduced from Buonanno et al. [68] with permission).

than for males as a result of the higher doses received by women since they reside in microenvironments characterized by higher particle concentrations (i.e., during cooking activity). $ELCR_{UFP}$ trends for people living in southern Italy differ from those in northern Italy. In particular, $ELCR_{UFP}$ due to PAHs for females

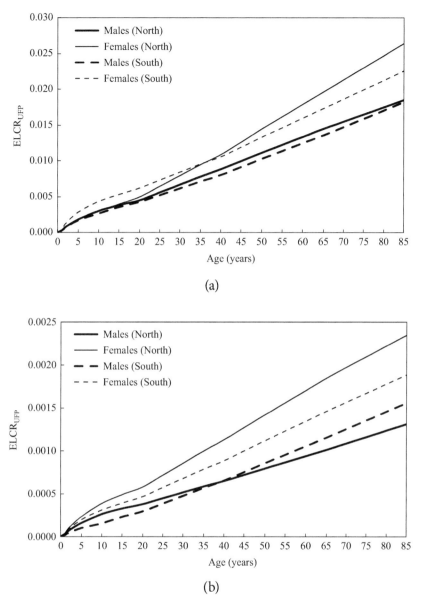

Figure 8.5 Cumulative $ELCR_{UFP}$ as function of the age for exposure to UFPs containing PAHs (a) and total heavy metals (b) (figure reproduced from Buonanno et al. [68] with permission).

were similar to those estimated for northern Italy, whereas the growth rate of $ELCR_{UFP}$ for males in southern Italy showed a different slope in the age range of 0–18 years. In particular, the increase in ELCR was slower than for males residing in northern Italy, which is likely due to the different daily time activity patterns of this group, who spent a negligible daily time percentage in microenvironments affected by cooking activities.

8.2.2 Population Exposed to Biomass-Burning Activities Indoors

The dose and risk data of the Italian population provided in section 8.2.1 do not take into account the possible effect of indoor biomass-fueled heaters (e.g., fireplaces or pellet stoves) since exposure measurements were performed in indoor environments where no biomass-fueled heaters were used. This could lead to an underestimation of indoor exposure to particle concentrations and their related PAHs/PM_{10} ratios during the wintertime, thereby reducing the estimated number of lung cancer cases attributed to air quality. To this end, in other research we have evaluated the exposure in indoor microenvironments to airborne particles emitted from biomass-burning systems employed in dwellings for heating purposes, including open fireplaces, closed fireplaces, and pellet stoves with automatic feeders. The dose of both sub- and supermicron particles received by the exposed population living in such dwellings was also evaluated. Moreover, the resulting lung cancer risk was estimated using the previously mentioned risk model taking into account the contribution of both sub- and supermicron particles. To this end, the mass fraction of carcinogenic compounds (heavy metals and PAHs) on PM_{10} emitted by biomass-burning devices under investigation was also measured.

8.2.2.1 Methodology

To estimate the risk received by population exposed to indoor heating systems, two different experimental analyses were performed:

1. Evaluation of the typical exposure of people to particle number, lung-deposited surface area, and PM_{10} concentrations in indoor microenvironments where heating systems are in operation
2. Evaluation of the mass fraction of carcinogenic compounds on PM_{10} emitted by wood and pellet combustion

The exposure to the different aerosol metrics in indoor microenvironments was measured through the following instruments:

- A diffusion charger particle counter (DiscMini, Matter Aerosol AG), which is a compact handheld particle counter based on a diffusion charging technique able to measure particle number concentration (N), lung-deposited particle surface area concentration (sum of the alveolar- and tracheobronchial-deposited particle surface area concentrations, hereinafter referred to as S_{Alv+TB}), and average diameter of particles ranging in size from 10 to 700 nm
- A handheld laser photometer (DustTrak Model 8534, TSI Inc.) able to measure PM_1, $PM_{2.5}$, PM_{10}, and total PM mass concentration fractions

The evaluation of the chemical composition of PM_{10} emitted by wood and pellet combustion phenomena was performed by collecting PM_{10} samples and performing a post hoc chemical analysis. To this end, the following equipment was used:

- A gravimetric sampler made up of a volumetric rotating pump (Zambelli 6000 Plus, equipped with temperature and atmospheric pressure sensors to measure normalized sampling volume) and a Zambelli PM_{10} impactor (working at a nominal fixed flow rate of 2.3 $m^3\,h^{-1}$ according to EN 12341 [90]) to collect particulate matter on a quartz filter for post hoc chemical analysis and PM_{10} mass concentration evaluation
- An Ultra Trace gas chromatograph coupled with a TSQ mass spectrometer (Thermo Fischer Scientific) to perform gas chromatography–mass spectrometry (GC/MS) analyses on PM samples
- A Triga Mark II nuclear reactor (ENEA-Casaccia Laboratories) for the PM sample irradiation

Three different heating systems were considered in the survey: open fireplaces, closed fireplaces, and pellet stoves with automatic feeders. In particular, 30 dwellings (10 per heating system) were involved in the experimental campaign. Particle measurements were performed in the room of the dwelling where the heating system was placed; in particular, the DiscMini and the DustTrak were placed on a desk at a distance of about 2 m from the source. To characterize the exposure to particles, the following procedure was considered: (1) 30–60 minutes of background concentrations in the room when the heating system was turned off and no other particle sources were in operation (e.g., cooking or candles) and (2) 2–4 hours of measurement during the combustion phenomena of the heating system with no other particle sources in operation. Measurements were performed through the DiscMini and the DustTrak considering a 1-second sampling time.

For both measurements performed during background and combustion periods, the owners were asked to conduct the dwellings as they typically did in terms of internal doors (open/closed) and biomass feeding rate. No restriction in terms of wood/pellet quality and its water content was given to the owners to take into account the real variability of fuel quality and combustion conditions. The dwellings considered in the survey were characterized by different volumes/floor surfaces to include different exposure conditions; moreover, the ventilation of all the dwellings under investigation relied only on natural ventilation: the authors point out that this represents the typical ventilation system installed in Italian dwellings [87, 93].

To check whether particle concentrations measured during combustion periods were statistically larger than those characteristic of background periods, a statistical analysis of the data was performed. In particular, a preliminary normality test (Shapiro-Wilk test) was carried out to evaluate the statistical distribution of the data. Since the assumption of Gaussian distribution was not met, a nonparametric test (Kruskal-Wallis test [94]) was adopted considering a significance level of 99% (a p value lower than 0.01).

To evaluate the mass fraction of carcinogenic compounds (As, Cd, Ni, and BaP) on PM_{10}, particulate matter was gravimetrically collected on a filter. Gravimetric measurements were performed in a 20-m^3 room (with doors and windows closed) equipped with an open fireplace for 4 hours. The fuel (wood or pellet) was burned in the open fireplace and continuously fed during the experiment. Three combustion tests were carried out for each type of fuel (wood and pellet). Thus, three particle-laden quartz filters were obtained for each biomass type to take into account the different type/quality of the biomass typically burned for heating purposes. All the filters were weighted according to the gravimetric procedure in ambient air [28, 91] to obtain the PM_{10} concentrations, whereas the fraction of As, Cd, Ni, and BaP was obtained through specific procedures characteristic of PAH and heavy metal analyses.

PAHs were determined using the GC/MS technique through the isotopic dilution method on the basis of a robust procedure reported in Paolini et al. [95]. The inorganic composition was investigated by a nuclear nondestructive technique: the Instrumental Neutron Activation Analysis [96, 97]. Major details on the methodology adopted for the chemical analyses are reported in Stabile et al. [17].

The typical dose received by people residing in indoor microenvironments where biomass heating systems are in operation was evaluated by means of the concentration levels measured during the experimental campaign. In particular, the extra doses were evaluated to highlight the additional exposure (and thus the additional dose) to airborne particles with respect to the background concentrations, that is, the concentrations characteristic of dwellings not equipped with biomass-burning heating systems. The hourly extra doses in terms of total particle surface area (expressed as the sum of alveolar and tracheobronchial contributions) and PM_{10} were obtained as [74, 98]

$$\delta_{Alv+TB\_(h)} = IR \cdot \left[S_{Alv+TBcombustion} - S_{Alv+TBbackground} \right] \quad (mm^2\ h^{-1}) \qquad (5)$$

$$\delta_{PM_{10}\_(h)} = IR \cdot \left[PM_{10combustion} - PM_{10background} \right] \cdot DF_{PM_{10}} \quad (mg\ h^{-1}) \qquad (6)$$

where IR ($m^3\ h^{-1}$) is the inhalation rate (0.45 $m^3\ h^{-1}$ for people performing sitting activities [74, 98]) and $DF_{PM_{10}}$ represents the deposition fraction of PM_{10} in the lungs (a function of the activity, age, and particle diameter D_p; here, a constant value of 0.2 was assumed). The total daily extra dose received for a typical exposure of the Italian population was obtained multiplying the hourly doses $\delta_{Alv+TB\_(h)}$ and $\delta_{PM_{10}\_(h)}$ by the typical daily exposure time (T) to heating system emissions (roughly 8 h d^{-1}; http://www.istat.it):

$$\delta_{Alv+TB} = \delta_{Alv+TB\_(h)} \cdot T \quad (mm^2\ day^{-1}) \qquad (7)$$

$$\delta_{PM_{10}} = \delta_{PM_{10}\_(h)} \cdot T \quad (mg\ day^{-1}) \qquad (8)$$

On the basis of the extra dose values and the amount of carcinogenic compounds, the ELCR due to the exposure in indoor environments where heating systems are run was evaluated. In particular, the extra ELCR, that is, the risk related to the extra dose received by people exposed to aerosol emitted by biomass heating systems with respect to those not using them, was calculated through the model proposed by Sze-To et al. [25] and described in the previous sections. The hourly and lifetime (assumed as 70 years) extra ELCRs were evaluated as

$$\text{ELCR}_{extra\_(h)} = \frac{1}{BW}\left(\sum_{i}^{n} SF_i \cdot \frac{m_i}{\text{PM}_{10}}\right) \cdot \left[c_f \cdot \delta_{Alv+TB\_(h)} + \delta_{PM_{10}\_(h)}\right] \cdot \frac{1}{70} \quad \left(\text{h}^{-1}\right) \quad (9)$$

$$\text{ELCR}_{extra} = \text{ELCR}_{extra\_(h)} \cdot T \cdot 70 \cdot N_{day} = \frac{1}{BW}\left(\sum_{i}^{n} SF_i \cdot \frac{m_i}{PM_{10}}\right) \cdot \left[c_f \cdot \delta_{Alv+TB} + \delta_{PM_{10}}\right] \cdot N_{day}$$

$$(10)$$

where N_{day} is the heating period expressed in number of days per year (a function of the climate [99]). To evaluate the extra ELCR for a typical Italian population exposed to biomass-burning systems, a Monte Carlo simulation [100] was performed considering the variability of airborne particle dose values and mass fractions of carcinogenic compounds on PM_{10}; in particular, the probability distribution functions of the doses were obtained from the estimated extra dose data considering four equally spaced ranges, whereas the mass fractions of carcinogenic compounds on PM_{10} were expressed as mean value ± standard deviation after being checked for normality through the Shapiro-Wilk test. Constant values (i.e., uniform probability distribution functions) for IR and BW were adopted since no data were available. Similarly, since no detailed data on the biomass use are available, uniform probability distribution functions for N_{day} and T were adopted too: the authors point out that this hypothesis could represent a limit in the calculation that should be addressed in future studies.

8.2.2.2 Results

8.2.2.2.1 Exposure. Figure 8.6 reports an example of the particle number concentration trends measured in the indoor microenvironments during tests performed considering the burning phenomena of an open fireplace, a closed fireplace, and a pellet stove. The trends clearly show the initial background period characterized by constant concentrations (about 30 minutes) and followed by a combustion period with an increase in particle concentration in the environments. The greatest particle concentration increase was in the cases of wood combustion in an open fireplace and a smaller yet clear increase for closed fireplaces, whereas a minor (or negligible) increase was measured for wood combustion in pellet stoves with automatic feeders. This is likely due to the reduced air permeability of the stove allowing a negligible (for perfectly sealed stoves) or reduced stove-to-indoors particle exfiltration. Open fireplaces presented the higher concentration increase: peaks in concentrations occurred during the start-up phase as well as during biomass feeding periods, as also recognized by Salthammer et al. [101]. Closed fireplaces generally caused indoor concentrations lower than those typically measured for open fireplaces but still noticeable due to the non-negligible air permeability of the front doors. Moreover, frequent

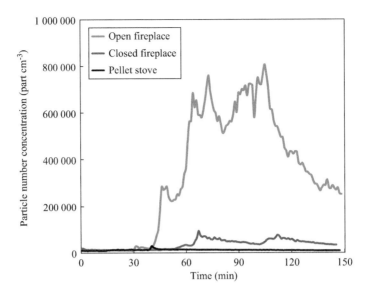

Figure 8.6 Examples of particle number concentration trends measured during the experimental campaigns for an open fireplace, a closed fireplace, and a pellet stove (figure reproduced from Stabile et al. [17] with permission).

peaks were recognized due to the door-opening periods during, once again, the start-up and wood feeding.

Nonetheless, the concentrations in the indoor microenvironments were also affected by the room/dwelling volume, building ventilation, fireplace/stove feeding, and so on. For this reason, the typical concentration indoors strongly varied on a case-by-case basis: as an example, Table 8.4 shows the ranges of median particle concentrations measured during the background and combustion periods for the three heating systems. Median particle concentrations during the combustion periods of wood in open fireplaces were in the range $0.18\text{–}4.33 \times 10^5$ part. cm^{-3}, $0.74\text{–}12.6 \times 10^2$ μm^2 cm^{-3}, and 24–552 $\mu g\ m^{-3}$ in terms of number, lung-deposited surface area, and PM_{10} concentrations, respectively. Similar values in terms of particle number concentrations during combustion periods were measured during tests on open and closed wood-burning stoves [101, 102]. Such values were quite high since they are similar to those measured during cooking activities in private dwellings [103] and significantly higher than those measured in indoor environments with no submicron particle sources [86, 87]. Exposure in indoor microenvironments with open fireplaces was evidently higher than those characteristic of closed fireplaces and pellet stoves. In particular, the lowest median particle concentrations were measured during pellet stove tests with maximum median particle number concentrations of about 2×10^4 part. cm^{-3}. Statistical comparisons between concentrations measured during background and combustion periods through nonparametric statistical tests showed that wood combustion phenomena in open and closed fireplaces caused statistically higher concentrations than background levels for all the particle metrics tested (for all the tests performed, or 10 of 10). On the other hand,

TABLE 8.4 Ranges of Median Particle Concentrations (Expressed as Min-Max) Measured During the Background and Combustion Periods of the 10 Tests per Heating System Under Investigation (Table Reproduced From Stabile, et al. [17] with Permission)

	Open Fireplaces		Closed Fireplaces		Pellet Stoves	
	Background	Combustion	Background	Combustion	Background	Combustion
N (part. cm^{-3})	$0.28–5.35 \times 10^4$	$0.18–4.33 \times 10^5$	$0.18–8.70 \times 10^4$	$0.03–1.34 \times 10^5$	$0.45–1.50 \times 10^4$	$0.49–2.03 \times 10^4$
S_{Ab+TB} (μm^2 cm^{-3})	$0.13–1.91 \times 10^2$	$0.74–12.6 \times 10^2$	$0.10–1.29 \times 10^2$	$0.14–4.14 \times 10^2$	$0.14–0.67 \times 10^2$	$0.17–0.68 \times 10^2$
PM_{10} (μg m^{-3})	17–143	24–552	6–150	29–227	14–49	16–70

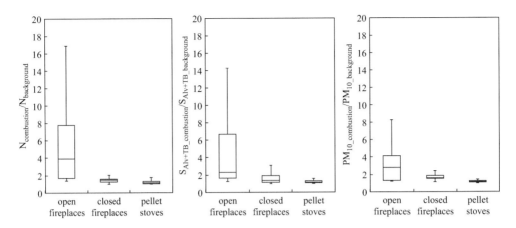

Figure 8.7 Statistics of the ratios between median concentrations measured during the combustion and background periods in terms of number, lung-deposited surface area (sum of alveolar and tracheobronchial contributions), and PM_{10} for the three heating systems under investigation. Box plots report fifth and 95th percentiles, first (Q_1) and third (Q_3) quartiles, and median value of the ratios. Upper (U) and lower (L) whiskers were evaluated as $U = Q_3 + 1.5 \times (Q_3 - Q_1)$ and $L = Q_1 - 1.5 \times (Q_3 - Q_1)$, respectively. Measurement data higher than the upper whisker or lower than the lower whisker were considered outliers and are not shown here (figure reproduced from Stabile et al. [17] with permission).

pellet combustion in pellet stoves caused significantly larger concentrations for number and lung-deposited surface area concentrations (eight of 10 tests) and for PM_{10} (five of 10 tests).

Figure 8.7 reports the statistics of the increase of the different airborne particle metric concentrations indoors. In particular, the increase was expressed as the ratio between the median concentrations measured during the combustion phenomena and the background period for all the tests performed. Median values were chosen on the basis of the typical non normal distribution of the concentration data collected during the combustion period. Both Table 8.4 and Figure 8.7 confirm the larger concentration increases measured for open fireplace systems for all particle metrics investigated (e.g., median ratio roughly equal to 4 and peaks up to 17 in terms of particle number concentrations) with respect to closed fireplaces and pellet stoves (median ratios in particle number concentrations lower than 2). An increase in supermicron particle concentrations (well described by the PM_{10} concentrations, ratio <2) was also measured for closed fireplaces and pellet stoves, showing a noticeable effect of such biomass heating systems on indoor air quality.

8.2.2.2.2 Dose.   Figure 8.8 shows the statistics of the hourly extra doses, in terms lung-deposited surface area and PM_{10}, received by people exposed to the three heating systems under investigation. Larger doses were obviously received by people exposed to aerosol produced during wood combustion in open fireplaces since median values equal to 56 $mm^2\ h^{-1}$ and 5 $\mu g\ h^{-1}$ in terms of lung-deposited surface area and PM_{10},

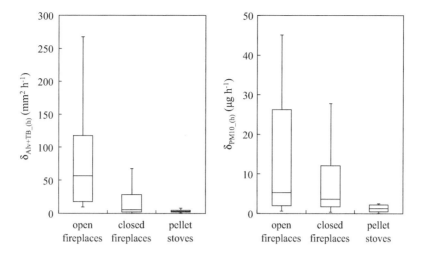

Figure 8.8 Statistics of the extradoses, in terms of surface area and PM_{10}, received by people standing in indoor microenvironments and exposed to biomass-burning generated particles. Box plots report fifth and 95th percentiles, first (Q1) and third (Q3) quartiles, and median value of the doses. Upper (U) and lower (L) whiskers were evaluated as $U = Q_3 + 1.5 \times (Q_3 - Q_1)$ and $L = Q_1 - 1.5 \times (Q_3 - Q_1)$, respectively. Measurement data higher than the upper whisker or lower than the lower whisker were considered outliers and are not shown here (figure reproduced from Stabile et al. [17] with permission).

respectively, were measured. Such lung-deposited surface area dose can be considered quite high considering that it is larger than the one typically received during other typical indoor and outdoor activities, such as exposure to cooking activity [103] and transportation microenvironments [74]. Lower median values were measured for closed fireplaces (about 5 mm² h⁻¹ and 4 μg h⁻¹) and pellet stoves (about 3 mm² h⁻¹ and 1 μg h⁻¹).

8.2.2.2.3 Risk. Table 8.5 summarizes the mass fraction of carcinogenic compounds on PM_{10} emitted by wood and pellet combustion phenomena. Data were reported as average and standard deviation after being checked for normality through the Shapiro-Wilk test. A negligible As amount was measured during wood combustion tests (the mass fraction corresponding to the As limit of detection is reported in Table 8.5), whereas it was found in PM_{10} emitted by pellet combustion. The larger fraction of carcinogenic compounds was due to the Ni for both wood and pellet combustion with a higher amount for pellet combustion (1.2×10^{-2} mg_{Ni}/mg_{PM10}). Larger concentrations of Cd were also found during pellet combustion tests, whereas higher amounts of B*a*P were measured during wood combustion tests. Such mass fractions were significantly larger (one or two orders of magnitude) than the typical values measured in Italian outdoor environments [68, 104]. When compared to mass fraction emitted by incinerator plants, higher values of B*a*P and Ni were measured for wood and pellet combustions, whereas lower amounts of As and Cd were detected [70]. Table 8.5 reports the *SF* of the mixture (*SF$_m$*), evaluated

TABLE 8.5   Mass Fractions of Carcinogenic Compounds on PM$_{10}$ (Expressed as mg/mg) Emitted by Wood and Pellet Combustion Phenomena and Corresponding SF of the Mixture (SF$_m$, Obtained Through a Monte Carlo Simulation) (Table Reproduced From Stabile et al. [17] With Permission)

	Wood	Pellet
m_{BaP}/PM_{10}	$6.2 \pm 0.7 \times 10^{-5}$	$4.0 \pm 0.3 \times 10^{-6}$
m_{As}/PM_{10}	$6.2 \pm 1.7 \times 10^{-8*}$	$9.0 \pm 1.8 \times 10^{-5}$
m_{Cd}/PM_{10}	$2.4 \pm 0.5 \times 10^{-5}$	$4.3 \pm 0.9 \times 10^{-4}$
m_{Ni}/PM_{10}	$7.2 \pm 1.4 \times 10^{-3}$	$1.2 \pm 0.2 \times 10^{-2}$
SF_m	$6.9 \pm 1.3 \times 10^{-3}$	$1.5 \pm 0.2 \times 10^{-2}$
Contribution to the SF_m	BaP = 4%, As = 0%, Cd = 2%, Ni = 94%	BaP < 1%, As = 9%, Cd = 18%, Ni = 73%

*Evaluated as the limit of detection.

through a Monte Carlo simulation, and the contributions of the four pollutants to such SF_m for both wood and pellet fuels. SF_m values for wood and pellet resulted in significantly larger (two and three orders of magnitude, respectively) than those typical of cooking-generated particulate matters (estimated by Sze-To et al. [25] on the basis of the data reported in He et al. [105]) and cigarette mainstream aerosols (five- to 10-fold, respectively [35]), whereas the values were comparable to the SF_m evaluated for incinerator plants [70]. The main contribution to the SF_m for both wood and pellet was due to the Ni (94% and 73% for wood and pellet, respectively), whereas a minor but not negligible contribution was recognized for Cd due to pellet combustion (<20%) and BaP due to wood combustion (4%). The authors point out that the emission of PAHs during wood combustion is due to the incomplete combustion processes characteristics of solid fuel [106]; therefore, their presence cannot be easily reduced. On the contrary, the presence of heavy metals is due to different reasons; indeed, some papers recognized a plant uptake of elements (including heavy metals) from soils in polluted sites [107]. Nonetheless, differences between biomass pellets and raw biomass were recognized in this and previous papers [108]. This should be due to the wood contamination occurring during the manufacturing processes [109–111], such as the use of chromated copper arsenate, a wood preservative. Therefore, the emission of heavy metals during wood and pellet combustion could be strongly reduced by providing ad hoc policy guidance for wood storage and pellet production.

Table 8.6 reports the lung cancer extra risk due to the exposure to the different heating systems on hourly (equation 9) and lifetime (equation 10) bases. In particular, ELCR$_{extra}$ values are given as most probable values and fifth 95th percentile ranges as obtained through the Monte Carlo simulation. To evaluate the lifetime risk, a heating period (N_{day} in equation 10) equal one-third of the year was considered a rough average of the different Italian heating periods. Larger risks are related to the exposure to open fireplaces due to the previously mentioned significantly larger exposures and doses. As an example, a 1-hour exposure to

TABLE 8.6   Hourly (ELCR$_{extra\_(h)}$) and Lifetime Risk (ELCR$_{extra}$) Due to Exposure to Particles Emitted by Combustion Phenomena. Data Expressed as Most Probable Risk and Corresponding Interval (Fifth to 95th Percentiles). Contributions of Each Carcinogenic Compound (BaP, As, Cd, and Ni) and Aerosol Metric (Surface Area vs. PM$_{10}$) to the Lifetime Extra Risk, Evaluated on the Most Probable Risk Value, Are Also Provided (Table Reproduced From Stabile et al. [17] with Permission)

	Open Fireplaces	Closed Fireplaces	Pellet Stove
ELCR$_{extra\_(h)}$	1.6×10^{-5}	1.9×10^{-6}	2.5×10^{-6}
	$(3.8 \times 10^{-6} - 1.6 \times 10^{-4})$	$(1.4 \times 10^{-8} - 2.5 \times 10^{-5})$	$(1.6 \times 10^{-7} - 1.0 \times 10^{-5})$
ELCR$_{extra}$	8.8×10^{-3}	1.1×10^{-3}	1.4×10^{-3}
	$(2.2 \times 10^{-3} - 9.0 \times 10^{-3})$	$(8.0 \times 10^{-6} - 1.4 \times 10^{-2})$	$(8.6 \times 10^{-5} - 5.7 \times 10^{-3})$
ELCR$_{extra}$_BaP	3.5×10^{-4}	4.2×10^{-5}	1.4×10^{-6}
ELCR$_{extra}$_As	$1.2 \times 10^{-6*}$	$*1.4 \times 10^{-7}$	1.5×10^{-4}
ELCR$_{extra}$_Cd	1.8×10^{-4}	2.1×10^{-5}	2.8×10^{-5}
ELCR$_{extra}$_Ni	8.3×10^{-3}	1.0×10^{-3}	1.2×10^{-3}
ELCR$_{extra}$_δ_{Alv+TB}	99.97%	99.93%	99.93%
ELCR$_{extra}$_δ_{PM10}	0.03%	0.07%	0.07%

*Evaluated as limit of the detection.

an open fireplace leads to a risk larger than the EPA's acceptable lifetime risk (10^{-5} [112]). The lifetime extra risks due to exposure to open fireplaces, closed fireplaces, and pellet stoves were 8.8×10^{-3}, 1.1×10^{-3}, and 1.4×10^{-3}, respectively. They were significantly larger than the EPA's acceptable lifetime risk (10^{-5}) and larger than the risk received at a receptor site of a waste-to-energy plant [70, 113] and 0.05- to 0.4-fold the lifetime overall risk of the Italian nonsmoking population not exposed to biomass heating systems, that is, roughly 2×10^{-2} [68, 104]. In particular, the risk due to exposure to open fireplaces is almost comparable to the one experienced by the Italian population in cooking and eating activities, which represent the main contributors to the overall risk of the Italian population. Therefore, the risk of the Italian nonsmoking population due to the exposure to indoor heating systems solely (and in particular to open fireplaces) cannot be neglected: as an example, an Italian nonsmoking person exposed to particles emitted by open fireplaces for 8 hours per day for roughly one-third of the year can get a risk of about 3×10^{-2}. The authors point out that even if the toxicity of the aerosol emitted by these devices (i.e., the SF_m) is larger than that of the conventional cigarette, the risk due to the exposure to biomass-fueled heating systems is one order of magnitude lower than that due to the inhalation of the cigarette mainstream aerosols due to the extremely larger doses received during smoking activities [35]. Closed fireplaces and pellet stoves present a risk almost one order of magnitude lower than that of an open fireplace; this is attributable to the reduced dose experienced by people exposed to such heating systems. The authors point out that the risk related to pellet stoves is slightly larger than that of closed fireplaces even if lower dose values are recognized; this is due to the higher "toxicity" (i.e., the SF_m) of the particles emitted by pellet stoves. As mentioned above, the main contribution to the SF_m and thus to the $ELRC_{extra}$ is due to the Ni: the lifetime $ELCR_{extra}$ due to the Ni solely (corresponding to the most probable value) is 8.3×10^{-3}, 1.0×10^{-3}, and 1.2×10^{-3} for open fireplaces, closed fireplaces, and pellet stoves, respectively. A minor risk, but still higher than the acceptable lifetime risk (10^{-5}), was also calculated for the other chemicals except for As in wood combustion and BaP in pellet combustion (see Table 8.6). Concerning the contribution of aerosol metrics to the lung cancer risk, as summarized in Table 8.6, the effect of the PM_{10} dose (δ_{PM10}) can be considered negligible (<0.1%) with respect to the lung-deposited surface area dose (δ_{Alv+TB}, >99.9%).

8.3 Conclusions

This chapter analyzed the particle-related lung cancer risk received by the typical the Italian population. To this end, a simplified lung cancer risk model taking into account the contribution of both sub- and supermicron particles was adopted. The risk of the typical Italian population related only to air quality aspect (i.e., not considering the smoking population) was roughly 2,000 new lung cancer cases per 100,000 persons with slight differences due to the different exposure scenarios between males and females. Such ELCR data are remarkably high since the ELCR value typically accepted is just 1 new lung cancer case per 100,000 persons. The higher contribution to the lung cancer risk is due to the indoor microenvironments due to both the high fraction of time spent therein and the high particle concentrations experienced by people; indeed, cooking and eating periods solely contribute to more than 50% of the total daily dose received by people. When the contribution of indoor heating systems is also taken into account, the dose and risk received by the exposed population can increase significantly; indeed, the exposure to open fireplaces all through the heating season can cause an extra risk of almost 1×10^{-2}.

Summarizing, then, the data provided here highlight the high contribution of indoor sources and activities with respect to outdoor ones. This is a key aspect to be considered since the environmental policies provided by regulatory authorities consider only outdoor and workplace environments, whereas exposure in home microenvironments is affected only by people's lifestyles and cannot be easily reduced.

References

1. Hinds WC. *Aerosol Technology*. 2nd ed. New York, NY: John Wiley & Sons; 1999.
2. Kulkarni P, Baron PA, Willeke K. *Aerosol Measurement: Principles, Techniques, and Applications*. 3rd ed. Haboken, New Jersey: John Wiley & Sons Inc; 2011.

3. Seinfeld JN, Pandis SN. *Atmospheric Chemistry and Physics: From Air Pollution to Climate Change*. 2nd ed. Haboken, New Jersey: John Wiley & Sons Inc; 1998.

4. Friedlander SK. *Smoke, Dust, and Haze: Fundamentals of Aerosol Dynamics*. 2nd ed. New York, NY: Oxford University Press; 2000.

5. Forastiere F, Agabiti N. Assessing the link between air pollution and heart failure. *Lancet*. 2013;382:1008–1010.

6. Pedone C, Scarlata S, Chiurco D, Conte ME, Forastiere F, Antonelli-Incalzi R. Association of reduced total lung capacity with mortality and use of health services, *Chest*. 2012;141:1025–1030.

7. Wang M, Beelen R, Stafoggia M, et al. Long-term exposure to elemental constituents of particulate matter and cardiovascular mortality in 19 European cohorts: results from the ESCAPE and TRANSPHORM projects. *Environ Int*. 2014;66:97–106.

8. Beelen R, Stafoggia M, Raaschou-Nielsen O, et al. Long-term exposure to air pollution and cardiovascular mortality: an analysis of 22 European cohorts. *Epidemiology*. 2014;25(3):368–78.

9. Beelen R, Raaschou-Nielsen O, Stafoggia M, et al. Effects of long-term exposure to air pollution on natural-cause mortality: an analysis of 22 European cohorts within the multicentre ESCAPE project. *Lancet*. 2014;383:785–795.

10. Pope CA III, Dockery DW. Health effects of fine particulate air pollution: lines that connect. *J Air Waste Manag Assoc*. 2006;56:709–742.

11. Clifford S, Mazaheri M, Salimi F, et al. Effects of exposure to ambient ultrafine particles on respiratory health and systemic inflammation in children. *Environ Int*. 2018;114:167–180.

12. Weichenthal S. Selected physiological effects of ultrafine particles in acute cardiovascular morbidity. *Environ Res*. 2012;115:26–36.

13. Chen X, Zhang L-W, Huang J-J, et al. Long-term exposure to urban air pollution and lung cancer mortality: a 12-year cohort study in northern China. *Sci Total Environ*. 2016;571:855–861.

14. Morawska L, Ayoko GA, Bae GN, et al Airborne particles in indoor environment of homes, schools, offices and aged care facilities: the main routes of exposure. *Environ Int*. 2017;108:75–83.

15. Salthammer T, Uhde E, Schripp T, et al. Children's well-being at schools: impact of climatic conditions and air pollution. *Environ Int*. 2016;94:196–210.

16. Wallace L, Ott W. Personal exposure to ultrafine particles. *J Expo Sci Environ Epidemiol*. 2011;21:20–30.

17. Stabile L, Buonanno G, Avino P, Frattolillo A, Guerriero E. Indoor exposure to particles emitted by biomass-burning heating systems and evaluation of dose and lung cancer risk received by population. *Environ Pollut*. 2018;235:65–73.

18. Pacitto A, Stabile L, Moreno T, et al. The influence of lifestyle on airborne particle surface area doses received by different Western populations. *Environ Pollut*. 2018;232:113–122.

19. Rizza V, Stabile L, Buonanno G, Morawska L. Variability of airborne particle metrics in an urban area. *Environ Pollut*. 2017;220(pt A):625–635.

20. Buonanno G, Fuoco FC, Stabile L. Influential parameters on particle exposure of pedestrians in urban microenvironments. *Atmos Environ*. 2011;45:1434–1443.

21. International Agency for Research on Cancer. *Outdoor Air Pollution a Leading Environmental Cause of Cancer Deaths*. Lyon: International Agency for Research on Cancer; 2013.

22. Loomis D, Grosse Y, Lauby-Secretan B, et al. The carcinogenicity of outdoor air pollution. *Lancet Oncol.* 2013;14:1262–1263.

23. International Agency for Research on Cancer. *IARC Monographs on the Evaluation of Carcinogenic Risks to Humans.* Lyon: International Agency for Research on Cancer; 2013.

24. International Commission on Radiological Protection. Human respiratory tract model for radiological protection. A report of a Task Group of the International Commission on Radiological Protection. *Ann ICRP.* 1994;24:1–482.

25. Sze-To GN, Wu CL, Chao CYH, Wan MP, Chan TC. Exposure and cancer risk toward cooking-generated ultrafine and coarse particles in Hong Kong homes. *HVAC&R Res.* 2012;18:204–216.

26. International Organization for Standardization. ISO/TR 27628:2007. Workplace atmospheres—ultrafine, nanoparticle and nano-structured aerosols—inhalation exposure characterization and assessment. Geneva: International Organization for Standardization; 2007.

27. DeCarlo PF, Slowik JG, Worsnop DR, Davidovits P, Jimenez JL. Particle morphology and density characterization by combined mobility and aerodynamic diameter measurements. Part 1: theory. *Aerosol Sci Technol.* 2004;38:1185–1205.

28. Buonanno G, Dell'Isola M, Stabile L, Viola A. Uncertainty budget of the SMPS-APS system in the measurement of PM 1, PM 2.5, and PM 10. *Aerosol Sci Technol.* 2009;43:1130–1141.

29. Buonanno G, Bernabei M, Avino P, Stabile L. Occupational exposure to airborne particles and other pollutants in an aviation base. *Environ Pollut.* 2012;170:78–87.

30. Buonanno G, Lall AA, Stabile L. Temporal size distribution and concentration of particles near a major highway. *Atmos Environ.* 2009;43:1100–1105.

31. Buonanno G, Morawska L, Stabile L. Particle emission factors during cooking activities. *Atmos Environ.* 2009;43:3235–3242.

32. Buonanno G, Morawska L, Stabile L. Exposure to welding particles in automotive plants. *J Aerosol Sci.* 2011;42:295–304.

33. Buonanno G, Scungio M, Stabile L, Tirler W. Ultrafine particle emission from incinerators: the role of the fabric filter. *J Air Waste Manag Assoc.* 2012;62:103–111.

34. Scungio M, Stabile L, Buonanno G. Measurements of electronic cigarette-generated particles for the evaluation of lung cancer risk of active and passive users. *J Aerosol Sci.* 2018;115:1.

35. Stabile L, Buonanno G, Ficco G, Scungio M. Smokers' lung cancer risk related to the cigarette-generated mainstream particles. *J Aerosol Sci.* 2017;107:41–54.

36. Buonanno G, Fuoco FC, Marini S, Stabile L. Particle resuspension in school gyms during physical activities. *Aerosol Air Qual Res.* 2012;12:803–813.

37. Morawska L, Afshari A, Bae GN, et al. Indoor aerosols: from personal exposure to risk assessment. *Indoor Air.* 2013;23:462–487.

38. Gold K, Yung SC, Holmes TD. A quantitative analysis of aerosols inside an armored vehicle perforated by a kinetic energy penetrator containing tungsten, nickel, and cobalt. *Mil Med.* 2007;172:393–398.

39. Holmes TD, Guilmette RA, Cheng YS, Parkhurst MA, Hoover MD. Aerosol sampling system for collection of capstone depleted uranium particles in a high-energy environment. *Health Phys.* 2009;96:221–237.

40. Oberdürster G. Toxicology of ultrafine particles: in vivo studies. *Phil Trans R Soc Lond A Math Phys Eng Sci.* 2000;358:2719–2740.

41. Sayes CM, Reed KL, Warheit DB. Assessing toxicology of fine and nanoparticles: comparing in vitro measurements to in vivo pulmonary toxicity profiles. *Toxicol Sci.* 2007;97:163–180.

42. Schmid O, Möller W, Semmler-Behnke M, et al. Dosimetry and toxicology of inhaled ultrafine particles. *Biomarkers.* 2009;14:67–73.

43. Kreyling WG, Semmler M, Moller W. Dosimetry and toxicology of ultrafine particles. *J Aerosol Med.* 2004;17:140–152.

44. Donaldson K, Seaton A. A short history of the toxicology of inhaled particles. *Particle Fibre Technol.* 2012;9:13–33.

45. Ketzel M, Berkowicz R. Modelling the fate of ultrafine particles from exhaust pipe to rural background: an analysis of time scales for dilution, coagulation and deposition. *Atmos Environ.* 2004;38:2639–2652.

46. Kumar P, Ketzel M, Vardoulakis S, Pirjola L, Britter R. Dynamics and dispersion modelling of nanoparticles from road traffic in the urban atmospheric environment—a review. *J Aerosol Sci.* 2011;42:580–603.

47. Asgharian B, Hofmann W, Bergmann R. Particle deposition in a multiple-path model of the human lung. *Aerosol Sci Technol.* 2001;34:332–339.

48. Price OT, Asgharian B, Miller FJ, Cassee FR, de Winter-Sorkina R. Multiple path particle dosimetry model (MPPD v 1.0): a model for human and rat airway particle dosimetry. Ver. 1.0. Bilthoven: National Institute for Public Health and the Environment; 2002.

49. Ott WR. Concepts of human exposure to air pollution. *Environ Int.* 1982;7:179–196.

50. Cattaneo A, Taronna M, Garramone G, et al. Comparison between personal and individual exposure to urban air pollutants. *Aerosol Sci Technol.* 2010;44:370–379.

51. Stafoggia M, Schneider A, Cyrys J, et al. Association between short-term exposure to ultrafine particles and mortality in eight European urban areas. *Epidemiology.* 2017;28:172–180.

52. European Union. *EU Directive 2008/50/EC of the European Parliament and of the Council of 21 May 2008 on Ambient Air Quality and Cleaner Air for Europe, 2008.* L 152/1. Brussels: European Parliament; 2008.

53. U.S. Environmental Protection Agency. *National Ambient Air Quality Standards for Particulate Matter, Part II. Final Rule.* 40 CFR Part 50. Washington, DC: U.S. Environmental Protection Agency; 2006.

54. Kaur S, Nieuwenhuijsen MJ, Colvile RN. Pedestrian exposure to air pollution along a major road in central London, UK. *Atmos Environ.* 2005;39:7307–7320.

55. Puustinen A, Hämeri K, Pekkanen J, et al. Spatial variation of particle number and mass over four European cities. *Atmospheric Environment, Atmos. Environ.* 2007;41:6622–6636.

56. Buonanno G, Stabile L, Morawska L. Personal exposure to ultrafine particles: the influence of time-activity patterns. *Sci Total Environ.* 2014;468–469:903–907.

57. Cattaneo A, Garramone G, Taronna M, Peruzzo C, Cavallo DM. Personal exposure to airborne ultrafine particles in the urban area of Milan. *J Phys Conf Ser.* 2009;151:012039

58. Hasenfratz D, Saukh O, Walser C, et al. Deriving high-resolution urban air pollution maps using mobile sensor nodes. *Pervasive Mobile Comput.* 2015;16:268–285.

59. Ramirez N, Cuadras A, Rovira E, Marce RM, Borrull F. Risk assessment related to atmospheric polycyclic aromatic hydrocarbons in gas and particle phases near industrial sites. *Environ Health Perspect.* 2011;119:1110–1116.

60. Baek SO, Field RA, Goldstone ME, Kirk PW, Lester JN, Perry R. A review of atmospheric polycyclic aromatic hydrocarbons: sources, fate and behavior. *Water Air Soil Pollut.* 1991;60:279–300.

61. World Health Organization. *International Programme on Chemical Safety. Environmental Health Criteria 211. Health Effects of the Interaction Between Tobacco Use and Exposure to Other Agents.* Geneva: World Health Organization; 1999.

62. European Union. *Directive 2004/107/EC of European Parliament and Council, of 15 December 2004 Relating to Arsenic, Cadmium, Mercury, Nickel and Polycyclic Aromatic Hydrocarbons in Ambient Air.* L 23/03. Brussels: European Parliament; 2004.

63. Expert Panel on Air Quality Standards. *Polycyclic Aromatic Hydrocarbons. Report for the Department of the Environment, Transport and the Regions.* Expert Panel on Air Quality Standards; 1999.

64. Commission on Environmental Health. *Environment for Sustainable Health Development: An Action Plan for Sweden.* Stockholm: Ministry of Health and Social Affairs; 1996.

65. Bostrom CE, Gerde P, Hanberg A, et al. Cancer risk assessment, indicators, and guidelines for polycyclic aromatic hydrocarbons in the ambient air. *Environ Health Perspect.* 2002;110(suppl 3):451–488.

66. Reche C, Viana M, Brines M, et al. Determinants of aerosol lung-deposited surface area variation in an urban environment. *Sci Total Environ.* 2015;517:38–47.

67. California Environmental Protection Agency. *Technical Support Document for Cancer Potency Factors: Methodologies for Derivation, Listing of Available Values, and Adjustments to Allow for Early Life Stage Exposures.* Sacramento: California Environmental Protection Agency; 2009.

68. Buonanno G, Giovinco G, Morawska L, Stabile L. Lung cancer risk of airborne particles for Italian population. *Environ Res.* 2015;142:443–451.

69. Pacitto A, Stabile L, Viana M, et al. Particle-related exposure, dose and lung cancer risk of primary school children in two European countries. *Sci Total Environ.* 2018;616–617:720–729.

70. Scungio M, Buonanno G, Stabile L, Ficco G. Lung cancer risk assessment at receptor site of a waste-to-energy plant. *Waste Manag.* 2016;56:207–215.

71. Scungio M, Stabile L, Rizza V, Pacitto A, Russi A, Buonanno G. Lung cancer risk assessment due to traffic-generated particles exposure in urban street canyons: a numerical modelling approach. *Science of The Total Environment, Sci Total Environ.* 2018;631–632:1109–1116.

72. Sophonsiri C, Morgenroth E. Chemical composition associated with different particle size fractions in municipal, industrial, and agricultural wastewaters. *Chemosphere.* 2004;55:691–703.

73. See SW, Balasubramanian R. Chemical characteristics of fine particles emitted from different gas cooking methods. *Atmos Envorin.* 2008;42:8852–8862.

74. Buonanno G, Giovinco G, Morawska L, Stabile L. Tracheobronchial and alveolar dose of submicrometer particles for different population age groups in Italy. *Atmospheric Environment, Atmos Environ.* 2011;45:6216–6224.

75. Bastone A, Soggiu ME, Vollono C, Masciocchi M, Rago G, Sellitri C. *Assessment Study on Inhalation Exposure to Atmospheric Pollution in Ferrara. Part 1.* Rome: Istituto Superiore di Sanità; 2003.

76. Bastone A, Soggiu ME, Vollono C, et al. *Lifestyles and Behaviour of Taranto, Massafra, Crispiano and Statte Populations For Inhalation Exposure Assessment to Atmospheric Pollution*. Rome: Istituto Superiore di Sanità; 2006.

77. Soggiu ME, Bastone A, Vollono C, Masciocchi M, Rago G, Sellitri C. *Study of Inhalation Exposure Assessment to Atmospheric Pollution in Ferrara. Second Phase*. Rome: Istituto Superiore di Sanità; 2005.

78. Soggiu ME, Vollono C, Bastone A. *Human Exposure Assessment to Environmental Contaminants: Exposure Scenarios*. Rome: Istituto Superiore di Sanità;2010.

79. U.S. Environmental Protection Agency. *Metabolically Derived Human Ventilation Rates: A Revised Approach Based Upon Oxygen Consumption Rates*. Washington, DC: U.S. Environmental Protection Agency; 2009.

80. Adams WC. *Measurement of Breathing Rate and Volume in Routinely Performed Daily Activities. Final Report. Contract No. A033-205*. Davis: Human Performance Laboratory, Physical Education Department, University of California, Davis;1993.

81. World Health Organization. *WHO Child Growth Standards: Methods and Development. Length/Height-for-Age, Weight-for-Age, Weight-for-Length, Weight-for-Height and Body Mass Index-for-Age*. Geneva: World Health Organization; 2006.

82. Zoppi G, Bressan F, Luciano A. Height and weight reference charts for children aged 2–18 years from Verona, Italy. *Eur J Clin Nutr*. 1996;50:462–468.

83. Masali, M. *L'Italia si misura: Vademecum antropometrico per il Design e l'Ergonomia. Vent'anni di ricerca (1990–2010)*. Milan: L'aeroplanino editore; 2011.

84. Stabile L, Jayaratne ER, Buonanno G, Morawska L. Charged particles and cluster ions produced during cooking activities. *Sci Total Environ*. 2014;497–498:516–526.

85. Buonanno G, Johnson G, Morawska L, Stabile L. Volatility characterization of cooking-generated aerosol particles. *Aerosol Sci Technol*. 2011;45:1069–1077.

86. Stabile L, Dell'Isola M, Russi A, Massimo A, Buonanno G. The effect of natural ventilation strategy on indoor air quality in schools. *Sci Total Environ*. 2017;595: 894–902.

87. Stabile L, Dell'Isola M, Frattolillo A, Massimo A, Russi A. Effect of natural ventilation and manual airing on indoor air quality in naturally ventilated Italian classrooms. *Building Environ*. 2016;98:180–189.

88. AIRTUM Working Group. *I Tumori in Italia—Rapporto 2014, Tumori multipli*. Milan: Italy; AIRTUM Working Group; 2014.

89. Forastiere F, Perucci CA, Arca M, Axelson O. Indirect estimates of lung cancer death rates in Italy not attributable to active smoking. *Epidemiology*. 1993;4: 502–510.

90. European Committee for Standardization. *Determination of the PM_{10} Fraction of Suspended Particulate Matter*. EN 12341. Brussels: European Committee for Standardization; 2001.

91. Buonanno G, Dell'Isola M, Stabile L, Viola A. Critical aspects of the uncertainty budget in the gravimetric PM measurements. *Measurement*. 2010;44:139–147.

92. Mokhtar M-A, Jayaratne R, Morawska L, Mazaheri M, Surawski N, Buonanno G. NSAM-derived total surface area versus SMPS-derived "mobility equivalent" surface area for different environmentally relevant aerosols. *J Aerosol Sci*. 2013;66:1–11.

93. d'Ambrosio Alfano F, Dell'Isola M, Ficco G, Palella BI, Riccio G. Experimental air-tightness analysis in Mediterranean buildings after windows retrofit. *Sustainability*. 2016;8:991–999.

94. Kruskal WH, Wallis WA. Use of ranks in one-criterion variance analysis. *J Am Stat Assoc.* 1952;47:583–621.

95. Paolini V, Guerriero E, Bacaloni A, Rotatori M, Benedetti P, Mosca S. Simultaneous sampling of vapor and particle-phase carcinogenic polycyclic aromatic hydrocarbons on functionalized glass fiber filters. *Aerosol Air Qual Res.* 2016;16:175–183.

96. Avino P, Carconi PL, Lepore L, Moauro A. Nutritional and environmental properties of algal products used in healthy diet by INAA and ICP-AES. *J Radioanal Nucl Chem.* 2000;244:247–252.

97. Capannesi G, Rosada A, Avino P. Elemental characterization of impurities at trace and ultra-trace levels in metallurgical lead samples by INAA. *Microchem J.* 2009;93-188–194.

98. Buonanno G, Morawska L, Stabile L, Wang L, Giovinco G. A comparison of submicrometer particle dose between Australian and Italian people. *Environmental Pollution, Environ. Pollut.* 2012;169:183–189.

99. International Organization for Standardization. *Hygrothermal Performance of Buildings—Calculation and Presentation of Climatic Data—Part 6: Accumulated Temperature Differences (Degree-Days).* ISO 15927-6. Geneva:; 2007.

100. Hammersley JM, Handscomb DC. *Monte Carlo Methods.* London: Chapman and Hall; 1964.

101. Salthammer T, Schripp T, Wientzek S, Wensing M. Impact of operating wood-burning fireplace ovens on indoor air quality. *Chemosphere.* 2014;103:205–211.

102. Carvalho RL, Jensen OM, Afshari A, Bergsøe NC. Wood-burning stoves in low-carbon dwellings. *Energy Buildings.* 2013;59:244–251.

103. Stabile L, Fuoco FC, Marini S, Buonanno G. Effects of the exposure to indoor cooking-generated particles on nitric oxide exhaled by women. *Atmos Environ.* 2015;103:238–246.

104. Buonanno G, Stabile L, Morawska L, Giovinco G, Querol X. Do air quality targets really represent safe limits for lung cancer risk? *Sci Total Environ.* 2017;580:74–82.

105. He C, Morawska L, Hitchins J, Gilbert D. Contribution from indoor sources to particle number and mass concentrations in residential houses. *Atmos Environ.* 2004;38:3405–3415.

106. Zosima AT, Tzimou-Tsitouridou RD, Nikolaki S, Zikopoulos D, Ochsenkuhn-Petropoulou MT. PM10 emissions and PAHs: the importance of biomass type and combustion conditions. *J Environ Sci Health Part A Tox Hazard Subst Environ Eng.* 2016;51:341–347.

107. Wang Q-R, Cui Y-S, Liu X-M, Dong Y-T, Christie P. Soil contamination and plant uptake of heavy metals at polluted sites in China. *J Environ Helath Sci Part A Tox Hazard Subst Environ Eng.* 2003;38:823–838.

108. Zhang W, Tong Y, Wang H, et al. Emission of metals from pelletized and uncompressed biomass fuels combustion in rural household stoves in China. *Sci Rep.* 2014;4:5611.

109. Chandrasekaran SR, Hopke PK, Rector L, Allen G, Lin L. Chemical composition of wood chips and wood pellets. *Energy Fuels.* 2012;26:4932–4937.

110. Noonan CW, Navidi W, Sheppard L, et al. Residential indoor PM2.5 in wood stove homes: follow-up of the Libby changeout program. *Indoor Air.* 2012;22:492–500.

111. Chen AY, Olsen T. Chromated copper arsenate–treated wood: a potential source of arsenic exposure and toxicity in dermatology. *Int J Womens Dermatol.* 2016;2:28–30.

112. U.S. Environmental Protection Agency. *Risk Assessment Guidance for Superfund: Volume I—Human Health Evaluation Manual (Part B, Development of Risk-Based Preliminary Remediation Goals).* Vol. 540/R-92/003.Washington, DC: U.S. Environmental Protection Agency; 1991.
113. Scungio M, Buonanno G, Arpino F, Ficco G. Influential parameters on ultra-fine particle concentration downwind at waste-to-energy plants. *Waste Manag.* 2015;38:157–163.

9

Lung Nodule Classification Based on the Integration of a Higher-Order Markov-Gibbs Random Field Appearance Model and Geometric Features

Ahmed Shaffie, Ahmed Soliman, Ali Mahmoud, Mohammed Ghazal, Hassan Hajjdiab, Robert Keynton, Guruprasad Giridharan, Adel Elmaghraby, Jasjit S. Suri, and Ayman El-Baz

Contents

9.1 Introduction

Lung cancer is the second most common cancer among men and women the world over. It is second only to prostate cancer in men and breast cancer in women. Moreover, it is considered the leading cause of cancer-related deaths among both genders in the United States, as the number of people who die each year of lung cancer is more than the number of people who die of breast and prostate cancers combined [1]. The number of patients suffering from lung cancer has recently increased significantly all over the world, increasing the motivation for developing accurate and fast diagnostic tools to detect lung cancer earlier in order to increase the patient's survival rate. Lung nodules are the first indication to start diagnosing lung cancer. Lung nodules can be benign (normal subjects) or malignant (cancerous subjects). Figure 9.1 shows some samples of benign and malignant lung nodules.

Histological examination through biopsies is considered the gold standard for the final diagnosis of pulmonary nodules as malignant or benign. Even though resection of pulmonary nodules is the ideal and most reliable way for diagnosis, there

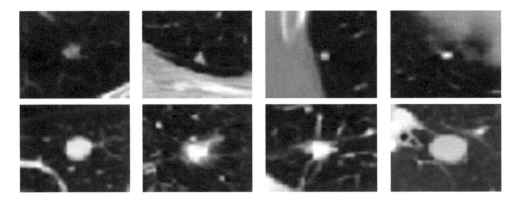

Figure 9.1 Sample two-dimensional (2D) axial projection for benign (first row) and malignant (second row) lung nodules.

is a crucial need for developing noninvasive diagnostic tools to eliminate the risks associated with the surgical procedure.

In general, there are several imaging modalities used to diagnose the pulmonary nodules, including chest radiography (X-ray), magnetic resonance imaging (MRI), positron emission tomography (PET), and computed tomography (CT). Some researchers prefer to use MRI to avoid exposing the patient to ionizing radiation, which has a negative effect and gives the potential to increase lifetime cancer risk [2]. Diffusion-weighted MRI has been reported to be used for lung cancer diagnosis, as it could be used to qualitatively check the high b value images and apparent diffusion coefficient (ADC) maps in addition to quantitatively generating the mean and median tumor ADCs [3]. However, CT and PET scans are the most widely used modalities for the diagnosis and staging of lung cancer. A CT scan is more likely to show lung tumors than other modalities because of its high resolution and clear contrast compared with other modalities. It can also show the size, shape, and accurate position of any lung tumor. We focus on and utilize the CT scan in our study, as it is considered a routine procedure for patients who have lung cancer and has ability to provide high-resolution pulmonary anatomical details.

Recently, much research has tried to develop computer-aided diagnostic (CAD) systems to classify detected lung nodules to detect lung cancer earlier. Sun et al. [4] studied the feasibility of using deep learning algorithms for benign/malignant classification on the Lung Image Database Consortium (LIDC) data set. Radiologists provided marks that they used to segment the nodules on each CT slice. After rotating and down sampling, they collected 174,412 samples, 52 by 52 pixels each, and the corresponding ground truth. They designed and implemented three deep learning algorithms: deep belief networks (DBNs), convolutional neural network (CNN), and stacked denoising autoencoder (SDAE). They compared the performance of deep learning algorithms with traditional CADx systems by designing a scheme with 28 image features and support vector machine (SVM). The accuracies of CNN, SDAE, and DBNs were 0.7976, 0.7929, and 0.8119, respectively; the accuracy of their designed traditional CADx was 0.7940, which was lower than DBNs and CNN. Shen et al. [5] studied the problem of classification of lung nodules as benign or malignant using CT images. They focused on modeling raw nodule patches without any prior definition of nodule morphology. They proposed a hierarchical learning framework based on multiscale CNNs to capture nodule heterogeneity by extracting discriminative features from alternatingly stacked layers. Their framework used multiscale nodule patches to learn a set of known features simultaneously by concatenating response neuron activations gotten at the last layer from each input scale. They evaluated the proposed method on CT images from the LIDC data set, which provides nodule annotations as being benign or malignant. Likhitka et al. [6] proposed a framework modeled into four steps: image enhancement, segmentation, feature extraction, and classification. For lung nodule diagnosis, they used the nodule size, nodule spine values, structure, and volume as input features for the SVM classifier to distinguish between benign and malignant nodules. An unsupervised spectral clustering algorithm has been studied by Wei et al. [7] to classify benign and malignant nodules. They constructed a new Laplacian matrix in their algorithm using local kernel regression models and incorporating a regularization term that can deal with the out-of-sample problem. To verify the accuracy of their algorithm, they assembled a ground-truth data set from the LIDC data set including 375 malignant and 371 benign lung nodules. Another study by Nishio et al. [8] analyzed 73 lung nodules from 60 sets of CT images. They performed contrast-enhanced CT in 46 CT examinations. They used images from the LUNGx Challenge, which does not have the ground truth of the nodules; this is why radiologists constructed a surrogate ground truth. Their method was based on novel patch-based feature extraction using principal component analysis, pooling operations, and image convolution. They compared their method to three other systems for the extraction of nodule features: histogram of CT density, 3D random local binary pattern, and local binary pattern on three orthogonal planes. They analyzed the probabilistic outputs of the systems and surrogate ground truth using the receiver operating characteristic (ROC) curve and the area under the curve (AUC). Given the ground truth, AUCs were as follows: histogram of CT density, 0.640; 3D random local binary pattern, 0.725; local binary pattern on three orthogonal planes, 0.688; and their method, 0.837. A set of handcrafted features has been used by Wang et al. [9] to reduce the false-positive rate and deep feature fusion for the nonmedical training. Their results show that the deep fusion feature can achieve sensitivity and specificity of 69.3% and 96.2% at 1.19 false positives per image compared to public data sets. An SVM-based CAD system used by Dhara et al. [10] focused on the classification of benign and malignant nodules using SVM. Nodules were segmented using a semiautomated technique that needed only a seed point from the user. They computed shape-, margin-, and texture-based features to represent the nodules. They determined a set of relevant features as a second step for an efficient representation of nodules in the feature space. They validated their classification method on 891 nodules of the LIDC data set. They evaluated the performance of the classification using AUC. They got AUCs of 0.9505, 0.8822, and 0.8488, respectively, for three different configurations of data sets. Song et al. [11] developed three types of deep neural networks (CNN, DNN, and SAE) for lung cancer calcification. They used those networks on the CT image classification task with some modification for the benign and malignant lung nodules. They evaluated those networks on the LIDC data set. The experimental results showed that the CNN network reached the best performance with an accuracy of 84.15%, specificity of 84.32%, and sensitivity of 83.96%. Shewaye et al. [12] proposed an automated system to diagnose benign or malignant nodules in CT images. Experimental results were illustrated using a combination of histogram and geometric lung nodule image features and different linear and nonlinear discriminant classifiers. They experimentally validated their proposed approach on the LIDC data set. Classification results were 93% correctly classified as benign and 82% correctly classified as malignant. A fusion framework between PET and CT features has been proposed by Guo et al. [13]. They applied SVM to train a vector of CT texture features and PET heterogeneity feature to improve the diagnosis and staging for lung cancer. They included in their study 32 subjects with lung nodules (19 males, 13 females, ages 70 ± 9 years) who underwent PET/CT scans.

The existing methods for the classification of lung nodules have the following limitations: (1) some methods depend on Hounsfield Unit (HU) values as the appearance descriptor without taking any spatial interaction into consideration, (2) most of the reported accuracies are low compared to the clinically accepted threshold, and (3) some of the methods depend only on raw data and disregard morphological information. The proposed framework overcomes the previously mentioned limitations through the integration of a novel appearance feature using seventh-order higher-order Markov-Gibbs random field (MGRF) that takes into account 3D spatial interaction between the nodule's voxels and geometrical features extracted from the segmented lung nodule with the deep autoencoder (AE) to achieve high classification accuracy.

9.2 Methods

The proposed framework presents a new automated noninvasive clinical diagnostic system for the early detection of lung cancer by classification of the detected lung nodule as benign or malignant. It integrates appearance and geometrical information derived from a single CT scan to significantly improve the accuracy, sensitivity, and specificity of early lung cancer diagnosis (Figure 9.2). In the CT markers method, two types of features are integrated: appearance and geometric. The appearance feature is modeled using an MGRF that is used to relate the joint probability of the nodule appearance and the energy of repeated patterns in the 3D scans in order to describe the spatial inhomogeneities in the lung nodule. The new higher seventh-order MGRF model is developed to have the ability to model the existing spatial inhomogeneities for both small and large detected pulmonary nodules. Geometric features are extracted from the binary segmented nodules to describe the pulmonary nodule geometry. Details of the framework's main components are given below.

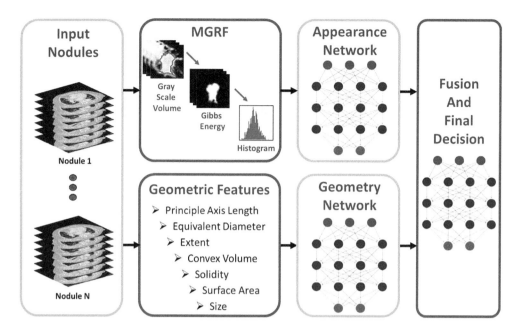

Figure 9.2   Lung nodule classification framework.

9.2.1 Appearance Features Using MGRF Energy

Since the HU values of the spatial distribution differ from benign nodules to malignant ones, the smoother the homogeneity the nodule is, the more likely it is benign. Describing the visual appearance features using the MGRF model will distinguish between benign and malignant nodules showing high distinctive features (see Figure 9.3). To describe the textural appearance of pulmonary nodules, Gibbs energy values are calculated using the seventh-order MGRF model to distinguish between benign and malignant nodules because these values show the interaction between the voxels and their neighbors [14] (see Figure 9.4). Let $\mathbb{Q} = \{0,\dots,Q-1\}$ denote a finite set of signals (HU values) in the lung CT scan, $s : \mathbb{R}^3 \to \mathbb{Q}$, with signals $\mathbf{s} = \left[s(r) : r = (x, y, z) \in \mathbb{R}^3 \right]$. The interaction graph, $\Gamma = \left(\mathbb{R}^3, \mathbb{E} \right)$, quantifies the signal probabilistic dependencies in the images with nodes at voxels, $r \in \mathbb{R}^3$, that are connected with edges $(r, r') \in \mathbb{E} \subseteq \mathbb{R}^3 \times \mathbb{R}^3$. An MGRF of images is defined by a Gibbs probability distribution

$$\Upsilon = \left[\Upsilon(\mathbf{s}) : \mathbf{s} \in \mathbb{Q}^{|\mathbb{R}|} ; \sum_{\mathbf{s} \in \mathbb{Q}^{|\mathbb{R}|}} \Upsilon(\mathbf{s}) = 1 \right] \tag{1}$$

factored over a set $\mathbb{C}$ of cliques in Γ supporting nonconstant factors, logarithms of which are Gibbs potentials [15]. To make modeling more efficient at describing the visual appearance of different nodules in the lung CT scans, the seventh-order MGRF

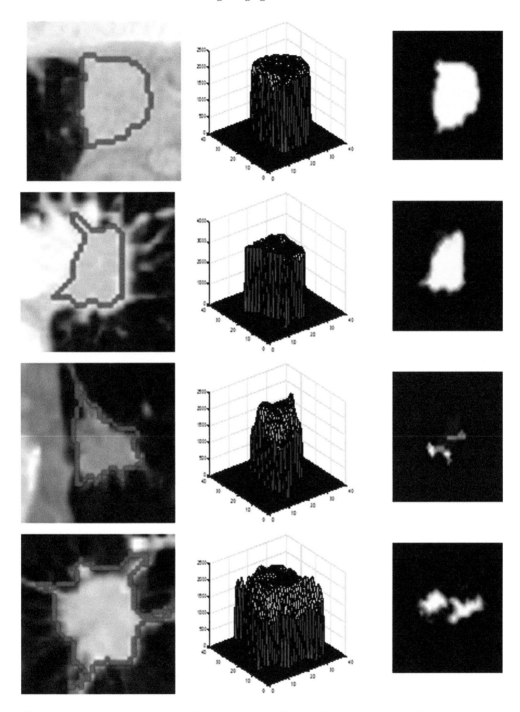

Figure 9.3 2D axial projection for two benign (first and second rows) and two malignant (third and fourth rows) lung nodules (a) along with their 3D visualization of Hounsfield values (b) and their calculated Gibbs energy (c).

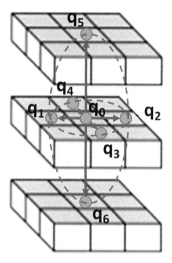

Figure 9.4   The seventh-order clique. Signals $q_0, q_1, \ldots, q_6$ are at the central pixel and its six central-symmetric neighbors at the radial distance r. Note that the selection of the neighborhood geometry takes into account the nodule's sphericity.

models the voxel's partial ordinal interaction within a radius r rather than modeling the pairwise interaction as in the second-order MGRF.

Let a translation-invariant seventh-order interaction structure on $\mathbb{R}$ be represented by A, $A \geq 1$, families, $\mathbb{C}_a$; $a = 1, \ldots, A$, of seventh-order cliques, $\mathbf{c}_{a:r} \in \mathbb{C}_a$, of the same shape and size. Every clique is associate with a certain voxel (origin), $r = (x, y, z) \in \mathbb{R}^3$, supporting the same (7)-variate scalar potential function, $V_a : \mathbb{Q}^7 \to (-\infty, \infty)$

The Gibbs probability distribution for this contrast/offset- and translation-invariant MGRF is

$$\Upsilon_7(\mathbf{s}) = \frac{1}{Z}\phi(\mathbf{s})\exp\left(-E_7(\mathbf{s})\right) \tag{2}$$

where $E_{7:a}(\mathbf{s}) = \sum_{\mathbf{c}_{a:r} \in \mathbb{C}_a} V_{7:a}\left(g(r') : r' \in \mathbf{c}_{a:r}\right)$ and $E_7(\mathbf{s}) = \sum_{a=1}^{A} E_{7:a}(\mathbf{s})$ denote the Gibbs energy for each individual and all the clique families, respectively; Z is a normalization factor; and $\phi(\mathbf{s})$ is a core distribution. The calculated Gibbs energy, $E_7(\mathbf{s})$, will be used to discriminate between benign and malignant tissues and gives an indication of malignancy. While a high potential of malignancy is indicated by lower energy, a high potential to be benign is indicated by higher energy. To calculate $E_7(\mathbf{s})$, the Gibbs potentials for the seventh-order model are calculated using the maximum likelihood estimates (MLEs) by generalizing the analytical approximation [16, 17]

$$V_{7:a}(\xi) = \frac{F_{7:a:\text{core}}(\xi) - F_{7:a}(\xi \,|\, \mathbf{s}^\circ)}{F_{7:a:\text{core}}(\xi)\left(1 - F_{7:a:\text{core}}(\xi)\right)}; \tag{3}$$

ALGORITHM 1   Learning the Seventh-Order MGRF Appearance Model

---

1. Given a training malignant nodules $\mathbf{g}^\circ$, find the empirical nodule ($l = 1$) and background ($l = 0$) probability distributions, $\mathbf{F}_{l:7:r}(\mathbf{g}^\circ) = \left[F_{l:7:r}(\beta \mid \mathbf{g}^\circ) : \beta \in \mathbb{B} \right]$ of the local binary pattern (LBP)-based descriptors for different clique sizes $r \in \{1, \ldots, r_{max}\}$ where the top size $r_{max} = 10$ in our experiments below.

2. Compute the empirical distributions $\mathbf{F}_{7:r:core} = \left[F_{7:r:core}(\beta) : \beta \in \mathbb{B} \right]$ of the same descriptors for the core independent random field (IRF) $\psi(\mathbf{g})$, e.g., for an image, sampled from the core.

3. Compute the approximate MLE of the potentials:

$$V_{l:7:r}(\beta) = \frac{F_{7:r:core}(\beta) - F_{l:7:r}(\beta \mid \mathbf{g}^\circ)}{F_{7:r:core}(\beta) \cdot \left(1 - F_{7:r:core}(\beta)\right)}$$

4. Compute partial Gibbs energies of the descriptors for equal and all other clique-wise signals over the training image for the clique sizes $r = 1, 2, \ldots, 10$ to choose the size ρ_l, making both the energies the closest one to another.

---

where $a = 1, \ldots, A$; $\xi \in \vartheta_7$, $\mathbf{s}^\circ$ denotes the training malignant nodule images, ξ denotes a numerical code of a particular seventh-order relation between the 7 signals on the clique, ϑ_7 is a set of these codes for all seventh-order signal co-occurrences, $F_{7:a}(\mathbf{s}^\circ)$ is an empirical marginal probability of the relation ξ; $\xi \in \vartheta_7$ over the seventh-order clique family $\mathbb{C}_{7:a}$ for $\mathbf{s}^\circ$, and $F_{7:a:core}(\xi)$ is the core probability distribution.

The proposed seventh-order MGRF appearance model is summarized in Algorithm 1.

9.2.2 Geometric Features

As lung nodules have different geometric characteristics based on whether they are malignant or benign, accounting for these differences as a discriminating feature helps differentiate between the different nodule types in the classification process. A set of seven geometric features are extracted from the nodule's binary mask (provided by a radiologist). The following geometric features are calculated: volume, surface area, convex volume, solidity, equivalent diameter, extent, and principal axis length. In order to calculate solidity, a convex hull C is defined around the segmented nodule, and the ratio between the volume of the voxels in C and the total volume of the segmented nodule is calculated. Then, in order to calculate extent, the bounding box around the segmented nodule is used, and the dimensions are named *dimx*, *dimy*, and *dimz*. To calculate extent, the proportion of the volume of the voxels in the bounding cube to the volume of the voxels of the segmented nodule is calculated. Principal axis length is defined as the largest dimension of the bounding cube (*max(dimx, dimy, dimz)*).

These features complement each other to come up with a final score for malignancy classification. To extract these features accurately without being dependent on scan accusation parameters, such as pixel spacing and slice thickness, a volume of interest (VOI) of size $40 \times 40 \times 40$ mm^3 that is centered around the center of each nodule is extracted and resampled to be an isotropic in the x-, y-, and z-directions.

9.2.3 Nodule Classification Using Autoencoders

Our CADx system utilizes a feed-forward deep neural network to classify the pulmonary nodules, whether malignant or benign. The implemented deep neural network comprises a two-stage structure of stacked AE.

The first stage consists of two AE-based classifiers—one classifier for appearance and one for geometry—that are used to give an initial estimation for the probabilities of the classification and that are augmented together to be considered as the input for the second-stage AE to give the final estimation of the classification probabilities (see Figure 9.1 for more details).

AE is employed in order to diminish the dimensionality of the input data (1,000 histogram bins for the Gibbs energy image in the network of the appearance) with multilayerd neural networks to get the most discriminating features by greedy unsupervised pretraining.

After the AE layers, a softmax output layer is stacked in order to refine the classification by reducing the total loss for the training labeled input.

For each AE, let $W = \left\{ W_j^e, W_i^d : j = 1,\ldots,s; i = 1,\ldots,n \right\}$ refer to a set of column vectors of weights for encoding (E) and decoding (D) layers and let T denote vector transposition. The AE changes the n-dimensional column vector $u = [u_1, u_n]^T$ into an s-dimensional column vector $h = [h_1, h_s]^T$ of hidden features such that $s < n$ by nonlinear uniform transformation of s weighted linear combinations of input where $\sigma(.)$ is a sigmoid function with values from [0, 1], $\sigma(t) = \dfrac{1}{1+e^{-t}}$.

Our classifier is constructed by stacking AE, which consists of three hidden layers with the softmax layer for the appearance network; the first hidden layer reduces the input vector to 500 level activators, while the second hidden layer continues the reduction to 300 level activators that are reduced to 100 after the third layer. The geometry network consists of the softmax layer only, as the input scale is not large enough to use AE with multiple hidden layers, like the appearance network (only nine geometric features), that computes the probability of being malignant or benign through the equation

$$p(c; W_{o:c}) = \frac{e^{\left(W_{o:c}^T h^3 \right)}}{e^{\left(\sum_1^c W_{o:c}^T h^3 \right)}} \tag{4}$$

where $C = 1, 2$ denotes the class number, $W_{o:c}$ is the weighting vector for the softmax for class c, and h^3 are the output features from the last hidden layer (the third layer) of the AE. In the second stage, the output probability obtained from the softmax of the appearance and geometry analysis networks are fused together and fed to another softmax layer to give the final classification probability.

9.3 Experimental Results

To train and test our proposed CADx system, the well-known LIDC data set is used. This data set consists of 1,018 thoracic CT scans that have been collected from 1,010 patients from seven academic centers. After removing the scans with slice thickness greater than 3 mm and the scans with inconsistent slice spacing, a total of 888 CT scans became available for testing and evaluating our CADx system [18]. The LIDC CT scans are associated with an XML file to provide a descriptive annotation and radiological diagnosis for the lung lesions, such as segmentation, shape, texture, and malignancy. All this information was provided by four thoracic radiologists in a two-phase image annotation process. In the first phase, each radiologist independently reviewed all cases, and this phase is called the blind read phase, as each radiologist gives an opinion regardless of the decisions of the other radiologists. The second phase is the final phase, as each radiologist gives a final decision after checking the decisions of the other three radiologists, and this phase is also called the unblinded phase, as all the annotations were made available to all the radiologists before giving their final annotation decision. The radiologists divided the lesions into two groups: nodules and nonnodules. We focused on the ≥ 3 mm nodules, as they have malignancy scores that vary from 1 (benign) to 5 (malignant) and a well-defined contour annotated by the radiologists.

We trained our CAD system on a randomly selected sample of nodules. In order to be sure that the data were almost balanced, we used 413 benign and 314 malignant nodules. For each nodule, the union of the four radiologists' masks is combined to obtain the final nodule mask that we used in our experiments. A VOI of size $40 \times 40 \times 40 \, mm^3$, measured around the center of the nodule's combined mask, is extracted for each nodule. The final diagnosis score of each nodule that we decided to work on is evaluated by calculating the average of the diagnosis scores for the four radiologists.

The system is evaluated by randomly dividing the data set into two parts: 70% for training and 30% for testing. The classification accuracy is described in terms of different measurement metrics, namely, the specificity, sensitivity, precision accuracy, and AUC. We reported the accuracy of the appearance model and the geometric model separately and for the complete fused system to highlight the effect of each model on the overall system (Table 9.1).

TABLE 9.1   Classification Results in Terms of Sensitivity, Specificity, Accuracy, Precession, and AUC for Different Feature Groups

	Evaluation Metrics				
	Sens.	Spec.	Acc.	Prec.	AUC
Geometric	76.64	84.68	80.73	82.83	87.20
Appearance	93.55	87.20	89.91	84.47	96.66
Comb. Features	**92.22**	**92.19**	**92.20**	**89.25**	**96.70**

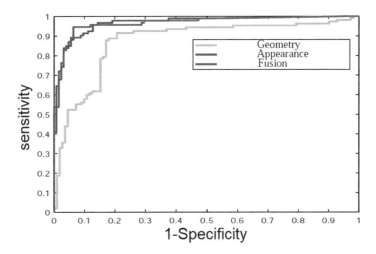

Figure 9.5   ROC for different feature classifications and the combined ones.

TABLE 9.2   Comparison Between Our Proposed System and Four Other Recent Nodule Classification Techniques in Terms of Sensitivity, Specificity, and Accuracy

		Metric		
		Sensitivity	Specificity	Accuracy
Method	Kumar et al. [19]	83.35	–	75.01
	Hua et al. [20]	73.30	78.70	–
	Krewer et al. [21]	85.71	94.74	90.91
	Jiang et al. [22]	86.00	88.50	–
	Our system	**92.22**	**92.19**	**92.20**

Figure 9.5 shows the ROC curve for each module and for the fused system, as it is considered a powerful tool to evaluate the discrimination of binary outcomes (benign or malignant). The curve is created by plotting the sensitivity against the specificity at diffident threshold settings. The area under the ROC curve was 0.96, 0.87, and 0.97 for the appearance model, geometric model, and fused system, respectively. Moreover, Table 9.2 provides a comparison between our proposed system and four other recent nodule classification techniques in terms of sensitivity, specificity, and accuracy.

9.4 Conclusion

In conclusion, this chapter introduced a novel framework for the classification of lung nodules by modeling the nodules' appearance features using a novel higher-order MGRF in addition to geometric features. The classification results obtained from a set of 727 nodules collected from 467 patients confirm that the proposed framework holds the promise for the early detection of lung cancer. A quantitative comparison with recently developed diagnostic techniques highlights the advantages of the proposed framework over state-of-the-art ones. These promising results encourage us to model new shape features using spherical harmonic analysis and include it in the proposed framework to reach the clinically accepted accuracy threshold, which is ≥95%. Moreover, we plan to file an institutional review board protocol in the future and locally collect data at our site to test on subjects who have malignant or benign nodules with biopsy confirmations.

This work could also be applied to various other applications in medical imaging, such as the kidney, the heart, the prostate, and the retina.

One application is renal transplant functional assessment. Chronic kidney disease affects about 26 million people in the United States, with 17,000 transplants being performed each year. In renal transplant patients, acute rejection is the leading cause of renal dysfunction. Given the limited number of donors, routine clinical posttransplantation evaluation is of immense importance in helping clinicians initiate timely interventions with appropriate treatment and thus prevent graft loss. In recent years, an increased area of research has been dedicated to developing noninvasive CAD systems for renal transplant function assessment, utilizing different image modalities (e.g., ultrasound, CT, and MRI). Accurate assessment of renal transplant function is critically important for graft survival. Although transplantation can improve a patient's well-being, there is a potential posttransplantation risk of kidney dysfunction that, if not treated in a timely manner, can lead to the loss of the entire graft and even patient death. Thus, accurate assessment of renal transplant function is crucial for the identification of proper treatment. In recent years, an increased area of research has been dedicated to developing noninvasive image-based CAD systems for the assessment of renal transplant function. In particular, dynamic and diffusion MRI-based systems have been clinically used to assess transplanted kidneys with the advantage of providing information on each kidney separately. For more details about renal transplant functional assessment, see the following works: [23–40] and [40–48].

The heart is also an important application to this work. The clinical assessment of myocardial perfusion plays a major role in the diagnosis, management, and prognosis of ischemic heart disease patients. Thus, there have been ongoing efforts to develop automated systems for the accurate analysis of myocardial perfusion using first-pass images [49–65].

Another application for this work could be the detection of retinal abnormalities. Most ophthalmologists depend on visual interpretation for the identification of diseases types. However, inaccurate diagnosis will affect the treatment procedure and may lead to fatal results. Hence, there is a crucial need for CAD systems that yield highly accurate results. Optical coherence tomography has become a powerful modality for the noninvasive diagnosis of various retinal abnormalities, such as glaucoma, diabetic macular edema, and macular degeneration. The problem with diabetic retinopathy is that the patient is not aware of the disease until the changes in the retina have progressed to a level that treatment tends to be less effective. Therefore, automated early detection could limit the severity of the disease and assist ophthalmologists in investigating and treating it more efficiently [66, 67].

Abnormalities of the lung could also be another promising area of research and a related application to this work. Radiation-induced lung injury is the main side effect of radiation therapy for lung cancer patients. Although higher radiation doses increase radiation therapy's effectiveness for tumor control, this can lead to lung injury, as a greater quantity of normal lung tissue is included in the treated area. Almost one-third of patients who undergo radiation therapy develop lung injury following radiation treatment. The severity of radiation-induced lung injury ranges from ground-glass opacities and consolidation at the early phase to fibrosis and traction bronchiectasis in the late phase. Early detection of lung injury will thus help improve management of the treatment [68–111].

This work can also be applied to other brain abnormalities, such as dyslexia and autism. Dyslexia is one of the most complicated developmental brain disorders that affect children's learning abilities. Dyslexia leads to the failure to develop age-appropriate reading skills despite a normal intelligence level and adequate reading instructions. Neuropathological studies have revealed an abnormal anatomy of some structures, such as the corpus callosum, in dyslexic brains. Much work in the literature has aimed to develop CAD systems for diagnosing such disorders, along with other brain disorders [112–134].

This work could also be applied to the extraction of blood vessels from phase contrast magnetic resonance angiography (MRA). Accurate cerebrovascular segmentation using noninvasive MRA is crucial for the early diagnosis and timely treatment of intracranial vascular diseases [117, 118, 135, 136].

References

1. American Cancer Society. *Cancer Facts and Figures.* Atlanta, GA: American Cancer Society; 2017.
2. Brazauskas KA, Ackman JB, Nelson B. Surveillance of actionable pulmonary nodules in children: the potential of thoracic MRI. *Insights Chest Dis.* 2016. Available at: http://insightsinchestdiseases.imedpub.com/surveillance-of-actionable-pulmonary-nodules-in-children-the-potential-of-thoracic-mri.php?aid=8342.
3. Wu LM, Xu JR, Hua J, et al. Can diffusion-weighted imaging be used as a reliable sequence in the detection of malignant pulmonary nodules and masses? *Magn Reson Imaging.* 2013;31(2)235–246.
4. Sun W, Zheng B, Qian W. Computer aided lung cancer diagnosis with deep learning algorithms. In: *Medical Imaging 2016: Computer-Aided Diagnosis.* Vol. 9785. Bellingham, WA: International Society for Optics and Photonics; 2016:97850Z.
5. Shen W, Zhou M, Yang F, Yang C, Tian J. Multi-scale convolutional neural networks for lung nodule classification. In: *International Conference on Information Processing in Medical Imaging.* New York, NY: Springer; 2015:588–599.
6. Likhitkar MVK, Gawande U, Hajari MKO. Automated detection of cancerous lung nodule from the computed tomography images. *IOSR J Comput Eng.* 2014;16(1):5–11.
7. Wei G, Ma H, Qian W, et al. Lung nodule classification using local kernel regression models with out-of-sample extension. *Biomed Signal Process Control.* 2018;40:1–9.
8. Nishio M, Nagashima C. Computer-aided diagnosis for lung cancer: usefulness of nodule heterogeneity. *Acad Radiol.* 2017;24(3):328–336.

9. Wang C, Elazab A, Wu J, Hu Q. Lung nodule classification using deep feature fusion in chest radiography. *Comput Med Imaging Graph*. 2017;57:10–18.

10. Dhara AK, Mukhopadhyay S, Dutta A, Garg A, Khandelwal N. A combination of shape and texture features for classification of pulmonary nodules in lung CT images. *J Digit Imaging*. 2016;29(4):466–475.

11. Song Q, Zhao L, Luo X, Dou X. Using deep learning for classification of lung nodules on computed tomography images. *J Healthcare Eng*. 2017; 2017:1–7.

12. Shewaye TN, Mekonnen AA. Benign-malignant lung nodule classification with geometric and appearance histogram features. arXiv preprint. arXiv:1605.08350, 2016.

13. Guo N, Yen R-F, El Fakhri G, Li Q. SVM based lung cancer diagnosis using multiple image features in PET/CT. In: *Nuclear Science Symposium and Medical Imaging Conference (NSS/MIC), 2015 IEEE*. New York, NY: IEEE; 2015:1–4.

14. Liu N, Soliman A, Gimel'farb G, El-Baz A. Segmenting kidney DCE-MRI using 1st-order shape and 5th-order appearance priors. In: *International Conference on Medical Image Computing and Computer-Assisted Intervention*. New York, NY: Springer; 2015:77–84.

15. Blake A, Kohli P, Rother C. *Markov Random Fields for Vision and Image Processing*. Cambridge, MA: MIT Press; 2011.

16. Gimel'farb G, Farag A. Texture analysis by accurate identification of simple Markovian models. *Cybernet Syst Anal*. 2005;41(1):27–38.

17. El-Baz A, Gimel'farb G, Suri JS. *Stochastic Modeling for Medical Image Analysis*. Boca Raton, FL: CRC Press; 2015.

18. Armato SG, McLennan G, Bidaut L, et al. The Lung Image Database Consortium (LIDC) and Image Database Resource Initiative (IDRI): a completed reference database of lung nodules on CT scans. *Med Phys*. 2011;38(2):915–931.

19. Kumar D, Wong A, Clausi DA. Lung nodule classification using deep features in CT images. In: *IEEE 12th Conference on Computer and Robot Vision (CRV), 2015*. 2015:133–138.

20. Hua K-L, Hsu C-H, Hidayati SC, Cheng H-W, Chen Y-J. Computer-aided classification of lung nodules on computed tomography images via deep learning technique. *OncoTargets Ther*. 2015;8.

21. Krewer H, Geiger B, Hall LO, et al. Effect of texture features in computer aided diagnosis of pulmonary nodules in low-dose computed tomography. In: *IEEE International Conference on Systems, Man, and Cybernetics (SMC)*. 2013:3887–3891.

22. Jiang H, Ma H, Qian W, Wei G, Zhao X, Gao M. A novel pixel value space statistics map of the pulmonary nodule for classification in computerized tomography images. In: *Engineering in Medicine and Biology Society (EMBC), 39th Annual International Conference of the IEEE*. 2017:556–559.

23. Ali AM, Farag AA, El-Baz A. Graph cuts framework for kidney segmentation with prior shape constraints. In: *Proceedings of International Conference on Medical Image Computing and Computer-Assisted Intervention (MICCAI'07)*. Vol. 1. 2007:384–392.

24. Chowdhury AS, Roy R, Bose S, Elnakib FKA, El-Baz A. Non-rigid biomedical image registration using graph cuts with a novel data term. In: *Proceedings of IEEE International Symposium on Biomedical Imaging: From Nano to Macro (ISBI'12)*. 2012:446–449.

25. El-Baz A, Farag AA, Yuksel SE, El-Ghar MEA, Eldiasty TA, Ghoneim TA. Application of deformable models for the detection of acute renal rejection. In: Farag AA, Suri JS, eds. *Deformable Models*. Vol. 1. New York, NY: Springer; 2007:293–333.

26. El-Baz A, Farag A, Fahmi R, Yuksel S, El-Ghar MA, Eldiasty T. Image analysis of renal DCE MRI for the detection of acute renal rejection. In: *Proceedings of IAPR International Conference on Pattern Recognition (ICPR'06)*. 2006:822–825.

27. El-Baz A, Farag A, Fahmi R, et al. A new CAD system for the evaluation of kidney diseases using DCE-MRI. In: *Proceedings of International Conference on Medical Image Computing and Computer-Assisted Intervention (MICCAI'08)*. 2006:446–453.

28. El-Baz A, Gimel'farb G, El-Ghar MA. A novel image analysis approach for accurate identification of acute renal rejection. In: *Proceedings of IEEE International Conference on Image Processing (ICIP'08)*. 2008:1812–1815.

29. El-Baz A, Gimel'farb G, El-Ghar MA. Image analysis approach for identification of renal transplant rejection. In: *Proceedings of IAPR International Conference on Pattern Recognition (ICPR'08)*. 2008:1–4.

30. El-Baz A, Gimel'farb G, El-Ghar MA. New motion correction models for automatic identification of renal transplant rejection. In: *Proceedings of International Conference on Medical Image Computing and Computer-Assisted Intervention (MICCAI'07)*. 2007:235–243.

31. Farag A, El-Baz A, Yuksel S, El-Ghar MA, Eldiasty T. A framework for the detection of acute rejection with dynamic contrast enhanced magnetic resonance imaging. In: *Proceedings of IEEE International Symposium on Biomedical Imaging: From Nano to Macro (ISBI'06)*. 2006:418–421.

32. Khalifa F, Beache GM, El-Ghar MA, et al. Dynamic contrast-enhanced MRI-based early detection of acute renal transplant rejection. *IEEE Trans Med Imaging*. 2013;32(10):1910–1927.

33. Khalifa F, El-Baz A, Gimel'farb G, El-Ghar MA. Non-invasive image-based approach for early detection of acute renal rejection. In: *Proceedings of International Conference Medical Image Computing and Computer-Assisted Intervention (MICCAI'10)*. 2010:10–18.

34. Khalifa F, El-Baz A, Gimel'farb G, Ouseph R, El-Ghar MA. Shape-appearance guided level-set deformable model for image segmentation. In: *Proceedings of IAPR International Conference on Pattern Recognition (ICPR'10)*. 2010:4581–4584.

35. Khalifa F, El-Ghar MA, Abdollahi B, Frieboes H, El-Diasty T, El-Baz A. A comprehensive non-invasive framework for automated evaluation of acute renal transplant rejection using DCE-MRI. *NMR Biomed*. 2013;26(11):1460–1470.

36. Khalifa F, El-Ghar MA, Abdollahi B, Frieboes HB, El-Diasty T, El-Baz A. Dynamic contrast-enhanced MRI-based early detection of acute renal transplant rejection. In: *2014 Annual Scientific Meeting and Educational Course Brochure of the Society of Abdominal Radiology (SAR'14)*. 2014:1855912.

37. Khalifa F, Elnakib A, Beache GM, et al. 3D kidney segmentation from CT images using a level set approach guided by a novel stochastic speed function. In: *Proceedings of International Conference Medical Image Computing and Computer-Assisted Intervention (MICCAI'11)*. 2011:587–594.

38. Khalifa F, Gimel'farb G, El-Ghar MA, et al. A new deformable model-based segmentation approach for accurate extraction of the kidney from abdominal CT images. In: *Proceedings of IEEE International Conference on Image Processing (ICIP'11)*. 2011:3393–3396.

39. Mostapha M, Khalifa F, Alansary A, Soliman A, Suri J, El-Baz A. Computer-aided diagnosis systems for acute renal transplant rejection: challenges and methodologies. In: El-Baz A, Saba L, Suri J, eds. *Abdomen and Thoracic Imaging*. New York, NY: Springer; 2014:1–35.

40. Shehata M, Khalifa F, Hollis E, et al. A new non-invasive approach for early classification of renal rejection types using diffusion-weighted MRI. In: *IEEE International Conference on Image Processing (ICIP)*. 2016:136–140.

41. Khalifa F, Soliman A, Takieldeen A, et al. Kidney segmentation from CT images using a 3D NMF-guided active contour model. In: *IEEE 13th International Symposium on Biomedical Imaging (ISBI)*. 2016:432–435.

42. Shehata M, Khalifa F, Soliman A, et al. 3D diffusion MRI-based CAD system for early diagnosis of acute renal rejection. In: *IEEE 13th International Symposium on Biomedical Imaging (ISBI)*. 2016:1177–1180.

43. Shehata M, Khalifa F, Soliman A, et al. A level set-based framework for 3D kidney segmentation from diffusion MR images. In: *IEEE International Conference on Image Processing (ICIP)*. 2015:4441–4445.

44. Shehata M, Khalifa F, Soliman A, et al. A promising non-invasive CAD system for kidney function assessment. In: *International Conference on Medical Image Computing and Computer-Assisted Intervention*. 2016:613–621.

45. Khalifa F, Soliman A, Elmaghraby A, Gimel'farb G, El-Baz A. 3D kidney segmentation from abdominal images using spatial-appearance models. *Comput Math Methods Med.* 2017;2017:1–10.

46. Hollis E, Shehata M, Khalifa F, El-Ghar MA, El-Diasty T, El-Baz A. Towards non-invasive diagnostic techniques for early detection of acute renal transplant rejection: a review. *Egypt J Radiol Nucl Med.* 2016;48(1):257–269.

47. Shehata M, Khalifa F, Soliman A, El-Ghar MA, Dwyer AC, El-Baz A. Assessment of renal transplant using image and clinical-based biomarkers. In: *Proceedings of 13th Annual Scientific Meeting of American Society for Diagnostics and Interventional Nephrology (ASDIN'17)*. 2017.

48. Shehata M, Khalifa F, Soliman A, El-Ghar MA, Dwyer AC, El-Baz A. Early assessment of acute renal rejection. In: *Proceedings of 12th Annual Scientific Meeting of American Society for Diagnostics and Interventional Nephrology (ASDIN'16)*. 2017.

49. Khalifa F, Beache G, El-Baz A, Gimel'farb G. Deformable model guided by stochastic speed with application in cine images segmentation. In: *Proceedings of IEEE International Conference on Image Processing (ICIP'10)*. 2010:1725–1728.

50. Khalifa F, Beache GM, Elnakib A, et al. A new shape-based framework for the left ventricle wall segmentation from cardiac first-pass perfusion MRI. In: *Proceedings of IEEE International Symposium on Biomedical Imaging: From Nano to Macro (ISBI'13)*. 2013:41–44.

51. Khalifa F, Beache GM, Elnakib A, et al. A new nonrigid registration framework for improved visualization of transmural perfusion gradients on cardiac first-pass perfusion MRI. In: *Proceedings of IEEE International Symposium on Biomedical Imaging: From Nano to Macro (ISBI'12)*. 2012:828–831.

52. Khalifa F, Beache GM, Firjani A, Welch KC, Gimel'farb G, El-Baz A. A new nonrigid registration approach for motion correction of cardiac first-pass perfusion MRI. In: *Proceedings of IEEE International Conference on Image Processing (ICIP'12)*. 2012:1665–1668.

53. Khalifa F, Beache GM, Gimel'farb G, El-Baz A. A novel CAD system for analyzing cardiac first-pass MR images. In: *Proceedings of IAPR International Conference on Pattern Recognition (ICPR'12)*. 2012:77–80.

54. Khalifa F, Beache GM, Gimel'farb G, El-Baz A. A novel approach for accurate estimation of left ventricle global indexes from short-axis cine MRI. In: *Proceedings of IEEE International Conference on Image Processing (ICIP'11)*. 2011:2645–2649.

55. Khalifa F, Beache GM, Gimel'farb G, Giridharan GA, El-Baz A. A new image-based framework for analyzing cine images. In: El-Baz A, Acahrya UR, Mirmehdi, Suri JS, eds. *Handbook of Multi Modality State-of-the-Art Medical Image Segmentation and Registration Methodologies.* Vol. 2. New York, NY: Springer; 2011:69–98.

56. Khalifa F, Beache GM, Gimel'farb G, Giridharan GA, El-Baz A. Accurate automatic analysis of cardiac cine images. *IEEE Trans Biomed Eng.* 2012;59(2):445–455.

57. Khalifa F, Beache GM, Nitzken M, Gimel'farb G, Giridharan, GA El-Baz A. Automatic analysis of left ventricle wall thickness using short-axis cine CMR images. In: *Proceedings of IEEE International Symposium on Biomedical Imaging: From Nano to Macro (ISBI'11).* 2011:1306–1309.

58. Nitzken M, Beache G, Elnakib A, Khalifa F, Gimel'farb G, El-Baz A. Accurate modeling of tagged CMR 3D image appearance characteristics to improve cardiac cycle strain estimation. In: *19th IEEE International Conference on Image Processing (ICIP).* 2012:521–524.

59. Nitzken M, Beache G, Elnakib A, Khalifa F, Gimel'farb G, El-Baz A. Improving full-cardiac cycle strain estimation from tagged CMR by accurate modeling of 3D image appearance characteristics. In: *9th IEEE International Symposium on Biomedical Imaging (ISBI).* 2012:462–465.

60. Nitzken MJ, El-Baz AS, Beache GM. Markov-Gibbs random field model for improved full-cardiac cycle strain estimation from tagged CMR. *J Cardiovasc Magn Reson.* 2012;14(1):1–2.

61. Sliman H, Elnakib A, Beache G, Elmaghraby A, El-Baz A. Assessment of myocardial function from cine cardiac MRI using a novel 4D tracking approach. *J Comput Sci Syst Biol.* 2014;7:169–173.

62. Sliman H, Elnakib A, Beache GM, et al. A novel 4D PDE-based approach for accurate assessment of myocardium function using cine cardiac magnetic resonance images. In: *Proceedings of IEEE International Conference on Image Processing (ICIP'14).* 2014:3537–3541.

63. Sliman H, Khalifa F, Elnakib A, Beache GM, Elmaghraby A, El-Baz A. A new segmentation-based tracking framework for extracting the left ventricle cavity from cine cardiac MRI. In: *Proceedings of IEEE International Conference on Image Processing (ICIP'13).* 2013:685–689.

64. Sliman H, Khalifa F, Elnakib A, et al. Myocardial borders segmentation from cine MR images using bi-directional coupled parametric deformable models. *Med Phys.* 2013;40(9):1–13.

65. Sliman H, Khalifa F, Elnakib A, et al. Accurate segmentation framework for the left ventricle wall from cardiac cine MRI. In: *Proceedings of International Symposium on Computational Models for Life Science (CMLS'13).* 2013:287–296.

66. Eladawi N, Elmogy MM, Ghazal M, et al. Classification of retinal diseases based on OCT images. *Front Biosci (Landmark J).* 2017;23:247–264.

67. ElTanboly A, Ismail M, Shalaby A, et al. A computer aided diagnostic system for detecting diabetic retinopathy in optical coherence tomography images. *Med Phys.* 2017:44(3):914–923.

68. Abdollahi B, Civelek AC, Li X-F, Suri J, El-Baz A. PET/CT nodule segmentation and diagnosis: a survey. In: Saba L, Suri JS, eds. *Multi Detector CT Imaging.* New York, NY: Taylor & Francis; 2014:639–651.

69. Abdollahi B, El-Baz A, Amini AA. A multi-scale non-linear vessel enhancement technique. In: *Engineering in Medicine and Biology Society, EMBC, 2011 Annual International Conference of the IEEE.* 2011:3925–3929.

70. Abdollahi B, Soliman A, Civelek A, Li X-F, Gimel'farb G, El-Baz A. A novel Gaussian scale space-based joint MGRF framework for precise lung segmentation. In: *Proceedings of IEEE International Conference on Image Processing (ICIP'12).* 2012:2029–2032.

71. Abdollahi B, Soliman A, Civelek A, Li X-F, Gimel'farb G, El-Baz A. A novel 3D joint MGRF framework for precise lung segmentation. In: *Machine Learning in Medical Imaging*. New York, NY: Springer; 2012:86–93.

72. Ali AM, El-Baz AS, Farag AA. A novel framework for accurate lung segmentation using graph cuts. In: *Proceedings of IEEE International Symposium on Biomedical Imaging: From Nano to Macro (ISBI'07)*. 2007:908–911.

73. El-Baz A, Beache GM, Gimel'farb G, Suzuki K, Okada K. Lung imaging data analysis. *Int J Biomed Imaging*. 2013;2013:1–3.

74. El-Baz A, Beache GM, Gimel'farb G, et al. Computer-aided diagnosis systems for lung cancer: challenges and methodologies. *Int J Biomed Imaging*. 2013;2013:1–46.

75. El-Baz A, Elnakib A, Abou El-Ghar A, Gimel'farb G, Falk R, Farag A. Automatic detection of 2D and 3D lung nodules in chest spiral CT scans. *Int J Biomed Imaging*. 2013;2013:1–11.

76. El-Baz A, Farag AA, Falk R, La Rocca R. A unified approach for detection, visualization, and identification of lung abnormalities in chest spiral CT scans. In: *International Congress Series*. Vol. 1256. New York, NY: Elsevier; 2003:998–1004.

77. El-Baz A, Farag AA, Falk R, La Rocca R. Detection, visualization and identification of lung abnormalities in chest spiral CT scan: phase-I. In: *Proceedings of International Conference on Biomedical Engineering*. 2002.

78. El-Baz A, Farag A, Gimel'farb G, Falk R, El-Ghar MA, Eldiasty T. A framework for automatic segmentation of lung nodules from low dose chest CT scans. In: *Proceedings of International Conference on Pattern Recognition (ICPR'06)*. 2006:611–614.

79. El-Baz A, Farag A, Gimel'farb G, Falk R, El-Ghar MA. A novel level set-based computer-aided detection system for automatic detection of lung nodules in low dose chest computed tomography scans. *Lung Imaging Comput Aided Diagn*. 2011;10:221–238.

80. El-Baz A, Gimel'farb G, Abou El-Ghar M, Falk R. Appearance-based diagnostic system for early assessment of malignant lung nodules. In: *Proceedings of IEEE International Conference on Image Processing (ICIP'12)*. 2012:533–536.

81. El-Baz A, Gimel'farb G, Falk R. A novel 3D framework for automatic lung segmentation from low dose CT images. In: El-Baz A, Suri JS, eds. *Lung Imaging and Computer Aided Diagnosis*. New York, NY: Taylor & Francis; 2011:1–16.

82. El-Baz A, Gimel'farb G, Falk R, El-Ghar M. Appearance analysis for diagnosing malignant lung nodules. In: *Proceedings of IEEE International Symposium on Biomedical Imaging: From Nano to Macro (ISBI'10)*. 2010:193–196.

83. El-Baz A, Gimel'farb G, Falk R, El-Ghar MA. A novel level set-based CAD system for automatic detection of lung nodules in low dose chest CT scans. In: El-Baz A, Suri JS, eds. *Lung Imaging and Computer Aided Diagnosis*. New York, NY: Taylor & Francis; 2011:221–238.

84. El-Baz A, Gimel'farb G, Falk R, El-Ghar MA. A new approach for automatic analysis of 3D low dose CT images for accurate monitoring the detected lung nodules. In: *Proceedings of International Conference on Pattern Recognition (ICPR'08)*. 2008:1–4.

85. El-Baz A, Gimel'farb G, Falk R, El-Ghar MA. A novel approach for automatic follow-up of detected lung nodules. In: *Proceedings of IEEE International Conference on Image Processing (ICIP'07)*. 2007:v–501.

86. El-Baz A, Gimel'farb G, Falk R, El-Ghar MA. A new CAD system for early diagnosis of detected lung nodules. In: *IEEE International Conference on Image Processing, 2007*. 2007:ii–461.

87. El-Baz A, Gimel'farb G, Falk R, El-Ghar MA, Refaie H. Promising results for early diagnosis of lung cancer. In: *Proceedings of IEEE International Symposium on Biomedical Imaging: From Nano to Macro (ISBI'08)*. 2008:1151–1154.

88. El-Baz A, Gimel'farb GL, Falk R, Abou El-Ghar M, Holland T, Shaffer T. A new sto-chastic framework for accurate lung segmentation. In: *Proceedings of Medical Image Computing and Computer-Assisted Intervention (MICCAI'08)*. 2008:322–330.

89. El-Baz A, Gimel'farb GL, Falk R, Heredis D, Abou El-Ghar M. A novel approach for accurate estimation of the growth rate of the detected lung nodules. In: *Proceedings of International Workshop on Pulmonary Image Analysis*. 2008:33–42.

90. El-Baz A, Gimel'farb GL, Falk R, Holland T, Shaffer T. A framework for unsuper-vised segmentation of lung tissues from low dose computed tomography images. In: *Proceedings of British Machine Vision (BMVC'08)*. 2008:1–10.

91. El-Baz A, Gimel'farb G, Falk R, El-Ghar MA. 3D MGRF-based appearance modeling for robust segmentation of pulmonary nodules in 3D LDCT chest images. In: El-Baz A, Suri JS, eds. *Lung Imaging and Computer Aided Diagnosis*. New York, NY: Taylor & Francis; 2011:51–63.

92. El-Baz A, Gimel'farb G, Falk R, El-Ghar MA. Automatic analysis of 3D low dose CT images for early diagnosis of lung cancer. *Pattern Recogn.* 2009;42(6):1041–1051.

93. El-Baz A, Gimel'farb G, Falk R, et al. Toward early diagnosis of lung cancer. In: *Proceedings of Medical Image Computing and Computer-Assisted Intervention (MICCAI'09)*. 2009:682–689.

94. El-Baz A, Gimel'farb G, Falk R, El-Ghar MA, Suri J. Appearance analysis for the early assessment of detected lung nodules. In: El-Baz A, Suri JS, eds. *Lung Imaging and Computer Aided Diagnosis*. New York, NY: Taylor & Francis; 2011:395–404.

95. El-Baz A, Khalifa F, Elnakib A, et al. A novel approach for global lung registration using 3D Markov Gibbs appearance model. In: *Proceedings of International Conference Medical Image Computing and Computer-Assisted Intervention (MICCAI'12)*. 2012:114–121.

96. El-Baz A, Nitzken M, Elnakib A, et al. 3D shape analysis for early diagnosis of malignant lung nodules. In: *Proceedings of International Conference Medical Image Computing and Computer-Assisted Intervention (MICCAI'11)*. 2011:175–182.

97. El-Baz A, Nitzken M, Gimel'farb G, et al. Three-dimensional shape analysis using spherical harmonics for early assessment of detected lung nodules. In: El-Baz A, Suri JS, eds. *Lung Imaging and Computer Aided Diagnosis*. New York, NY: Taylor & Francis; 2011:421–438.

98. El-Baz A, Nitzken M, Khalifa F, et al. 3D shape analysis for early diagnosis of malignant lung nodules. In: *Proceedings of International Conference on Information Processing in Medical Imaging (IPMI'11)*. 2011:772–783.

99. El-Baz A, Nitzken M, Vanbogaert E, Gimel'Farb G, Falk R, Abo El-Ghar M. A novel shape-based diagnostic approach for early diagnosis of lung nodules. In: *2011 IEEE International Symposium on Biomedical Imaging: From Nano to Macro*. 2011:137–140.

100. El-Baz A, Sethu P, Gimel'farb G, et al. Elastic phantoms generated by microfluidics technology: validation of an imaged-based approach for accurate measurement of the growth rate of lung nodules. *Biotechnol J.* 2011;6(2):195–203.

101. El-Baz A, Sethu P, Gimel'farb G, et al. A new validation approach for the growth rate measurement using elastic phantoms generated by state-of-the-art microfluidics tech-nology. In: *Proceedings of IEEE International Conference on Image Processing (ICIP'10)*. 2010:4381–4383.

102. El-Baz E, Sethu P, Gimel'farb G, et al. Validation of a new imaged-based approach for the accurate estimating of the growth rate of detected lung nodules using real CT images and elastic phantoms generated by state-of-the-art microfluidics technology. In: El-Baz A, Suri JS, eds. *Lung Imaging and Computer Aided Diagnosis*. New York, NY: Taylor & Francis; 2011:405–420.

103. El-Baz A, Soliman A, McClure P, Gimel'farb G, El-Ghar MA, Falk R. Early assessment of malignant lung nodules based on the spatial analysis of detected lung nodules. In: *Proceedings of IEEE International Symposium on Biomedical Imaging: From Nano to Macro (ISBI'12)*. 2012:1463–1466.

104. El-Baz A, Yuksel SE, Elshazly S, Farag AA. Non-rigid registration techniques for automatic follow-up of lung nodules. In: *Proceedings of Computer Assisted Radiology and Surgery (CARS'05)*. New York, NY: Elsevier; 2005:1115–1120.

105. El-Baz AS, Suri JS, eds. *Lung Imaging and Computer Aided Diagnosis*. New York, NY: Taylor & Francis; 2011.

106. Soliman A, Khalifa F, Shaffie A, et al. Image-based CAD system for accurate identification of lung injury. In: *Proceedings of IEEE International Conference on Image Processing (ICIP'16)*. 2016:121–125.

107. Soliman A, Khalifa F, Dunlap N, Wang B, El-Ghar M, El-Baz A. An iso-surfaces based local deformation handling framework of lung tissues. In: *IEEE 13th International Symposium on Biomedical Imaging (ISBI)*. 2016:1253–1259.

108. Soliman A, Khalifa F, Shaffie A, et al. Detection of lung injury using 4D-CT chest images. In: *IEEE 13th International Symposium on Biomedical Imaging (ISBI)*. 2016:1274–1277.

109. Soliman A, Khalifa F, Shaffie A, et al. A comprehensive framework for early assessment of lung injury. In: *IEEE International Conference on Image Processing (ICIP)*. 2017:3275–3279.

110. Shaffie A, Soliman A, Ghazal M, et al. A new framework for incorporating appearance and shape features of lung nodules for precise diagnosis of lung cancer. In: *IEEE International Conference on Image Processing (ICIP)*. 2017:1372–1376.

111. Soliman A, Khalifa F, Shaffie A, et al. Image-based cad system for accurate identification of lung injury. In: *IEEE International Conference on Image Processing (ICIP)*. 2016:121–125.

112. Dombroski B, Nitzken M, Elnakib A, Khalifa F, El-Baz A, Casanova MF. Cortical surface complexity in a population-based normative sample. *Transl Neurosci*. 2014;5(1):17–24.

113. El-Baz A, Casanova M, Gimel'farb G, Mott M, Switwala A. An MRI-based diagnostic framework for early diagnosis of dyslexia. *Int J Comput Assist Radiol Surg*. 2008;3(3–4):181–189.

114. El-Baz A, Casanova M, Gimel'farb G, et al. A new CAD system for early diagnosis of dyslexic brains. In: *Proceedings of International Conference on Image Processing (ICIP'2008)*. 2008:1820–1823.

115. El-Baz A, Casanova MF, Gimel'farb G, Mott M, Switwala AE. A new image analysis approach for automatic classification of autistic brains. In: *Proceedings of IEEE International Symposium on Biomedical Imaging: From Nano to Macro (ISBI'2007)*. 2007:352–355.

116. El-Baz A, Elnakib A, Khalifa F, et al. Precise segmentation of 3-D magnetic resonance angiography. *IEEE Trans Biomed Eng*. 2012;59(7):2019–2029.

117. El-Baz A, Farag AA, Gimel'farb GL, El-Ghar MA, Eldiasty T. Probabilistic modeling of blood vessels for segmenting MRA images. In: *International Conference on Pattern Recognition (ICPR)*. 2006:917–920.

118. El-Baz A, Farag AA, Gimel'farb G, El-Ghar MA, Eldiasty T. A new adaptive probabilistic model of blood vessels for segmenting MRA images. In: *Medical Image Computing and Computer-Assisted Intervention—MICCAI 2006*. Vol. 4191. New York, NY: Springer; 2006:799–806.

119. El-Baz A, Farag AA, Gimel'farb G, Hushek SG. Automatic cerebrovascular segmentation by accurate probabilistic modeling of TOF-MRA images. In: *Medical Image Computing and Computer-Assisted Intervention—MICCAI 2005*. New York, NY: Springer; 2005:34–42.

120. El-Baz A, Farag A, Elnakib A, et al. Accurate automated detection of autism related corpus callosum abnormalities. *J Med Syst.* 2011;35(5):929–939.

121. El-Baz A, Farag A, Gimel'farb G. Cerebrovascular segmentation by accurate probabilistic modeling of TOF-MRA images. In: *Image Analysis.* Vol. 3540. New York, NY: Springer; 2005:1128–1137.

122. El-Baz A, Gimel'farb G, Falk R, El-Ghar MA, Kumar V, Heredia D. A novel 3D joint Markov-Gibbs model for extracting blood vessels from PC–MRA images. In: *Medical Image Computing and Computer-Assisted Intervention—MICCAI 2009.* Vol. 5762. New York, NY: Springer; 2009:943–950.

123. Elnakib A, El-Baz A, Casanova MF, Gimel'farb G, Switwala AE. Image-based detection of corpus callosum variability for more accurate discrimination between dyslexic and normal brains. In: *Proceedings of IEEE International Symposium on Biomedical Imaging: From Nano to Macro (ISBI'2010).* 2010:109–112.

124. Elnakib A, Casanova MF, Gimel'farb G, Switwala AE, El-Baz A. Autism diagnostics by centerline-based shape analysis of the corpus callosum. In: *Proceedings of IEEE International Symposium on Biomedical Imaging: From Nano to Macro (ISBI'2011).* 2011:1843–1846.

125. Elnakib A, Nitzken M, Casanova M, Park H, Gimel'farb G, El-Baz A. Quantification of age-related brain cortex change using 3D shape analysis. In: *21st International Conference on Pattern Recognition (ICPR).* 2012:41–44.

126. Mostapha M, Soliman A, Khalifa F, et al. A statistical framework for the classification of infant DT images. In: *IEEE International Conference on Image Processing (ICIP).* 2014:2222–2226.

127. Nitzken M, Casanova M, Gimel'farb G, et al. 3D shape analysis of the brain cortex with application to dyslexia. In: *18th IEEE International Conference on Image Processing (ICIP).* 2011:2657–2660.

128. El-Gamal FE, Elmogy MM, Ghazal M, et al. A novel CAD system for local and global early diagnosis of Alzheimer's disease based on PIB-PET scans. In: *2017 IEEE International Conference on Image Processing (ICIP).* 2017:3270–3274.

129. Ismail M, Soliman A, Ghazal M, et al. A fast stochastic framework for automatic MR brain images segmentation. *PloS One.* 12(11):e0187391.

130. Ismail MM, Keynton RS, Mostapha MM, et al. Studying autism spectrum disorder with structural and diffusion magnetic resonance imaging: a survey. *Front Hum Neurosci.* 2016;10:211.

131. Alansary A, Ismail M, Soliman A, et al. Infant brain extraction in t1-weighted MR images using BET and refinement using LCDG and MGRF models. *IEEE J Biomed Health Inform.* 2016;20(3):925–935.

132. Ismail M, Barnes G, Matthew M, et al. A new deep-learning approach for early detection of shape variations in autism using structural MRI. In: *2017 IEEE International Conference on Image Processing (ICIP).* 2017:1057–1061

133. Ismail M, Soliman A, ElTanboly A, et al. Detection of white matter abnormalities in MR brain images for diagnosis of autism in children. In: *2016 IEEE 13th International Symposium on Biomedical Imaging (ISBI).* 2016:6–9.

134. Ismail M, Mostapha M, Soliman A, et al. Segmentation of infant brain MR images based on adaptive shape prior and higher-order MGRF. In: *2015 IEEE International Conference on Image Processing (ICIP).* 2015:4327–4331.

135. El-baz A, Shalaby A, Taher F, et al. Probabilistic modeling of blood vessels for segmenting magnetic resonance angiography images. In: *Medical Research Archive—MRA*. KEI; 2017;7(5). ISSN 2375-1924. Available at: https://www.journals.ke-i.org/index.php/mra/article/view/1031. Date accessed: February 19, 2019.

136. Chowdhury AS, Rudra AK, Sen M, Elnakib A, El-Baz A. Cerebral white matter segmentation from MRI using probabilistic graph cuts and geometric shape priors. In: *Proceedings of IEEE International Conference on Image Processing (ICIP'10)*. 2010:3649–3652.

10

Smoking Cessation and Lung Cancer Screening Programs: The Rationale and Method to Integration

Meghan Cahill, Brooke Crawford O'Neill, Kimberly Del Mauro, Courtney Yeager, and Bradley B. Pua

Contents

10.1 Background

The American Cancer Society estimates that there will be 234,030 new lung and bronchus cancer diagnoses in 2018 alone, a recognizable increase from the 221,200 estimate in 2015 [1, 2]. Despite the increase in the estimated number of new diagnoses, lung cancer incidence and death rates continue to decline, decreasing 45% among males since 1990 and 19% among females since 2002. Unfortunately, lung cancer continues to remain the leading cause of all cancer-related deaths in the United States [1].

The majority of lung cancer patients presenting with advanced disease has strongly contributed to a 5-year survival rate of less than 18% [1]. Therefore, significant attention has been placed on screening for early detection as a means of reducing related morbidity and mortality [3, 4]. Detection at an early, localized stage improves prognosis and increases the 5-year survival rate to over 50%, compared to survival of less than 5% at distant stages [1]. However, many previously studied screening techniques, such as chest radiography, with or without sputum analysis, have not resulted in a survival benefit [5, 6]. The Prostate, Lung, Colorectal, and Ovarian Cancer Screening Trial, a randomized trial published in 2011, reinforced these findings, showing no difference in lung cancer mortality when screening with chest radiograph compared to usual care [7]. On the contrary, studies involving low-dose computed tomography (LDCT) have shown great value with regard to early detection of lung cancer with decreased mortality.

In 1999, it was established by the Early Lung Cancer Action Program (ELCAP) that the increased sensitivity of LDCT proved beneficial for detection of small non-calcified nodules and early-stage cancers [8]. Following, in 2006, the International Early Lung Cancer Action Program (I-ELCAP) reported that the vast majority of lung cancers detected by LDCT were in clinical stage I and thus more likely to be curable by surgical resection. This was demonstrated by an observed increase in 10-year survival from 88% to 92% for individuals with stage I cancer who underwent surgical resection within 1 month after diagnosis. Conversely, the few who did not receive treatment died within 5 years [9]. Five years later, the expansive 2011 National Lung Screening Trial (NLST), funded by the National Cancer Institute, solidified the need for screening recommendations in high-risk populations by determining that screening with LDCT, compared to chest radiography, significantly reduced lung cancer mortality by 20% among patients at high risk for developing lung cancer [10].

With mounting evidence confirming the benefits of lung-cancer screening with LDCT, the U.S. Preventive Services Task Force (USPSTF) released an updated recommendation in early 2014 [4]. The recommendation encouraged annual LDCT screening for high-risk adults—individuals aged 55–80 years with a 30-pack-year smoking history or greater who either are current smokers or have quit within the past 15 years. However, according to data collected from the Lung Cancer Screening Registry in 2016 [11], among the estimated 7.6 million individuals eligible for screening in the United States, only 1.9% were screened. Therefore, while the decline in cancer mortality can be partially attributed to lung cancer screening, the increase in awareness around associated health hazards and the significant reductions in smoking over the past two decades have likely made a far greater contribution.

While screening is an important component in reducing lung cancer–related mortality, targeting cigarette smoking, one of the strongest risk factors for development of lung cancer, is of vital importance. Not only does cigarette smoking remain the leading preventable cause of premature disease and death worldwide, in the United States it is the largest risk factor for lung cancer and accounts for 85% of all cases [3], [12]. Since the landmark 1964 Surgeon General's report *Smoking and Health*, adult smoking rates in the United States have decreased from 43% to 15.5% [12, 13]. However, an estimated 37.8 million adults continue to remain dependent on cigarettes, and, in consequence, more than 16 million Americans currently live with a smoking-related disease. Furthermore, one out of every five deaths annually are attributed to cigarette smoking, with an alarming 127,700 annual deaths accredited to smoking-related lung cancer [14]. Beyond the causal relationship that has been established between smoking and lung cancer, it has been determined that secondhand smoke also causes disease in never-smokers. The risk of developing lung cancer increases by 20% to 30% among nonsmokers who are exposed to secondhand smoke at home or at work, and each year, more than 7,300 lung cancer deaths are due to secondhand smoke [15].

With a total of 135,033 lung cancer deaths occurring annually due to cigarette smoking, including secondhand smoke exposure [14], interventions that target smoking habits can thus continue to serve an influential role in decreasing lung cancer burden. Therefore, as lung cancer screening programs continue to be developed, partnership with existing tobacco cessation programs or incorporation of these cessation services can offer a unique avenue for decreasing lung cancer mortality. This chapter discusses the impact of smoking cessation on lung cancer burden and the evidence supporting the addition of smoking cessations interventions to lung cancer screening programs and reviews approaches for implementation and potential barriers, including the additive value of the role of nonphysician clinicians to the process.

10.2 The Impact of Smoking Cessation

Published in 2005, the Lung Health Study (LHS) was the first randomized control trial to demonstrate the benefits of smoking cessation on mortality [16, 17]. A total of 5,887 current smokers with mild to moderate airway obstruction were included in the study and randomized to partake in a 10-week smoking cessation program or to the usual-care group, which did not include a cessation-related intervention. After following patients for 14.5 years, not only were all-cause mortality rates determined to be significantly higher in the usual-care group compared to the intervention group (10.38 per 1,000 person-years vs. 8.83 per 1,000 person-years; $p = 0.03$), but the findings were even more striking when stratified by smoking habit (6.04 per 1,000 person-years in sustained quitters vs. 7.77 per 1,000 person-years in intermittent quitters vs. 11.09 per 1,000 person-years in continuing smokers; $p < 0.001$). The difference in mortality rates among the three behavioral groups demonstrates a significant benefit to maintaining abstinence while suggesting a dose–response type of relationship [16].

Earlier studies performed in the United Kingdom as follow-up to the U.K. Doctor's Study in 1976 [18, 19], addressed the effects of smoking cessation on lung cancer burden with regard to age of cessation and quit time. For individuals who stopped smoking well into middle age, the majority of excess risk of lung cancer attributable to smoking was avoided, yet those who stopped before middle age avoided more than 90% of excess risk. More specifically, the cumulative risks of lung cancer by age 75 in men were 10%, 6%, 3%, and 2% for those who stopped smoking at 60, 50, 40, and 30 years of age, respectively, as compared to 16% in current smokers. Although these findings clearly demonstrate the benefits associated with smoking cessation at earlier ages, they also reinforce the notion that smoking cessation, at any age, reduces the risk of developing lung cancer and, likely, related mortality.

Recent studies examining smoking-related, all-cause mortality have confirmed the results of the previous LHS and U.K. Doctor's study. In 2013, a prospective, nationally representative study by Jha et al. [20] explored the 21st-century hazards of smoking and benefits of cessation at various ages in the United States. This study examined data from the National Health Interview Survey to measure mortality differences between current, former, and never-smokers. Jha et al. found a reduction in life expectancy among current smokers by more than 10 years compared to never-smokers. However, among those who quit smoking prior to the age of 40 years, risk of death associated with continued smoking was reduced by 90%. Although the benefits experienced by older adults were not as great, a reduction in excess risk of death remained. Even individuals who quit at 45–54 years of age gained 6 years of life compared to those who continued smoking. However, it is important to note that these results may underestimate the true population benefit of smoking cessation due to the potential bias introduced by reverse causality, or the "ill-quitter effect," an effect that occurs when individuals with smoking-related illness or other comorbidities quit smoking because of their illness [20, 21]. A 2018 case control study expanded on the Hong Kong Lifestyle and Mortality study by examining the effects of quit time and age of quitting on mortality using a proportional mortality study design [21]. This study found that longer durations of smoking cessation and quitting at a younger age were associated with progressively lower overall mortality rates, confirming the previously mentioned reports. Additionally, these findings were consistent with those pertaining to lung cancer mortality rates as well, with the exception of individuals quitting less than 5 years prior to death, again likely due to the ill-quitter effect, which can undermine the benefits of smoking cessation.

In addition to reducing the risk of developing lung cancer, early smoking cessation has also been found to increase survivability for individuals with diagnosed lung cancer regardless of histologic subtype [22]. Specifically, among patients diagnosed with non–small-cell lung cancer (NSCLC), Ferketich et al. [23] demonstrated a stage-specific survival benefit regarding smoking cessation. While never-smokers with stage I or II disease had significantly lower hazard rates for all-cause mortality compared to current smokers with the same disease staging, former smokers with stage IV disease who quit more than a year ago also had a survival benefit compared to current smokers. Furthermore, among those with early-stage NSCLC, Zhou et al. [24] reported a survival advantage for former smokers with a greater quit time (≥9 years prior to diagnosis) compared to current smokers. Ebbert et al. [25] reported similar findings among women.

Delving further, Warren et al. [26] explored the benefits of recent cessation at time of diagnosis from a subset of former smokers on overall and disease-specific survival. Their investigation demonstrated an increased risk in 5-year overall mortality and lung cancer mortality among current smokers compared to recent quit and former smokers. These data, accompanied by the previously mentioned studies, suggest a reversible effect of smoking in lung cancer patients despite length of cessation. However, a 2018 study by Japuntich et al. [27] contradicts this notion. Although this study reported a near 30% reduction in hazard of death from lung cancer among never-smokers compared to current smokers, Japuntich and his colleagues did not find a significant difference in survival among long-term, medium-term, or short-term quitters compared to current smokers. With conflicting data on the survival benefits of increased quit time, it is important to reiterate the potential impact of both abstinence and early cessation in regard to tobacco use.

Smoking cessation has also been found to reduce the risk of complications and enhance the quality of life after surgical resection. Comparing current to never-smokers, a study looking at primary lung cancer resections from the Society of Thoracic Surgeons General Thoracic Surgery Database found that the risk for major pulmonary complications increased significantly between the two groups (adjusted odds ratio [OR] = 1.08; p = 0.03) [28]. While there was no significant difference between former and never-smokers, the risk among former smokers decreased with longer quit time. Regarding postsurgical quality of life, current smokers suffered impairments in physical, social, and role functioning at 12 months compared to individuals who quit smoking after diagnosis but prior to surgery. The former smokers experienced returns to baseline in all three measures by 12 months [29]. While both studies mentioned suggest further benefits of smoking cessation, the quality-of-life study by Balduyck et al. [16] implies the potential for benefits at even later time points, such as after diagnosis, by allowing quicker returns to presurgical quality of life.

Studies have also examined the relationship between smoking persistence after diagnosis and the risk of developing a second primary lung cancer. A retrospective study by Richardson et al. [30] found that quitting smoking within 6 months of treatment initiation for small-cell lung cancer decreased an individual's relative risk for developing a second primary lung cancer given at least 2 years of remission posttherapy. These results were supported by a 2010 study looking at the effect of smoking cessation on prognosis [31]. Parsons et al. [31] found that among continued smokers, the hazard for development of a second primary tumor was 4.31 (95% confidence interval [CI] = 1.09–16.98) times the hazard among those who did not continue smoking, indicating that this persistent behavior is associated with poorer cancer-related prognoses.

With an estimated 6%–14% of total health care expenditures in the United States attributable to smoking [32], understanding smoking cessation as a cost-effective preventive service is essential. Utilizing a computer simulation model, Tsevat et al. [33] estimated that if the number of cigarettes smoked were reduced by half, the life expectancy of smokers and the general population would increase by 1.2–2.8 years and 0.4 years, respectively. Furthermore, studies exploring community-based cessation programs have proved promising in regard to cost-effectiveness [34–36]. Tran et al. [36] modeled the cost-effectiveness of a community, pharmacy-based cessation program, describing cost-effectiveness ratios as similar to ratios that would be achieved with vaccination and childhood safety programs, programs that are long standing and well established in preventive medicine [36].

10.3 The Evidence on Integration of Smoking Cessation and Lung Cancer Screening

It has previously been demonstrated that a smoker's readiness to quit is influenced by involvement with lung cancer screening [16]. Data from a prospective study by Taylor et al. [37] showed that among those enrolled in the NLST, more individuals expressed readiness to quit after receiving their CT screening result as compared to reports collected prior to screening. Similar results were reported by Ostroff et al. [38], who found that while 73.9% of active smokers enrolled in ELCAP felt that their enrollment in the screening program made them think about quitting, 89% of participants who recently quit or reduced their smoking habit reported that the program greatly influenced their behavior change. Therefore, it is clear that comprehensive lung cancer screening programs provide a unique opportunity for not only implementation but also utilization of smoking cessation interventions. The inherent "teachable moment" that presents within the structure of such programs allows for an opportunity to influence an individual's motivation and ability to make positive behavior changes [37–40].

With a high false-positive rate, communication of lung cancer screening results is thought to instigate further consideration of smoking cessation and provide an opportune time for related interventions [16]. This effect has been previously explored by Tammemägi et al. [40], who found that a strong inverse relationship exists between the severity of results delivered and the potential for continued smoking [40]. Specifically, Lung Screening Study (LSS) participants in the NLST with screening results that were suspicious for lung cancer were less likely to continue smoking than participants with normal screening results (OR = 0.66; 95% CI = 0.61–0.72; $p < 0.001$). This effect was also observed to vary by age. Taylor et al. [37] reported that more LSS participants than in the NLST sample, under 64 years of age, were ready to stop smoking after receiving an abnormal screening result compared to those with normal results ($p = 0.02$). However, there was no association found between readiness to stop smoking and screening results in participants 64 years or older. Additionally, the relationship between severity of results and smoking cessation was further emphasized by a follow-up study on the Danish Lung Cancer Screening Trial, a randomized control trial examining the effects of LDCT [41]. Ashraf et al. [41] found that among participants with positive screening results, the smoking cessation rate was significantly greater than among participants with negative results (17.7% vs. 10.6%; $p = 0.04$). Furthermore, Townsend et al. [42], after conducting a 3-year longitudinal study following current and former smokers through a series of annual screenings, discovered that the number of abnormal scans received influenced smoking cessation. Abstinence rates among this study population were 19.8%, 24.2%, 28%, and 41.9% for smokers with zero, one, two, and three abnormal screens, respectively. Results reflecting a teachable moment for smoking cessation among those presenting for lung cancer screening are further corroborated by a recent 2017 study by Brain et al. [43]. Odds of smoking cessation was ascertained among a subset of high-risk, current smokers from the U.K. Lung Cancer Screening pilot trial who were randomized to either the intervention group (LDCT scan) or the control group (usual care). Similar to the above studies, these findings demonstrate a significant increase in odds of smoking cessation at long-term follow-up (up to 2 years) among patients with positive scans compared to patients who received negative results or individuals in the control group who did not receive a scan.

On the contrary, several studies have failed to demonstrate a significant relationship between severity of results and smoking cessation [37, 38]. Van der Aalst et al. [44]

reported that within a subcohort of patients from the Dutch–Belgian Randomized Controlled Lung Cancer Screening Trial (NELSON trial), there was no statistically significant difference between abstinence rates and screening results. The study did find, however, that on 2-year follow-up, participants with only negative screens made significantly fewer attempts to quit smoking than participants whose screens required at least one follow-up scan ($p = 0.016$). While the effects of the teachable moment are clear among individuals with a positive scan, the lack of association or potential negative association between screening results and smoking cessation among those with negative scans compared to the former individuals is noteworthy. There is valid concern surrounding receipt of negative results providing an individual with a "license to smoke" or false reassurance that may lead to behavior reflective of risk compensation, or the risk homeostasis theory—a behavioral theory suggesting that with decreases in perceived risk, an individual will partake in subsequent, risk-taking behavior [45]. However, the additional findings indicating a significant relationship between quitting smoking and screening participation provides evidence against the effect of risk compensation [43]. Nevertheless, the need for integration of cessation interventions into lung cancer screening programs to deliver adequate counseling, especially in regard to risk compensation, should be reiterated.

While the potential for integration of these two interventions is obvious, understanding the cost-effectiveness of such is essential to rationalize implementation. By utilizing an actuarial model based on the screening efficacy of previous, well-established studies, Villanti et al. [46] compared the cost-effectiveness of annual lung cancer screening with varying intensities of smoking cessation interventions. This study concluded that while LDCT screening in high-risk populations was highly cost effective on its own, the addition of cessation interventions improved program cost-effectiveness. Whereas the accepted cost-effectiveness threshold for screening in 2012 was $109,000 per quality-adjusted life year (QALY) gained, the estimated cost per QALY gained for screening alone was $28,240. With the addition of smoking-related behavioral therapy or behavior therapy plus pharmacotherapy, the estimated cost per QALY gained decreased to $23,185 and $16,718, respectively.

10.4 Strategies and Obstacles for Implementation

Although the literature remains scarce, there are a handful of studies that describe their experiences with existing programs that have combined lung cancer screening and smoking cessation interventions [47–50]. Pua et al. [16] categorized these programs into two models: independent and integrated. The independent model is defined as a program in which participants are referred to a financially independent third party for smoking cessation treatment either via referrals to outside, person-to-person programs (e.g., counselors or smoking cessation programs) or by distribution of self-help material that contains information on smoking cessation and where to go for assistance. Comparatively, the integrated model is when the party administering the smoking cessation intervention is financially tied to that administering the lung cancer screening.

Clark et al. [47] investigated the efficacy of a smoking cessation intervention implemented within a lung cancer screening program at the Mayo Clinic. This program exemplified the independent model of integration by offering written materials or a list of 10 Internet sites (e.g., Nicotine Anonymous) that provided resources related to smoking cessation to current smokers. Of the smokers randomized to their respective self-help intervention, biochemically confirmed smoking abstinence rates at the 1-year follow-up did not significantly differ between either group (5% in the Internet listings group and 10% in the written materials group; $p = 0.166$). Furthermore, these abstinence rates were comparable to the annual spontaneous quit rate in the general population, suggesting that self-help materials may not be effective and/or sufficient in increasing abstinence rates. However, further analysis indicated that Internet-based resources may be more likely to influence smoking habits. With 68% of individuals who received the list of Internet resources attempting to quit compared to 48% who received written materials ($p = 0.01$), it was proposed that a more tailored approach to providing resources may improve the efficacy of the intervention.

However, it is possible that tailored information may not suffice. In 2012, van der Aalst et al. [50] reported on a randomly selected sample from the NELSON trial who participated in a similar study regarding distribution of self-help material as a smoking cessation intervention. Within this subcohort, participants were provided with either a brochure or tailored smoking cessation information. Again, abstinence rates did not differ between groups, nor did the spontaneous quit rate of the general adult population, despite applying a more tailored approach. As these results corroborate prior findings by Clark et al. [47], it is plausible that simply providing smokers with self-help guides about smoking cessation, whether universal or tailored, does not positively influence cessation.

More recent studies appear to have shifted toward exploration of the integrated model. While the limited size and number of these studies continue to hinder direct comparisons between models and model-specific programs, they do provide insight into factors that may make a program or model more favorable than another. For example, in 2012, Ferketich et al. [48] examined the feasibility of delivering a combined (pharmacotherapy plus counseling), comprehensive abstinence intervention during a lung cancer screening program and the importance of timing for delivering the intervention in relation to the LDCT scan. This two-arm pilot study, one arm receiving the intervention before the LDCT scan and the other arm receiving the same intervention after the LDCT scan, found that receiving the intervention prior to the LDCT scan induced higher abstinence rates at 4-month and 6-month follow-up as compared to the ALDCT group receiving the intervention after the scan. Although statistical analysis was precluded due to the small sample size, these findings suggest clinical significance regarding feasibility, efficacy, and timing of an intensive treatment program and the need for further investigation.

Even more recently, Taylor et al. [51] conducted a pilot study to determine the feasibility and efficacy of an intensive telephone-counseling tobacco abstinence program within a lung cancer screening setting. Current smokers were enrolled in this study from three geographically diverse lung cancer screening programs, asked to complete pre- and post-LDCT and 3-month follow-up telephone assessments, and randomized to the intervention group (up to six sessions of telephone counseling with a trained cessation counselor) or the usual-care group. Quit rates at three months post-randomization were 17.4% in the intervention arm and 4.3% in the usual-care arm ($p < 0.05$). Another randomized-controlled trial conducted by Marshall et al. [52] suggested the importance and efficacy of intensive smoking cessation programs as well as the need to tailor programs to the target population. Heavy smokers from the Queensland Lung Cancer Screening study were randomized to either the control group, which included distribution of printed quit materials and quitline contact details, or the intervention group, which received the same materials as the control group plus one in-person counseling session and audio quit materials. Despite the feasibility of implementation, this study did not find a significant difference in quit rates between the two study arms. These null findings may be a result of implementing a program without regard for the targeted population, as individuals with heavy smoking histories likely require more intensive services.

In light of the previously mentioned studies, it is imperative that several local factors be addressed prior to implementation of a smoking cessation program. Such factors include performance of a needs assessment, availability of resources, and the logistics behind incorporating tobacco treatment into a functioning lung screening program.

10.4.1 Needs Assessment

Prior to implementation of a new program or expansion of an existing program, it is important to assess whether there is a need for the services being offered. With approximately 70% of all smokers expressing a desire to quit and nearly half of the LSS participants in the NLST reported as current smokers [40, 53], integration of smoking cessation and lung cancer screening programs provides a great opportunity to reach the targeted population and to assist with fulfilling their desires around cessation. Additionally, while half of all smokers expressing a desire to quit attempt to actually do so each year, the majority of attempts are unaided, and only 4%–7% of smokers who attempt to quit maintain abstinence for at least 1 year [53, 54]. Therefore, not only is the need for integration of both interventions clear, but the active demand, or request for services, is also likely to be significant. The USPSTF Final Recommendation Statement: Lung Cancer Screening, 2013 is further evidence that there is a need for integration [3]. It states that "all persons enrolled in a screening program should receive smoking cessation interventions . . . [and] the USPSTF encourages incorporating such interventions into the screening program." Furthermore, national coverage decision by the Centers for Medicare and Medicaid Services on lung cancer screening also requires that smoking cessation interventions be offered to current smokers receiving LDCT scans for lung cancer screening. Consequently, addressing the needs of lung cancer screening participants for tobacco dependence treatment, whether or not the individual is actively seeking assistance, is essential and will ultimately assist with program engagement and/or maintenance in order to facilitate long-term abstinence.

Increasing access to a variety of smoking cessation services is a valid means of addressing equitably the needs of a population that seeks such services yet lacks the resources to aid in utilization (e.g., financial resources or means of transportation). With significant evidence supporting the benefit of nicotine replacement therapy (NRT) on abstinence rates [55, 56], ubiquitous access for those in need should be a fundamental goal of smoking cessation programs. However, access to and uptake of NRT are limited due to financial and physical barriers. By assessing the needs of a community, barriers preventing access to treatment can be addressed, and the utilization of services will likely follow. Prior to the addition of NRT to the Minnesota QUITPLAN Helpline in 2002, telephone counseling via state and national quitlines was widely available, yet limited quitlines offered pharmacological therapy, and only 10 quitlines offered this service at no cost to at least some of their callers. In 2002, the Minnesota Partnership for Action Against Tobacco began providing NRT at no cost to the callers of the Minnesota QUITPLAN Helpline, employing the established reach of the quitline to increase NRT access to their callers. The addition of free NRT to their program increased participation from 155 to 679 callers per month. Additionally, the proportion of participants enrolling in multisession counseling and NRT significantly increased 66.6% and 40.0%, respectively. Abstinence rates also increased post-NRT, with 30-day abstinence at 6 months increasing 8.2% and, ultimately, resulting in an eightfold increase in program impact [57].

10.4.2 Resource Availability

Many resources are available for smokers in the United States seeking or considering cessation, including quitlines, self-help materials, support groups, and pharmacotherapy. Despite the breadth of existing programs, it is common that cessation services are underutilized [16, 58]. It also appears to have become regular practice for primary health care providers to not offer these services and, as a result, miss a crucial opportunity to provide cessation counseling to patients. Data from the 2001–2004 National Ambulatory Medical Care Survey [59] uncovered that nearly one-third of all patients surveyed did not have tobacco use information included in their chart. Additionally, 81% of smokers disclosed not having received related counseling from a physician during an office visit. Since it is likely that this lack of care partially explains the underutilization of tobacco cessation services, employing nurse practitioners and other nonphysician clinicians may increase resource availability and reach and assist in providing more comprehensive care with regard to treatment for tobacco dependence.

In fact, incorporating a multidisciplinary team of physicians and nonphysician clinicians into lung cancer screening programs is essential to enhancing the capabilities and strength of each program. With appropriate training, nonphysician clinicians can function as tobacco treatment specialists in order to minimize the disparity between treatment availability and utilization. The U.S. Public Health Service Clinical Practice

Guideline defines a tobacco treatment specialist as someone whose primary profes-
sional role relates to tobacco dependence treatment and possesses the skills, knowledge,
and training to provide effective interventions [60]. While this guideline suggests that
any provider type with sufficient training can fulfill this role, those with a background
in counseling may be better suited as a tobacco treatment specialist. Clinicians with
training in mental health, social work, and/or psychology will be able to provide further support for any psychosocial needs that may present during program evolvement,
such as anxiety or distress related to screening and/or tobacco cessation. However,
many of these providers (e.g., mental health counselors, social workers, or psycholo-
gists) must collaborate with the patient's primary health care provider or make referrals to another provider for prescription cessation medications [16]. Although their
expertise may or may not be in mental health counseling, nurse practitioners trained
in tobacco cessation can also effectively fulfill the position of tobacco treatment specialist. Nurse practitioners are able to write patient orders and provide prescriptions
for cessation medications at time of treatment, which may positively affect treatment
compliance due to increased convenience for the patient and provider.

The Association for the Treatment of Tobacco Use and Dependence (ATTUD), an
organization dedicated to the promotion of and access to evidence-based tobacco
treatment, has established the standards for the core competencies, training, and cre-
dentialing of tobacco treatment specialists [61]. It is highly recommended that any
clinician offering tobacco cessation interventions complete an ATTUD-accredited
tobacco treatment training program. Due to the specialized training and necessary
increase in allotted time per patient visit, nonphysician tobacco treatment specialists
are able to offer more intensive treatment than the brief counseling interventions
typically offered by a primary health care provider. Intensive treatments are usually
longer in duration and might include comprehensive biopsychosocial assessments,
tobacco use history, multisession counseling, individualized quit plans, group support, and follow-up care. Behavioral counseling interventions that include problem
solving, skills training, and support have been shown to be effective in the treatment of tobacco dependence [16]. For individuals not yet ready to quit smoking,
motivational interviewing should be utilized and may be an effective way to initiate
an attempt. As illustrated by studies previously mentioned [37–42], including LDCT
results in the discussion of tobacco cessation may also be a useful tool in increasing
one's readiness to quit.

The context of a lung cancer screening program offers a unique and beneficial
setting for which smoking cessation can be implemented. With a network of clinicians, ranging from the referring physician to the tobacco treatment specialist, there
are many opportunities to reinforce the importance of abstinence and cessation and
provide individualized support for patients. As mentioned, specialized tobacco cessation services offered by lung cancer screening programs should include patient
history assessments, multisession counseling, support groups, and follow-up care as
well as prescriptions or referrals for pharmacotherapy to all active smokers, including
patients who are not yet ready to quit. However, primary health care providers are
not the only individuals missing the opportunity to provide cessation-related care.
According to Ostroff et al. [62], while lung cancer screening sites believe promotion

of smoking cessations to be of high priority, many sites are not adequately providing cessation treatment aside from asking patients routine questions about current smoking status and advising current smokers to quit. Out of a nationwide sample of 93 lung cancer screening sites, only 57%–60% are routinely providing cessation counseling or referring smokers to a quitline. Also of concern, only 37% are routinely recommending cessation medications to patients. With perceived lack of patient motivation to quit, limited time, and lack of staff training as the most commonly mentioned barriers to delivering comprehensive treatment, assessments regarding resource availability are a necessity, especially in regard to size and adequacy of the specialized treatment team.

10.4.3 Treatment Approach

Maintaining engagement in screening and abstinence programs is fundamental to the purpose of such interventions. Therefore, most lung cancer screening programs utilize a program coordinator or nurse navigator to guide patients through the process, making the progression from initial visit to follow-up and/or treatment as seamless as possible. Additionally, it is common practice for this individual to meet with patients prior to their screening to partake in a shared decision-making visit. During this visit, the nurse navigator will assess the individual's smoking history, and, together, the clinician and the patient will discuss the risks and benefits of screening. When a current smoker is identified, a conversation regarding the harms of smoking and the benefits of cessation should be introduced. Despite the patient's readiness to quit, a referral to treatment should be given and contact by the tobacco treatment specialist initiated. If the program follows the independent model, the referral will be to an outside specialist and/or program, while under the independent model, the nurse navigator will refer directly to their program's tobacco treatment specialist [16].

As proposed by Clark et al. [47], creating individualized cessation treatment may improve a program's chances of success. Therefore, by first assessing one's motivation and readiness to quit, the tobacco treatment specialist can utilize the principles of the transtheoretical model of change (Figure 10.1) and appropriately tailor their discussions and treatments to the patient's needs [16, 63]. An initial outreach should be made to the patient addressing what services and resources the program offers. For individuals who are at the precontemplation or contemplation stage, motivational interviewing should be implemented to engage with smokers who are not yet ready to quit or are intending to quit in the future but not yet ready to take action. Smokers who are interested in quitting are invited for an in-person comprehensive assessment. At that point, the individuals who choose to participate in the cessation program may either be referred back to their primary health care provider for minimally intensive treatment, or be offered 8–12 individual counseling sessions, depending on the intensity of treatment required (Figure 10.2) [64]. For patient convenience and to increase compliance, counseling can be offered in person or via telephone, and additional services should be offered. These service may include but not be limited

Precontemplation	**Contemplation**	**Preparation**	**Action**	**Maintenance**
Not intending to take action in the next 6 months	Intending to take action in the next 6 months	Ready to take action in the next 30 days	Have made overt lifestyle changes in the past 6 months	Doing a new behavior for more than 6 months

Figure 10.1 Transtheoretical Model of Change [63]. This figure depicts the theoretical process an individual undergoes when making a behavior change, such as smoking cessation. Although this model is explained as a progressive, unidirectional process, the transition between stages may be more fluid or bidirectional for many individuals.

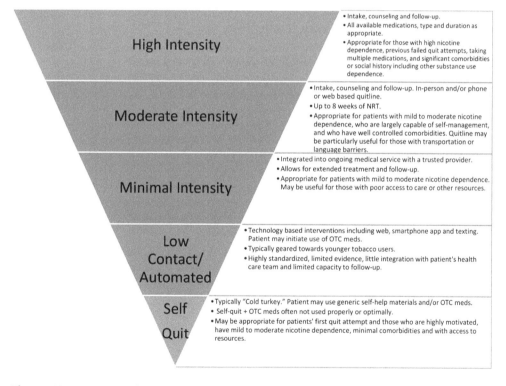

High Intensity
- Intake, counseling and follow-up.
- All available medications, type and duration as appropriate.
- Appropriate for those with high nicotine dependence, previous failed quit attempts, taking multiple medications, and significant comorbidities or social history including other substance use dependence.

Moderate Intensity
- Intake, counseling and follow-up. In-person and/or phone or web based quitline.
- Up to 8 weeks of NRT.
- Appropriate for patients with mild to moderate nicotine dependence, who are largely capable of self-management, and who have well controlled comorbidities. Quitline may be particularly useful for those with transportation or language barriers.

Minimal Intensity
- Integrated into ongoing medical service with a trusted provider.
- Allows for extended treatment and follow-up.
- Appropriate for patients with mild to moderate nicotine dependence. May be useful for those with poor access to care or other resources.

Low Contact/ Automated
- Technology based interventions including web, smartphone app and texting. Patient may initiate use of OTC meds.
- Typically geared towards younger tobacco users.
- Highly standardized, limited evidence, little integration with patient's health care team and limited capacity to follow-up.

Self Quit
- Typically "Cold turkey." Patient may use generic self-help materials and/or OTC meds.
- Self-quit + OTC meds often not used properly or optimally.
- May be appropriate for patients' first quit attempt and those who are highly motivated, have mild to moderate nicotine dependence, minimal comorbidities and with access to resources.

Figure 10.2 Approaches to Tobacco Cessation Treatment [64]. This figure describes the different intensity levels of tobacco cessation treatment our group offers. This approach was adopted from the Tobacco Treatment Specialist Certification (CTTS) Program developed by the ACT Center for Tobacco Treatment, Education, and Research at the University of Mississippi Medical Center.

to information and/or prescriptions for pharmacotherapy, available support groups, and skills training workshops [16].

While a primary benefit of integrated programs is the ability to better tailor their approach based on the needs of individual patients, this model type requires a demanding amount of financial capital, staff, space, and time. Therefore, until more definitive research is published, the extent of integration realized between lung cancer screening and tobacco cessation programs will continue to depend on the resources available.

References

1. American Cancer Society. Cancer facts and figures. 2018. Atlanta, GA: American Cancer Society; 2018.
2. American Cancer Society. Cancer facts and figures. 2015. Atlanta, GA: American Cancer Society; 2015.
3. Humphrey L, Deffebach M, Pappas M, et al. *Screening for Lung Cancer: Systematic Review to Update the U.S. Preventive Services Task Force Recommendation Statement.* Evidence synthesis no. 105. AHRQ publication no. 13-05196-EF-1. Rockville, MD: Agency for Healthcare Research and Quality; 2013.
4. Moyer VA. Screening for lung cancer: U.S. Preventive Services Task Force recommendation statement. *Ann Intern Med.* 2014;160(5):330–338.
5. Marcus PM, Bergstralh EJ, Fagerstrom RM, et al. Lung cancer mortality in the Mayo Lung Project: impact of extended follow-up. *J Natl Cancer Inst.* 2000;92(16):1308–1316.
6. Frost JK, Ball WC, Levin ML, et al. Early lung cancer detection: results of the initial (prevalence) radiologic and cytologic screening in the Johns Hopkins study. *Am Rev Respir Dis.* 1984;130(4):549–554.
7. Oken MM, Hocking WG, Kvale PA, et al. Screening by chest radiograph and lung cancer mortality: the Prostate, Lung, Colorectal, and Ovarian (PLCO) randomized trial. *J Am Med Assoc.* 2011;306:1865–1873.
8. Henschke CI, McCauley DI, Yankelevitz DF, et al. Early Lung Cancer Action Project: overall design and findings from baseline screening. *Lancet.* 1999;354:99–105.
9. International Early Lung Cancer Action Program Investigators, Henschke CI, Yankelevitz DF, et al. Survival of patients with stage I lung cancer detected on CT screening. *N Engl J Med.* 2006;355(17):1763–1771.
10. National Lung Screening Trial Research Team, Aberle DR, Adams AM, et al. Reduced lung-cancer mortality with low-dose computed tomographic screening. *N Engl J Med.* 2011;365(5):395–409.
11. Pham D, Bhandari S, Oechsli M, Pinkston CM, Kloecker GH. Lung cancer screening rates: data from the lung cancer screening registry [abstract]. In: 2018 ASCO Annual Meeting, June 1–5, 2018. Chicago, IL. *J Clin Oncol.* 2018:6504.
12. U.S. Department of Health and Human Services. *The Health Consequences of Smoking—50 Years of Progress: A Report of the Surgeon General.* Atlanta, GA: U.S. Department of Health and Human Services, Centers for Disease Control and Prevention, National Center for Chronic Disease Prevention and Health Promotion, Office on Smoking and Health; 2014.
13. Centers for Disease Control. Current cigarette smoking among adults in the United States. Available at: https://www.cdc.gov/tobacco/data_statistics/fact_sheets/adult_data/cig_smoking/index.htm. Accessed March 24, 2018.

14. Centers for Disease Control. Tobacco-related mortality. Available at: https://www.cdc.gov/tobacco/data_statistics/fact_sheets/health_effects/tobacco_related_mortality/index.htm. Accessed March 24, 2018.

15. Centers for Disease Control. Health effects of secondhand smoke. Available at: https://www.cdc.gov/tobacco/data_statistics/fact_sheets/secondhand_smoke/health_effects/index.htm. Accessed March 24, 2018.

16. Pua BB, Dou E, O'Connor K, Crawford CB. Integrating smoking cessation into lung cancer screening programs. *Clin Imaging*. 2016;40:302–306.

17. Anthonisen NR, Skeans MA, Wise RA, et al. The effects of a smoking cessation intervention on 14.5-year mortality: a randomized clinical trial. *Ann Intern Med*. 2005;142(4):233–239.

18. Peto R, Darby S, Deo H, Silcocks P, Whitley E, Doll R. Smoking, smoking cessation, and lung cancer in the UK since 1950: combination of national statistics with two case-control studies. *BMJ*. 2000;321(7257):323–329.

19. Doll R, Peto R, Wheatley K, Gray R, Sutherland I. Mortality in relation to smoking: 40 years' observations on male British doctors. *BMJ*. 1994;309:901–911.

20. Jha P, Ramasundarahettige C, Landsman V, et al. 21st-century hazards of smoking and benefits of cessation in the United States. *N Engl J Med*. 2013;368(4):341–350.

21. Mai Z, Ho S, Lo C, Wang M, Peto R, Lam T. Mortality reduction from quitting smoking in Hong Kong: population-wide proportional mortality study. *Int J Epidemiol*. 2018. Available at: http://doi.org/10.1093/ije/dyx267.

22. Lewis DR, Check DP, Caporaso NE, Travis WD, Devesa SS. US lung cancer trends by histologic type. *Cancer*. 2014;120(18):2883–2892.

23. Ferketich AK, Niland JC, Mamet R, et al. Smoking status and survival in the national comprehensive cancer network non-small cell lung cancer cohort. *Cancer*. 2013;119(4):847–853.

24. Zhou W, Heist RS, Liu G, et al. Smoking cessation before diagnosis and survival in early stage non-small cell lung cancer patients. *Lung Cancer*. 2006;53(3):375–380.

25. Ebbert JO, Williams BA, Sun Z, et al. Duration of smoking abstinence as a predictor for non–small-cell lung cancer survival in women. *Lung Cancer*. 2005;47(2):165–172.

26. Warren GW, Kasza KA, Reid ME, Cummings KM, Marshall JR. Smoking at diagnosis and survival in cancer patients. *Int J Cancer*. 2013;132:401–410.

27. Japuntich SJ, Kumar P, Pendergast J, et al. Smoking status and survival among a national cohort of lung and colorectal cancer patients. *Nicotine Tob Res*. 2018. Available at: https://doi.org/10.1093/ntr/nty012.

28. Mason DP, Subramanian S, Nowicki ER, et al. Impact of smoking cessation before resection of lung cancer: a Society of Thoracic Surgeons General Thoracic Surgery Database study. *Ann Thorac Surg*. 2009;88(2):362–370 [discussion 370–371].

29. Balduyck B, Sardari NP, Cogen A, et al. The effect of smoking cessation on quality of life after lung cancer surgery. *Eur J Cardiothorac Surg*. 2011;40(6):1432–1438.

30. Richardson GE, Tucker MA, Venzon DJ, et al. Smoking cessation after successful treatment of small-cell lung cancer is associated with fewer smoking-related second primary cancers. *Ann Intern Med*. 1993;119(5):383–390.

31. Parsons A, Daley A, Begh R, Aveyard P. Influence of smoking cessation after diagnosis of early stage lung cancer on prognosis: systematic review of observational studies with meta-analysis. *BMJ*. 2010. Available at: http://dx.doi.org/10.1136/bmj.b5569.

32. Tai EW, Guy GP Jr, Steele CB, Henley SJ, Gallaway MS, Richardson LC. Cost of tobacco-related cancer hospitalizations in the U.S., 2014. *Am J Prev Med*. 2018. Available at: https://doi.org/10.1016/j.amepre.2017.12.004.

33. Tsevat J. Impact and cost-effectiveness of smoking interventions. *Am J Med.* 1992;93(1A):43S–47S.

34. Levy DE, Klinger EV, Linder JA, et al. Cost-effectiveness of a health system-based smoking cessation program. *Nicotine Tob Res.* 2017;19(12):1508–1515.

35. An LC, Schillo BA, Kavanaugh AM, et al. Increased reach and effectiveness of a state-wide tobacco quitline after the addition of access to free nicotine replacement therapy. *Tob Control.* 2006;15:286–293.

36. Tran MT, Holdford DA, Kennedy DT, Small RE. Modeling the cost-effectiveness of a smoking-cessation program in a community pharmacy practice. *Pharmacotherapy.* 2002;22(12):1623–1631.

37. Taylor KL, Sanderson L, Zincke N, Mehta L, McGuire C, Gelmann E. Lung cancer screening as a teachable moment for smoking cessation. *Lung Cancer.* 2007;56:125–134.

38. Ostroff JS, Buckshee N, Mancuso CA, Yankelevitz DF, Henschke CI. Smoking cessation following CT screening for early detection of lung cancer. *Prev Med.* 2001;33:613–621.

39. McBride CM, Emmons KM, Lipkus IM. Understanding the potential of teachable moments: the case of smoking cessation. *Health Educ Res.* 2003;18(2):156–170.

40. Tammemägi MC, Berg CD, Riley TL, Cunningham CR, Taylor KL. Impact of lung cancer screening results on smoking cessation. *J Natl Cancer Inst.* 2014;106(6). Available at: http://dx.doi.org/10.1093/jnci/dju084.

41. Ashraf H, Tønnesen P, Holst Pedersen J, Dirksen A, Thorsen H, Døssing M. Effect of CT screening on smoking habits at 1-year follow-up in the Danish Lung Cancer Screening Trial. *Thorax.* 2009;64:388–392.

42. Townsend CO, Clark MM, Jett JR, et al. Relation between smoking cessation and receiving results from three annual spiral chest computed tomography scans for lung carcinoma screening. *Cancer.* 2005;103:2154–2162.

43. Brain K, Carter B, Lifford KJ, et al. Impact of low-dose CT screening on smoking cessation among high-risk participants in the UK Lung Cancer Screening Trial. *Thorax.* 2017. Available at: http://doi.org/10.1136/thoraxjnl-2016-209690.

44. van der Aalst CM, van Klaveren RJ, van den Bergh KAM, Willemsen MC, de Koning HJ. The impact of a lung cancer CT screening result on smoking abstinence. *Eur Respir J Express.* 2011;37(6):1466–1473.

45. Eaton LA, Kalichman SC. Risk compensation in HIV prevention: implications for vaccines, microbicides, and other biomedical HIV prevention technologies. *Curr HIV/AIDS Rep.* 2007;4(4):165–172.

46. Villanti AC, Jiang Y, Abrams DB, Pyenson BS. A cost-utility analysis of lung cancer screening and the additional benefits of incorporating smoking cessation interventions. *PLoS One.* 2013;8(8):1–11.

47. Clark MM, Cox LS, Jett JR, et al. Effectiveness of smoking cessation self-help materials in a lung cancer screening population. *Lung Cancer.* 2004;44:13–21.

48. Ferketich AK, Otterson GA, King M, Hall N, Browning KK, Wewers ME. A pilot test of a combined tobacco dependence treatment and lung cancer screening program. *Lung Cancer.* 2012;76(2):211–215.

49. Filippo L, Principe R, Cesario A, et al. Smoking cessation intervention within the framework of a lung cancer screening program: preliminary results and clinical perspectives from the "Cosmos-II" trial. *Lung.* 2015;193:147–149.

50. van der Aalst CM, de Koning HF, van der Bergh KAM, Willemsen MC, va Klaveren RJ. The effectiveness of a computer-tailored smoking cessation intervention for participants in lung cancer screening: a randomized controlled trial. *Lung Cancer.* 2012;76:204–210.

51. Taylor KL, Hagerman CJ, Luta G, et al. Preliminary evaluation of a telephone-based smoking cessation intervention in the lung cancer screening setting: a randomized clinical trial. *Lung Cancer.* 2017;108:242–246.

52. Marshall HM, Courtney DA, Passmore LH, et al. Brief tailored smoking cessation counseling in a lung cancer screening program is feasible: a pilot randomized controlled trial. *Nicotine Tob Res.* 2016;18(7):1665–1669. Available at: http://doi.org/10.1093/ntr/ntw010.

53. Fiore MC, Jaén CR, Baker TB, et al. *Treating Tobacco Use and Dependence: 2008 Update. Clinical Practice Guideline.* Rockville, MD: U.S. Department of Health and Human Services, Public Health Service; 2008.

54. Hurt RD, Ebbert JO, Hays JT, McFadden DD. Preventing lung cancer by treating tobacco dependence. *Clin Chest Med.* 2011;32:645–657.

55. Stead LF, Perera R, Bullen C, et al. Nicotine replacement therapy for smoking cessation. *Cochrane Database of Systematic Reviews* 2012;(11). Available at: http://doi.org/10.1002/14651858.CD000146.pub4.

56. Wadgave U, Nagesh L. Nicotine replacement therapy: an overview. *Int J Health Sci (Qassim).* 2016;10930:425–435.

57. An LC, Schillo BA, Kavanaugh AM, et al. Increased reach and effectiveness of a statewide tobacco quitline after the addition of access to free nicotine replacement therapy. *Tob Control.* 2006;15:286–293. Available at: http://doi.org/10.1136/tc.2005.014555.

58. Shiffman S. Smoking-cessation treatment utilization: the need for a consumer perspective. *Am J Prev Med.* 2010;38:S382–S384.

59. Ferketich AK, Khan Y, Wewers ME. Are physicians asking about tobacco use and assisting with cessation? Results from the 2001–2004 National Ambulatory Medical Care Survey (NAMCS). *Prev Med.* 2006;43:472–476.

60. Clinical Practice Guideline Treating Tobacco U, Dependence Update Panel L, Staff. A clinical practice guideline for treating tobacco use and dependence: 2008 update. A U.S. Public Health Service report. *Am J Prev Med.* 2008;35:158–176.

61. Association for the Treatment of Tobacco Use and Dependence. Why join ATTUD? Available at: https://www.attud.org/index.php. Accessed March 24, 2018.

62. Ostroff JS, Copeland A, Borderud SP, Li Y, Shelley DR, Henschke CI. Readiness of lung cancer screening sites to deliver smoking cessation treatment: current practices, organizational priority, and perceived barriers. *Nicotine Tob Res.* 2016;18(5):1067–1075.

63. Prochaska JO, Redding CA, Evers KE. The transtheoretical model and stages of change. In: Glanz K, Rimer BK, Viswanath K, eds. *Health Behavior and Health Education: Theory, Research, and Practice.* 4th ed. San Francisco, CA: Jossey-Bass; 2008:97–121.

64. University of Mississippi Medical Center. *Tobacco Treatment Specialist Certification (CTTS) Program: Workshop Manual 2017B.* Jackson, MS: University of Mississippi Medical Center; 2017.

11

Automatic Lung Segmentation and Interobserver Variability Analysis

Joel C. M. Than, Norliza M. Noor, Luca Saba,
Omar M. Rijal, Rosminah M. Kassim,
Ashari Yunus, Chuen R. Ng, and Jasjit S. Suri

Contents

11.1 Introduction

Lung diseases such as tuberculosis, lower respiratory infections, chronic obstructive pulmonary disease, and lung cancer are among the top 10 causes of death worldwide [1]. There are an estimated 9.5 million deaths annually from causes related to lung disease. This is one-sixth of the total annual deaths worldwide [1]. In the United States, lung disease is the third-leading cause of death, and lung disease–related deaths are on the rise [2]. An estimated 400,000 Americans die from lung disease–related cases annually [3].

Interstitial lung Disease (ILD) is a broad category of diseases that share common physiologic and radiologic properties that can be caused by exposure to hazardous materials [4–6]. These disorders mostly have a common trait of progressive scarring or fibrosis of the lung tissue, which decreases oxygen gas exchange at the lungs. In ILD, lung volumes can be reduced, decreasing the lungs' diffusing capacity [7]. The diagnosis of ILD by clinicians is based on the interpretation of the high-resolution computed tomography (HRCT) from CT images.

Computer-aided diagnosis (CADx) systems serve a complementary role to radiologists. CADx helps by providing a "second opinion" to a radiologist [8]. Since looking at large numbers of CT images is very laborious and can lead to fatigue, radiologists have an interest in implementing CADx-based systems for assistance in diagnostic evaluations. CADx systems can help in the classification of diseased areas and the quantification of their masses [9, 10]. Radiologists serve to validate and test these systems. Current medical regulatory requirements mandate human interaction to be present in a medical system for it to be clinically implemented [11].

Automated segmentation is one of the preliminary and crucial steps in the development of a CADx system to help radiologists [12]. Most automated lung segmentation systems are evaluated through a comparison of their segmented regions with lung segmentations or manual tracings done by a lung expert. For this chapter, the diagram in Figure 11.1 shows an overview of the two major components used in this

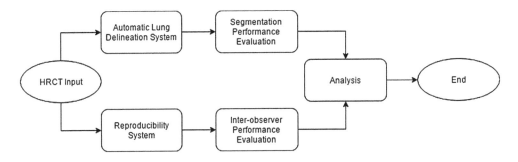

Figure 11.1 Overview flow diagram of systems utilized.

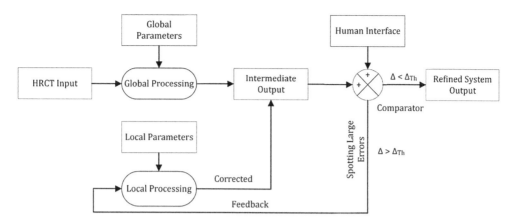

Figure 11.2 Flow diagram of automated lung segmentation system (ALDS) (used with permission).

study. The first component is an automatic lung segmentation system, and the second component is the reproducibility system. In the lung segmentation system, its performance is evaluated, whereas in the reproducibility system, the three observers are evaluated.

The first focus of this study is the automated lung segmentation system (Automatic Lung Delineation System [ALDS]) that is paired with a human interaction system, which is all part of Figure 11.1 and is shown in Figure 11.2 [13]. This system utilizes an initial automated lung segmentation using a threshold-based strategy combined with morphology and is termed global processing. Human interaction was introduced in the form of the manual tracing done by a trained individual, termed an observer. The human interaction was then compared with the initial segmentation output. This helps to catch large deviations and correct them by using a secondary automated lung segmentation based on a texture paradigm, termed local processing. The texture paradigm mentioned here involves the use of the texture property of entropy. An entropy filter was used as an additional segmentation method. Other segmentation techniques used widely include but are not limited to thresholding [14], active contours [15], region growing [16], and texture-based methods [17].

Since the human interaction mentioned thus far is in itself a source of error, there could exist two sources of variability [18]. The first variability is intraobserver variability, where the same observer may be inconsistent in the measurement of the lung [19]. The second variability is the interobserver difference that the system shows when more than one observer is introduced. The observers' manual tracing is considered the gold standard or ground truth (GT). As the system is not definitive, it is especially important to study the variability from both sources. In addition, the process of tracing can be tedious and time consuming, which leaves room for variability from one observer to another [20]. For this study, there were three observers enlisted to perform manual tracings. This study used three observers because they can easily reach a majority decision when deciding the validity of a system since the number of observers is an odd number. Ideally, the more observers, the better. However, there were only three observers available to do manual tracings for this study.

The second focus of study is interobserver variability. It is beneficial to explore the effects of different observers in the ALDS segmentation system on the segmentation performance yielded. Interobserver variability is a growing factor signified by the numerous studies in different fields where the manual tracing relies on an input by an expert. Related studies have been done in different areas including, ventricular wall motion [21], carotid intima media thickness [22], pulmonary nodules [23, 24], lesions [10, 25], lung "honeycombing" [26], and tumors [27–29]. However, there are also various other studies that showed interobserver variability on lung borders produced from automated lung segmentation [30–33].

Thus, the goal of study is to investigate the interobserver variability in automated lung segmentation and its performance. The main contribution of this study is that it performs the interobserver analysis over a relatively large database of 96 patients, which introduces diversity to the study. The presence of patients from three main categories (healthy patients, ILD patients, and non-ILD patients) also increases the diversity of the patient data. Since the study uses three observers, it allows for the validation of the segmentation system and the study of the effect of introducing different human interaction with diverse data to a segmentation system. The main limitation of this study was that only interobserver variability was studied; intraobserver variability was not studied due to a lack of resources and time.

The first observer (Obs-1) is a novice radiologist pursing his medical residency with lesser experience, whereas both the second (Obs-2) and the third (Obs-3) observers are trained biomedical image scientists and have more experience. The interobserver variability was studied using various methods to see both visually and numerically the difference(s) of having multiple observers. The general statistics of the observers' tracings and the analysis of variance (ANOVA) was demonstrated in this study. Next, the performance of the automatic segmentation system compared to the three observers was demonstrated using the following performance measures: Dice Similarity Coefficient (DSC), Jaccard index, and Hausdorff distance. To determine the acceptability of an observer who has lesser experience, the Observer Deterioration Factor (ODF) was computed, which was shown to be less than 10% for each observer, which was an acceptable criterion for our analysis. The study here defines the rule of ODF being less than 10% based on the observer being able to perform at least a 90% similarity to that of an experienced observer in order to be accepted. The value of 90% here shows the same reliability and accuracy as that of an experienced observer.

One approach to observe the difference between observers figuratively is using the Bland-Altman (BA) plot. The BA plot uses the Bland-Altman method, which demonstrates the level of agreement between two methods measuring the same variable [34]. Statistically the difference between observers was shown using the t test, Mann-Whitney test, and chi-square test [35, 36]. The correlation and regression tests were also performed to show the agreement between observers. In Table 11.1, the

TABLE 11.1   Abbreviations Used in This Study and Their Definitions (Used with Permission)

Abbreviations	Definition
Obs	Observer
Obs-1	Observer 1
Obs-2	Observer 2
Obs-3	Observer 3
DSC	Dice Similarity Coefficient
JI	Jaccard index
ANOVA	Analysis of variance
HD	Hausdorff distance
ALDS	Automatic Lung Delineation System
BA	Bland-Altman
ILD	Interstitial lung disease

abbreviations used in this study are displayed for ease of understanding. The abbreviations listed here are the most commonly used throughout the text.

The limitation of this chapter is that it evaluates only the interobserver variability and not the intraobserver variability. This is due to the limited resources and time in this study. However, when more resources become readily available, the authors would like to investigate the intraobserver variability as well. For future works, the authors would like to evaluate the observer variability in a three-dimensional (3D) perspective since this study was limited to 2D analysis.

11.2 Materials and Methods

11.2.1 Data Acquisition and Patient Demographics

HRCT thorax images were obtained from the Department of Diagnostic Imaging of Kuala Lumpur Hospital with ethical clearance granted for 96 patients. Images were recorded using a Siemens Somatom Plus4 CT scanner from May 2011 to June 2012. Each slice was attained at 10–30-mm intervals of patients in the supine position during full suspended inspiration. All images were processed to be in the size of 512 by 512 pixels. For each patient, a senior radiologist determined the five slices to represent the disease based on anatomical landmarks. The anatomical landmarks for the five levels were as follows: level 1, aortic arch; level 2, trachea carina; level 3, pulmonary hilar; level 4, pulmonary venous confluence; and level 5, 1–2 cm above the dome of the right hemidiaphragm. The 96 patients consisted of 15 healthy (normal cases) and 81 diseased cases. The diseased cases consisted of ILD patients and non-ILD lung disease–related patients (non-ILD cases). There were 48 male patients and 48 female patients ages 18–90 years. Figures 11.3 and 11.4 show examples of normal and diseased lungs, respectively.

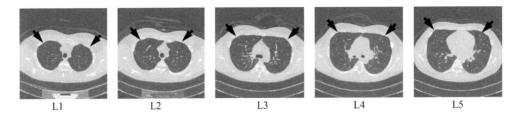

Figure 11.3   Five levels of HRCT lungs (normal) (used with permission).

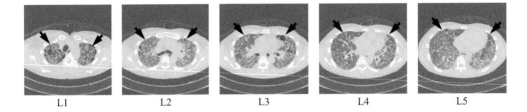

Figure 11.4   Five levels of HRCT lungs (abnormal) (used with permission).

11.2.2 ALDS

The ALDS was developed by members of the Advanced Diagnostics and Progressive Human Care (Diagnostics) Research Group in the UTM Razak School in collaboration with Global Biomedical Technologies, Inc. (Roseville, CA, USA), as shown in the flowchart in Figure 11.2 [13]. The system involves a global processing and a local processing. The global processing consisted of two types of threshold-based and morphology operations that include dilation and erosion. The first type of threshold method used was Otsu's threshold method, which finds the optimum threshold to separate the image into two classes for the variance between the classes to be minimum [37]. This threshold was applied to remove the body pixels from the surroundings. Second, an empirical threshold was used to separate the lung pixels from the body pixels. The global parameters included the threshold value of −324 HU, the structure element used for morphology operation, which was a "square" that is 3 × 3 pixels in size. This global processing yielded the initial segmentation.

11.2.2.1 Global Segmentation System
The idea behind the global system is to capture the shape of the lung by differentiating the lung from its background. The regional information has statistics associated with it that are based on Hounsfield units (HU) generated from the X-ray attenuation. These HU values have specific ranges for the lung region on a global scale. These HU can be well captured by considering a two-class paradigm. Thus, our objective is to develop a class segregation system that can pick up regional statistics considering the two-class problem. A simple approach can be a threshold criterion embedded with statistical means and standard deviations. A fast and robust

method, such as the classical Otsu threshold paradigm, can be adapted for our model development [37].

Even though such a threshold scheme may not be a novel contribution in the proposed work, it contributes as a component to fetch the global lung shape, incorporating deviations that are corrected by our novel feedback system, leading to final estimated accurate borders. Using such a framework, if ω_i represents the probability that the two classes are separated by threshold (t) and σ_i^2 represents the variance of the classes, the Otsu paradigm can lead to the formation of an equation for optimal threshold computation that is mathematically given as equation 1:

$$\sigma_\omega^2 = \omega_1(t)\sigma_1^2(t) + \omega_2(t)\sigma_2^2(t) \tag{1}$$

Thus, we can get the optimum threshold given by T_{opt} when it fits the criteria of the minimum variance of the classes in equation 2. With a given input image, such as Figure 11.5(a), using T_{opt}, it is possible to separate the nonbody, represented by black pixels, from the body, represented by white pixels, as shown in Figure 11.5(b):

$$\sigma_\omega^2 = \omega_1(T_{opt})\sigma_1^2(T_{opt}) + \omega_2(T_{opt})\sigma_2^2(T_{opt}) \tag{2}$$

To completely remove the background tissues, the global system requires an iterative process to establish a complete isolation of the lung region in the CT lung image. This iterative threshold was empirically determined based on the bias of the global Otsu threshold. Such a refinement ensured that all regions not relevant to the lung region were eradicated for quantification. We call this threshold T_{emp}, and it was defined for our database as 324 for our dynamic range. T_{emp} was applied, and the lung region is represented in the body as shown in Figure 11.5(c). The last stage of the global shape extraction system consisted of smoothing and cleaning using binary morphology. The binary morphology consisted of dilation followed by erosion. The results from morphological cleaning are shown in Figure 11.5(d). This consisted of a fundamental dilation and erosion equation expressed as equations 3 and 4, respectively:

$$I \oplus H = \left\{ z \in E \,|\, \left(H^S\right)_z \cap I \neq \varnothing \right\} \tag{3}$$

$$I \ominus H = \left\{ z \in E \,|\, H_z \subseteq I \right\} \tag{4}$$

where E is a Euclidean space or an integer grid and a binary image in E, H^S is the symmetric of H, $(H^S)_z$ is the translation of H^S by the vector z, H is the square structuring element (3×3 size), and H_z is the translation of H by the vector z.

Connected component analysis (CCA) was used to detect the lung region in the binary image shown in Figure 11.5(e). There should be two large regions, where one region is larger than the other. In some cases where the lungs are in close proximity,

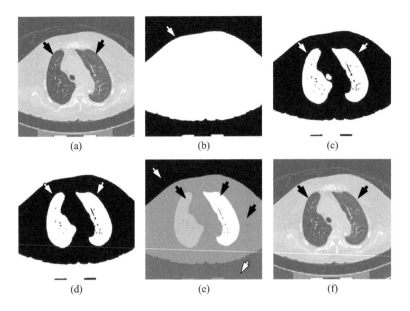

Figure 11.5 Overview of global processing: (a) Input image. (b) Mask image. (c) Iterative threshold output. (d) Morphological cleaning. (e) CCA. (f) Labeled image (used with permission).

they will be grouped as one. The region where the two lungs connect is usually the lowest pixel width of the lung region. To solve this, dynamic programming was done by calculating the lowest pixel width of each column to locate the region of separation. Pixels with the highest contrast were selected as the region of splitting between two lungs. Once two lungs were detected, erosion and dilation with the same structure element were again done to smoothen the boundary of the lungs, and the boundaries were labeled in green boundaries for the right and the left lung in Figure 11.5(f).

When the error criterion was exceeded, local processing was done on the initial segmentation. The error criterion was the error difference between the initial segmentation and the lung segmentation done by the lung image experts. Large errors would indicate poor segmentation. This would show that the particular lung analyzed is a diseased lung. This feature adds the ability of the segmentation system to detect possible erroneous segmentations and easily correct them. The local processing is a refined segmentation based on the texture property, entropy of the image, and morphology operations of dilation and erosion. This refined segmentation will deal with the segmentation that could not be done through the global processing.

11.2.2.2 Local Segmentation System

Segmentation of structures in medical images is challenging due to several factors, including anatomical differences, abnormalities, image noise, and differences in acquisition parameters [38]. As a result of the above challenges, it is always advisable to have a human trained system that can act as a tool to provide the correction to the global system challenges. Such a system was presented in Figure 11.2 using the control system analogy by providing the feedback to correct the global challenges using the local system. Local parameters mentioned in Figure 11.2 include the structure element used, which is a 3×3-pixel "square." The local system we provided uses the local characteristics of the lung region. Such characteristics had two motives: (1) to classify the normal versus diseased lungs and (2) to be able to automatically track the borders of the left and right lungs so that deviations can be traced against the human-trained system. Since the nature of the tissues in the diseased lung and normal lung could better be represented by aggressiveness of the tissue, we used the fundamental property of surface randomness to segregate the normal versus diseased lungs. Thus, we adapted a texture paradigm that had the property of tracing the tissues of diseased lungs compared to normal lungs. This texture was best adapted using the textured or entropy of the pixels in lung regions. We modeled this using entropy of the image, defined as equation 5:

$$Entropy = -\sum_i P_i \log_2 P_i \qquad (5)$$

where P_i is the probability that the difference between two adjacent pixels is equal to i and $\log_2$ is the base 2 logarithm.

This distinguishing feature led to the correction of global weakness. To bring back in the classical framework of morphology, we have to compute the regional characteristics of the lung region followed by binarization. The regional characteristics of the lung were split into two categories: one for undersegmentation and another for oversegmentation. Once the regional characteristics were determined, an empirical computed threshold can be applied. There are two possible thresholds. The first is for undersegmentation (ϑ_{Under}), and the other is for oversegmentation (ϑ_{Over}). Next, the same clinical noise reduction and CCA were applied. Although the feedback system offered the advantage of correction, it did require the automated spotting of the global system weakness. This can be done by the comparator system, which provides the human-trained system, which consisted of the database of human-trained borders from the human intervention system. The effect of the local system is shown in the shift of lung region symbolized by the green borders and arrow in Figure 11.6 when compared to the global system.

11.2.3 Manual Delineation

In this study, manual tracings by three observers were used to study the effect of having different tracers. The first observer is a novice trainer who is a resident in radiology under the guidance of a radiologist (L.S.) and therefore has less experience. The second and third observers (C.R.N. and J.C.M.T) are lung image scientists trained by a lung radiologist (A.Y.) and biomedical imaging scientist and experts

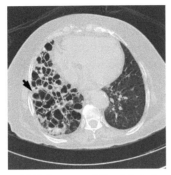 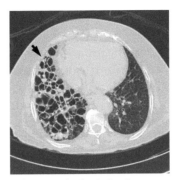

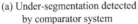

(a) Under-segmentation detected   (b) Correction by the local system
   by comparator system   using control feedback system

Figure 11.6   Feedback control system showing the segmentation correction using local system (used with permission).

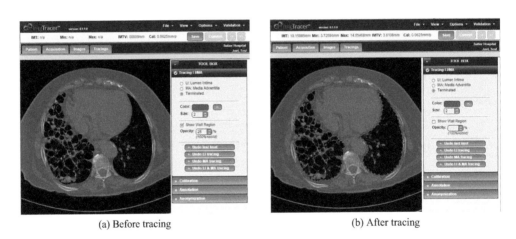

(a) Before tracing   (b) After tracing

Figure 11.7   ImgTracer system used for tracing the manual lung borders. (a) Web-based ImgTracer has loaded the CT lung image. (b) Boundary traced for lungs (courtesy of AtheroPoint, Roseville, CA, USA) (used with permission).

(J.S.S. and N.M.N.). All tracings were done independently using the same software, called ImgTracer (AtheroPoint, Roseville, CA, USA/Global Biomedical Technologies, Inc., Roseville, CA, USA), as shown in Figure 11.7.

11.2.4 Interobserver Analysis

Statistical analysis was done to compare the lung area from the tracings of observers and the lung area segmented using the ALDS. The lung area was calculated for each lung using segmentation borders and GT borders from the observers. The length of

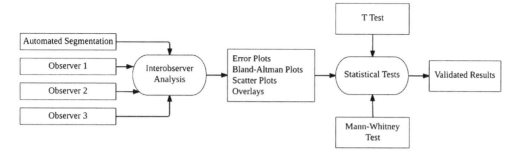

Figure 11.8   Interobserver variability system overview (used with permission).

each pixel was obtained from each DICOM header. The area was counted as shown in equation 6:

$$A = h \times l \qquad (6)$$

where h = height of the pixel (mm) and l = length in (mm). Area (A) is in mm². The interobserver analysis is the reproducibility component in Figure 11.1. The system used for the variability analysis in this research is shown in Figure 11.8. The inputs of this proposed system are the output from the ALDS system mentioned before and the three manual segmentations of the lungs from the three observers. These four inputs were analyzed with summary statistics, and the performances of the segmentation based on all three observers were compared. The summary statistics were calculated for both right lung and left lung area. This included the mean, variance, standard deviation (SD), relative standard deviation (RSD), standard error of the mean (SEM), minimum, maximum, and median. After this was completed, the error plots were drawn. The error plots included BA plots, regression plots, and overlays of the segmentation by the ALDS system together with manual segmentations by the three observers. The next step of the system was to evaluate the interobserver variability with a t test and a Mann-Whitney test. These two tests functioned to show the variability of the observers when compared to one another for both right and left lungs. Eventually, this leads to the validation of the variability tests between the observers.

11.3 Results

The results of the interobserver analysis are shown in the following four subsections. The general analysis subsection shows the summary statistics of the left lung and right lung. The second subsection shows the ALDS segmentation performance compared with all three observers. The third subsection presents the comparison of the three GTs where intervariability is in the form of BA plots and where one GT represents one axis. Finally, the final subsection shows the classification capability of the ALDS segmentation system to identify normal and diseased lungs based on the delineated GT lung area by all observers.

TABLE 11.2 Summary Statistics of the Manual Tracing Done by Three Observers for the Right Lung (Used with Permission)

Obs	Area of Right Lung (1,000 mm²)								
	Mean	95% CI	Var	SD	RSD	SEM	Med	Min	Max
Obs-1	10.542	10.261–10.823	9,461.206	3.076	0.029	0.143	10.459	1.123	19.491
Obs-2	10.427	10.151–10.702	9,113.126	3.019	0.029	0.140	10.334	1.117	19.773
Obs-3	10.421	10.147–10.696	9,041.789	3.007	0.029	0.140	10.295	1.116	19.727

Abbreviations: Obs, observer; CI, confidence interval; Var, variance; SD, standard deviation; RSD, relative standard deviation; SEM, standard error of the mean; Med, median; Min, minimum; Max, maximum.

TABLE 11.3 Summary Statistics of the Manual Tracing Done by Three Observers for the Left Lung (Used with Permission)

Obs	Area of Left Lung (1,000 mm²)								
	Mean	95% CI	Var	SD	RSD	SEM	Med	Min	Max
Obs-1	8.04917	7.831–8.268	5,704.412	2.388	0.0297	0.111	7.939	1.231	14.008
Obs-2	7.95435	7.740–8.169	5,515.769	2.349	0.0295	0.109	7.867	1.350	14.020
Obs-3	7.95556	7.742–8.169	5,454.474	2.335	0.0294	0.108	7.869	1.327	13.991

Abbreviations: Obs, observer; CI, confidence interval; Var, variance; SD, standard deviation; RSD, relative standard deviation; SEM, standard error of the mean; Med, median; Min, minimum; Max, maximum.

11.3.1 General Analysis

11.3.1.1 Area of Left and Right Lung Traced by Observers

Tables 11.2 and 11.3 show the variability between all three observers and the summary statistics of the right lung and left lung for all three observers (Obs). The means for Obs-2 and Obs-3 were very similar at 10,427 and 10,421 mm² for the right lung and 7,954.35 and 7,955.56 mm² for the left lung, respectively. Obs-1 had a higher mean than Obs-2 and Obs-3, with 10,542 mm² as a mean area for the right lung and 8,049.17 mm² for the left lung. The other parameters listed also differed in a similar manner.

11.3.1.2 Data Normality Test for Three Observer Tracings

The normality of the tracings from the three observers was also tested using the D'Agostino-Pearson test. The test computes a p value based on the coefficients of skewness and kurtosis. Obs-1 yielded a p value of 0.08 and Obs-2 a p value of 0.10, whereas Obs-3 yielded a p value of 0.08 for both right and left lungs. The p values of all three observers were above 0.05, which suggested normality for all three observers.

11.3.1.3 ANOVA Test Between Observers and Automated System (ALDS)

Further, an ANOVA test was also performed on the segmented lung area corresponding to the three observers and the automated system, as shown in

TABLE 11.4   ANOVA Calculation for the Right Lung Area Tracing Using Three Observers and the Automated Lung Area (Used with Permission)

Source	DF	Adj SS	Adj MS	F Value	p Value
Obs	3	5.65E+06	1.88E+06	0.204	0.893
Error	1,844	1.70E+10	9.22E+06		
Total	1,847	1.70E+10			

Abbreviations: Obs, observers; DF, degrees of freedom; Adj SS, adjusted sum of squares; Adj MS, adjusted mean square

TABLE 11.5   ANOVA Calculation for the Left Lung Area Tracing Using Three Observers and the Automated Lung Area (Used with Permission)

Source	DF	Adj SS	Adj MS	F Value	p Value
Obs	3	5.40E+06	1.80E+06	0.319	0.811
Error	1,844	1.04E+10	5.64E+06		
Total	1,847	1.04E+10			

Abbreviations: Obs, observers; DF, degrees of freedom; Adj SS, adjusted sum of squares; Adj MS, adjusted mean square.

Tables 11.4 and 11.5, respectively. The ANOVA test results show that the p value (0.893) for the right lung (Table 11.4) and the p value for the left lung (0.811) (Table 11.5) are above 0.05.

11.3.2 Performance Evaluation of ALDS Against Three Observers

11.3.2.1 Performance of ADLS Using the Jaccard Index and the DSC Against Three Observers
Next, the performance of the ALDS segmentation is shown when compared with three different observers. This is done by comparing the output of the ALDS segmentation with three different observers' manual tracings. The similarity of the ALDS segmentation compared to the GT from the observers is measured to evaluate the ALDS system performance. To do this, the study used the DSC and the Jaccard index for both left lung and right lung. The DSC and Jaccard index were calculated and are tabulated in Tables 11.6 and 11.7.

For the right lung, the DSC mean values were 97.25%, 98.58%, and 98.53%, and the Jaccard index mean values were 94.69%, 97.24%, and 97.15%, for Obs-1, Obs-2, and Obs-3, respectively. For the left lung, the DSC mean values were 96.70%, 98.21%, and 98.26%, and the Jaccard index mean values were 92.75%, 96.52%, and 96.62% for Obs-1, Obs-2, and Obs-3, respectively. The results show that for both the left lung and the right lung, Obs-2 and Obs-3 gave a higher similarity. This suggests that Obs-2 and Obs-3 managed to give relatively comparable performances of segmentation because they are more similar and have less variability between them compared to Obs-1.

TABLE 11.6 Performance Evaluation of ALDS Using the Right Lung (Used with Permission)

Level	DSC			Jaccard Index		
	Obs-1	Obs-2	Obs-3	Obs-1	Obs-2	Obs-3
L1	97.26	98.55	98.43	94.79	97.20	97.02
L2	97.35	98.66	98.58	94.87	97.37	97.21
L3	96.95	98.43	98.39	94.11	97.02	96.85
L4	96.75	98.39	98.44	93.74	96.86	96.95
L5	97.94	98.87	98.83	95.98	97.78	97.70
Mean	97.25	98.58	98.53	94.69	97.24	97.15

TABLE 11.7 Performance Evaluation of ALDS Using the Left Lung (Used with Permission)

Level	DSC			Jaccard Index		
	Obs-1	Obs-2	Obs-3	Obs-1	Obs-2	Obs-3
L1	97.54	98.71	98.70	95.23	97.47	97.46
L2	97.02	98.48	98.49	94.25	97.01	97.04
L3	96.30	98.30	98.37	92.91	96.67	96.80
L4	96.10	97.64	97.79	92.53	95.44	95.73
L5	96.59	97.96	97.99	93.48	96.06	96.09
Mean	96.70	98.21	98.26	93.66	96.52	96.62

11.3.2.2 Performance of ALDS Using Hausdorff Distance Against Three Observers
We adapted the Hausdorff distance (HD) as a metric for computing the performance of ALDS. Here, we compute the HD between the automated lung borders and the manually traced lung borders using three observers. Since HD in principle extracts the maximum distance from one point of the automated lung border to another point of the manual traced lung border, any difference between these two borders is amplified. When comparing the two lung borders, say, A and B, HD is mathematically expressed as $H(A, B)$ and computed mathematically according to equation 7 [39–42]:

$$H(A,B) = \max(h(A,B), h(B,A)) \tag{7}$$

and h (A, B) is expressed as equation 8:

$$h(A,B) = \max_{a \in A} \min_{b \in B} \| a - b \| \tag{8}$$

where $\| a - b \|$ is the underlying Euclidean distance between point a and point b. Point a is any point along the border A, and point b is any point along the border B. Therefore, $h(A, B)$ in essence ranks each point of the border A based on its nearest point on the border B and uses the largest distance or highest rank as the distance. Note that $h(B, A)$ is computed the same way as $h(A, B)$. Using the above formulation, HD was computed for the left and right lungs, shown in Table 11.8.

TABLE 11.8 HD Performance of ALDS on the Right and Left Lungs (Used with Permission)

	HD (mm)					
	Right Lung			Left Lung		
Level	Obs-1	Obs-2	Obs-3	Obs-1	Obs-2	Obs-3
L1	7.33	3.73	4.26	8.62	4.80	3.59
L2	18.31	11.43	12.71	15.54	8.92	9.55
L3	19.70	10.42	11.48	19.45	9.65	9.12
L4	26.62	11.87	12.02	19.83	11.23	11.06
L5	15.79	9.13	10.00	14.13	8.98	9.79
Mean	17.55	9.32	10.09	15.51	8.72	8.62

It can be seen that level 1 showed the lowest HD for all three observers for both right and left lungs. This suggests that level 1 has the highest segmentation quality. This concurs with the high DSC values represented in level 1 (Tables 11.6 and 11.7). This was just the opposite in level 4, where HD was largest, suggesting the highest difference between the three observers and the automated ALDS system. This again concurs with previous DSC values presented in Tables 11.6 and 11.7. Obs-2 and Obs-3 have the least amount of difference in the HD values and are relatively consistent for all levels (L1–L5) compared to Obs-1. Obs-1 showed the largest difference between Obs-1 and ALDS for all five levels for both left and right lungs. All this is very consistent with our assumptions because Obs-1 is the least trained and is a medical resident compared to the experienced Obs-2 and Obs-3.

11.3.2.3 The ODF and the Interpretation of HD Error for Evaluation of the Observers
On further inspection of the observers' HD values, 90% of tracings from Obs-2 and Obs-3 showed HD less than 20 mm, whereas Obs-1 showed HD less than 30 mm. The deviation of 10 mm corresponded to the lack of experience of Obs-1 compared to Obs-2 and Obs-3. To understand and quantify the tracing performance of Obs-1, we compute the degradation factor of Obs-1 with respect to the other two observers: Obs-2 and Obs-3. The ODF is mathematically expressed as the variability between the observer's HD errors (HDE) per unit lung maximum length. The maximum lung length (L_{max}) was computed as the maximum distance between any two pair of points along the lung boundary. The variability between the observers HDE is the difference of HDE between an observer who is being evaluated (say, A) against a reference observer (say, B). Mathematically, it is expressed as equation 9:

$$\text{ODF(A, B)} = \frac{\left| \text{HDE(A)} - \text{HDE(B)} \right|}{L_{max}} \times 100\% \qquad (9)$$

where HDE(A) is the HDE between ALDS borders and borders taken from Obs-A, while HDE(B) is correspondingly the HDE between ALDS borders and the borders from Obs-B. L_{max} is the mean of the maximum span of the lung space over all the images in the database. Using this concept, we can express ODF between Obs-1 and Obs-2, ODF(1, 2), and between Obs-1 and Obs-3, ODF(1, 3), as equations 10 and 11:

$$ODF(1, 2) = \frac{\left|HDE(\text{Obs-1 }) - HDE(\text{Obs-2 })\right|}{L_{\max}} \times 100\% \tag{10}$$

$$ODF(1, 3) = \frac{\left|HDE(\text{Obs-1 }) - HDE(\text{Obs-3})\right|}{L_{\max}} \times 100\% \tag{11}$$

where $L_{\max}$ is the maximum span of the lung space over the entire database, ODF(1, 2) represents the ODF of Obs-1 against Obs-2, and ODF(1, 3) represents the ODF of Obs-1 against Obs-3. One can now compute the stability of the observer's ability by giving the threshold value on ODF as per the assumption adapted in the medical industry for performance evaluation. Here, the stability of the system can be defined in a regulatory spirit where the medical device can be considered stable under average conditions. Such an assumption leads us to assume that a typical degradation of the performance should be less than 10%, which implies an accuracy of 90%. This means that the ODF should be less than 10% for a system to be accepted as stable; however, it has a potential for improvement under further training. Since both ODF(1, 2) and ODF(1, 3) are less than a threshold deterioration of 10%, this shows that Obs-1 is acceptable.

11.3.3 Interobserver Variability of Ground-Truth Lung Area

11.3.3.1 Correlation Coefficient and Regression Test Between Observers
Next, to demonstrate the similarity between observers, a correlation test and a regression test were done to evaluate the three relationships: Obs-1 versus Obs-2, Obs-1 versus Obs-3, and Obs-2 versus Obs-3. The correlation coefficient (CC) and R^2 coefficient from the region test are presented in Table 11.9. Both the CC and the R^2 coefficient for all relationships show an encouragingly high number that suggests a high degree of similarity across all the observers. One observation that can be noticed is that the Obs-2 versus Obs-3 relationship gave the highest CC value and R^2 value for both right and left lungs, suggesting that Obs-2 and Obs-3 are the most similar to each other.

TABLE 11.9   CC and R^2 Coefficient Between Observers (Used with Permission)

	Right Lung		Left Lung	
Obs	CC	R^2	CC	R^2
Obs-1 vs. Obs-2	0.9939	0.9878	0.9928	0.9857
Obs-1 vs. Obs-3	0.9941	0.9882	0.9928	0.9856
Obs-2 vs. Obs-3	0.9996	0.9992	0.9992	0.9985

11.3.3.2 BA Plots

The graphical comparison of the lung area traced by the three observers is done using BA plots for the right and left lungs, as shown in Figure 11.9. From the BA plots, it can be seen that the difference between the manual tracing of Obs-2 and Obs-3 is in a higher agreement compared to the difference between Obs-1 and Obs-3 and the difference between Obs-1 and Obs-3. This is due to the smaller two SD ranges of the difference between Obs-2 and Obs-3. This in turn shows that the variability between Obs-2 and Obs-3 is relatively lower than the variability between Obs-1 and Obs-2 and the variability between Obs-1 and Obs-3. The low variability means that Obs-2 and Obs-3 managed to produce more similar manual tracings over the different slices of HRCT. A similar behavior was observed for the left lung.

11.3.3.3 t test, Mann-Whitney Test, and Chi-Square Test Between
*   Three Observers and Its Interpretation*

Next, a two tailed *t* test and Mann-Whitney test were done to show the variability of the observers when compared to one another for both right and left lungs. Since there are three observers, there are three categories of relationships, as shown in Table 11.10. Both tests reveal that Obs-2 and Obs-3 have high similarity, with 0.98 and 0.99 for the *t* test and the Mann-Whitney test, respectively, for the right lung (Table 11.10). For the left lung, the values also reflect that of the right lung with 0.99 for both the *t* test and the Mann-Whitney test (Table 11.10). These high numbers indicate that the level of tracing can actually be achieved and be duplicated by another individual. For the cases of Obs-1 and Obs-2, the value of the *t* test and Mann-Whitney test are similar to each other at 0.57 and 0.50, respectively, for the right lung and 0.54 and 0.59, respectively, for left lung. The high *p* values reject the null hypothesis that the observers are completely different.

Besides the *t* test and Mann-Whitney test, a chi-square test was performed to evaluate the three observers, and the results are displayed in Table 11.10. The results from the chi-square test do not show in detail the difference between observers as shown in the *t* test and Mann-Whitney test; however, the results showed that there was a high level of similarity between observers. This can be seen from the *p* value of 0.239, which is more than 0.05 across all relationships between Obs-1, Obs-2, and Obs-3. The *p* value coincides with a contingency coefficient of 0.99 from

TABLE 11.10   *t* Test and Mann-Whitney Test of Interobserver Variability on Both Lungs (Used with Permission)

	Right Lung			Left Lung		
	t Test	Mann-Whitney Test	Chi-Square Test	*T* Test	Mann-Whitney Test	Chi-Square Test
Observer	*p* Value	*p* Value	*p* Value	*p* Value	*p* Value	*p* Value
Obs-1 vs. Obs-2	0.57	0.5	0.239	0.54	0.59	0.239
Obs-1 vs. Obs-3	0.55	0.48	0.239	0.55	0.59	0.239
Obs-2 vs. Obs-3	0.98	0.99	0.239	0.99	0.99	0.239

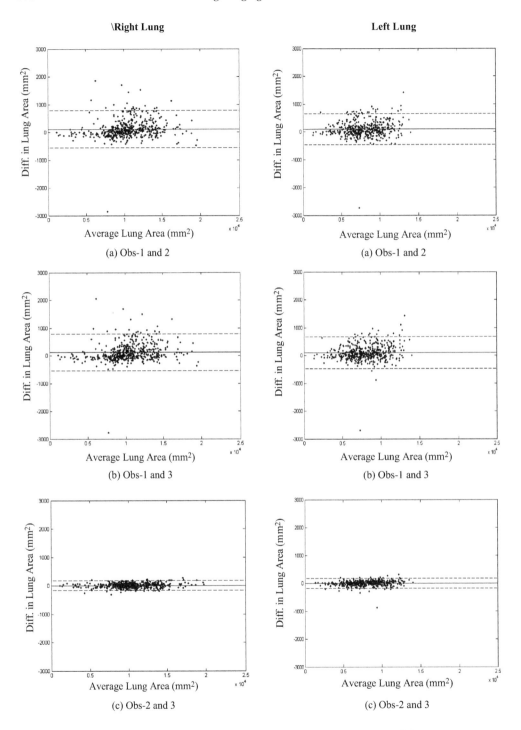

Figure 11.9   BA plots of different observers for the right lung and the left lung.

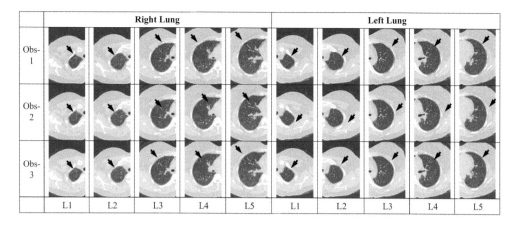

Figure 11.10 Overlay of segmentation (green borders) and three observers (red borders) for normal right lung and left lung (used with permission).

the chi-square test, which also suggests a high degree of association between the observers.

11.3.4 Interobserver Variability Between Diseased and Control Lungs

11.3.4.1 Area Quantification of Diseased Versus Controls Using Three Observers

The observations of the GT from all the observers were then compared to the ALDS segmentation visually in the form of overlays for normal cases in Figure 11.10 and for abnormal cases in Figure 11.11. The green boundaries represent the segmentation, and the red boundaries represent the GT from different observers. For normal cases, the similarity between the green borders and red borders are almost indistinguishable, indicating high similarity. This is because normal lungs are easier to segment due to clearer borders between lungs and body. For abnormal cases, the comparison is done

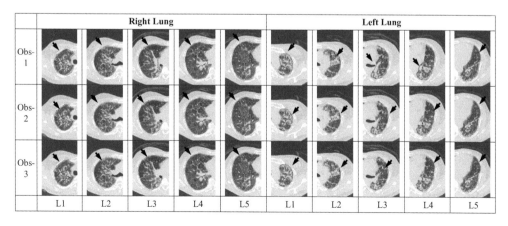

Figure 11.11 Overlay of segmentation (green) and three observers (red) borders for abnormal right lung and left lung (used with permission).

TABLE 11.11   Normal and Abnormal Lung Area from ALDS and GTs from Observers (Obs) for the Right Lung (Used with Permission)

Level	Normal Lung Average Area ($\times$ 1,000 mm^2)				Abnormal Lung Average Area ($\times$ 1,000 mm^2)			
	ALDS	Obs-1	Obs-2	Obs-3	ALDS	Obs-1	Obs-2	Obs-3
L1	7.152	8.0834	7.145	7.138	8.131	8.039	8.041	8.084
L2	8.610	9.706	8.557	8.536	9.766	9.762	9.773	9.706
L3	10.406	10.674	10.328	10.281	10.649	10.853	10.626	10.674
L4	11.566	11.641	11.526	11.466	11.522	11.972	11.649	11.641
L5	12.575	12.336	12.505	12.464	12.159	12.403	12.347	12.336
Mean	10.099	10.506	10.048	10.013	10.462	10.625	10.505	10.506

TABLE 11.12   Normal and Abnormal Lung Area from ALDS and GTs from Observers (Obs) for the Left Lung (Used with Permission)

Level	Normal Lung Average Area ($\times$ 1,000 mm^2)				Abnormal Lung Average Area ($\times$ 1,000 mm^2)			
	ALDS	Obs-1	Obs-2	Obs-3	ALDS	Obs-1	Obs-2	Obs-3
L1	6.452	6.419	6.445	6.422	7.199	7.204	7.192	7.251
L2	7.887	7.862	7.832	7.819	8.174	8.329	8.272	8.231
L3	9.333	9.219	9.272	9.228	8.433	8.698	8.440	8.486
L4	9.655	9.766	9.599	9.545	7.768	8.054	7.894	7.869
L5	9.273	9.288	9.228	9.204	7.214	7.411	7.371	7.374
Mean	8.546	8.537	8.501	8.469	7.765	7.949	7.842	7.850

as in Figure 11.11. For example, for Level 4 for the left lung, as shown in Figure 11.11, it can be seen that the green border is farther away from the red boundary and that the green region is smaller than the red region. The abnormal lungs can have complicated and more vague borders between the lungs and body region.

In Tables 11.11 and 11.12, the area of each level of segment is compared to that of the three observers for the right and left lungs. The area of the right lung is typically larger than that of the left lung because of the position of the heart [43]. The diseased lung area theoretically should be smaller than that of normal lungs [7]. However, in certain levels, the diseased lung could actually be a similar size with the GT signifying accurate segmentation. The disease may not be prevalent in certain levels, which would explain the good segmentation in those levels. In Tables 11.11 and 11.12, it can be seen that for certain levels, the area of the abnormal lungs is smaller than that of the normal lungs in Level 4 (L4) and Level 5 (L5) for Obs-2 and Obs-3 for the left lung. The variation between observers can be seen for the normal lung in Table 11.11, where Obs-1 has a higher mean area compared to Obs-2 and Obs-3.

11.3.4.2 Regression Plots of Diseased Versus Controls Using Three Observers
For all three observers, the regression plots indicate the abnormal right lung and left lung labeled "x" and normal right lung and left lung area labeled "o" in Figure 11.12.

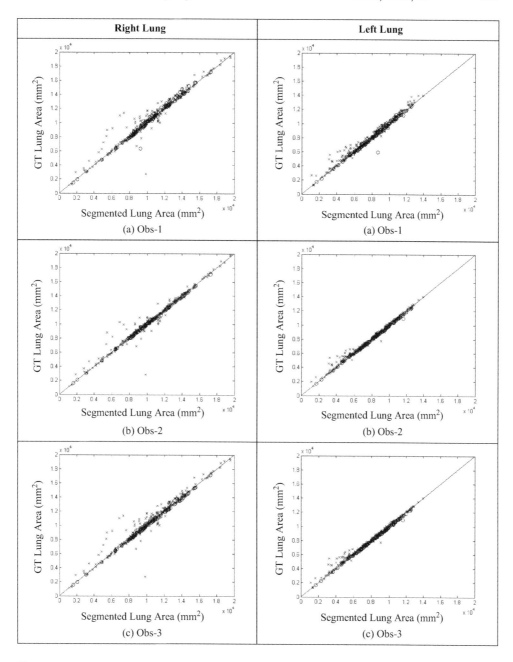

Figure 11.12   Regression plot of normal, labeled "o," and abnormal lung, labeled "x," for the right lung and the left lung (used with permission).

The trend line represents the ideal case where the segmented lung area is identical to that of GT lung area, indicating accurate segmentation. Deviation from the trend line would indicate poor segmentation. It is encouraging that most of the points are close to the trend line, signifying accurate segmentation.

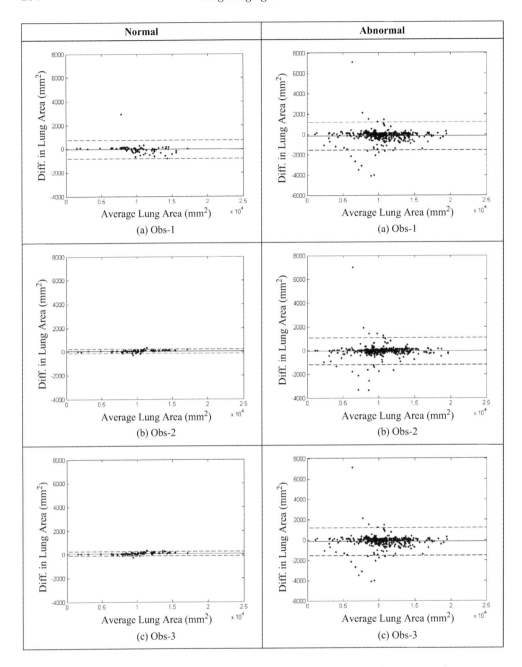

Figure 11.13 BA plot of normal lung and abnormal lung by three observers and segmentation for the right lung (used with permission).

However, from Figure 11.12, it can be seen that most of the large deviations from the trend line are points labeled "x," which are abnormal lungs. This feature is present in the analyses of all three observers. The abnormal lungs can be detected based on the large lung area difference between segmentation and GT for all three observers.

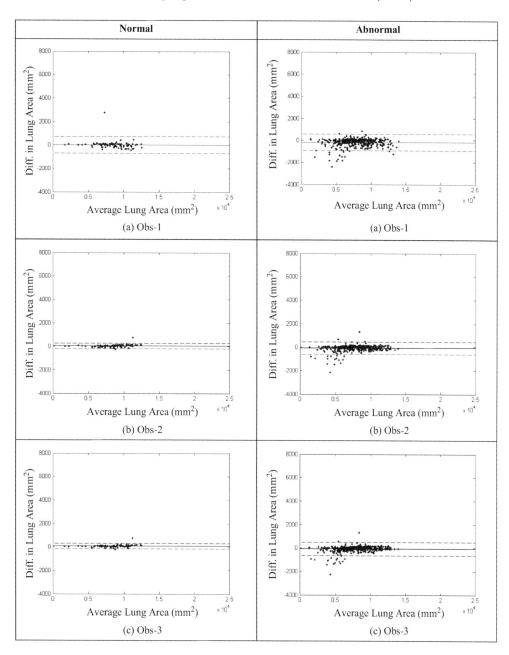

Figure 11.14   BA plot of normal lung and abnormal lung by three observers and segmentation for the left lung (used with permission).

The same feature is seen for the left lung. It is encouraging that all three observers exhibit the feature of abnormal lungs deviating from the trend line.

Graphical representations highlighting the differences between normal and abnormal lungs using BA plots for all three observers are shown in Figures 11.13 and 11.14. It is noticeable that the two standard deviation (2SD) ranges shown as the two dotted lines are larger in abnormal lungs compared to those of the normal lungs for both left and right lungs. This supports the notion that abnormal lungs are detected based on low similarity to that of the GT for all three observers. This difference can be seen in both left and right lungs.

11.4 Discussion

The purpose of this study was to investigate the interobserver variability in the analysis of lung segmentation and segmentation performance. From the "Results" section, we can visually see the high performance of the system for segmentation in the places where the manual borders of all three observers can be totally overlapped against the borders of the segmentation (green) (see Figure 11.10) and the high performance numbers summarized in Tables 11.6 and 11.7. The general statistics from Tables 11.2 and 11.3 show that Obs-1 is slightly different than Obs-2 and Obs-3. The BA plots in Figure 11.9 show that Obs-1 has a higher difference when compared with Obs-2 and Obs-3. When compared with Obs-3, Obs-2 has a smaller difference shown by the smaller 2SD ranges.

In terms of outliers, comparisons of Obs-1 versus Obs-2 and Obs-1 versus Obs-3 have more spread-out outliers as compared to the Obs-2 versus Obs-3 comparison, as seen for the right lung and the left lung in Figure 11.9. When the outliers are removed, the 2SD ranges decreased for all comparisons, suggesting that the observers are more in agreement. The decrease in 2SD ranges signifies that the observers show less variability when the outliers are removed. These outliers are actually samples of manual tracing that observers differ in. This difference can be due to a difference of opinion or an error in tracing. This is possible considering that manual tracing is not definitive and the process of tracing is a long and tedious process that may give rise to fatigue [20]. From the comparison 2SD ranges in Figure 11.9, it can be suggested that Obs-2 versus Obs-3 had the highest agreement, denoted by the smaller 2SD ranges. Thus, Obs-2 and Obs-3 are relatively similar and have less variability compared to Obs-1.

The effect of different observers on the system is shown by the difference in performance of segmentation, as shown in Tables 11.6 and 11.7. For the right lung, the DSC values were 97.25%, 98.58%, and 98.53% for Obs-1, Obs-2, and Obs-3, respectively. In terms of the Jaccard index for the right lung, the three observers yielded 94.69%, 97.24%, and 97.15% for Obs-1, Obs-2, and Obs-3, respectively. For the left lung, the DSC values were 96.70%, 98.21%, and 98.26% for Obs-1, Obs-2, and Obs-3, respectively. The Jaccard index values for the left lung were 92.75%, 96.52%, and 96.62% for Obs-1, Obs-2, and Obs-3, respectively. These values showed that the ALDS segmentation accuracy was still high for three observers with a small difference. This shows that the ALDS system was able to segment the lung with an acceptable accuracy for all three observers compared with their manual segmentations. This is of significance especially to validate that another observer could repeat the high performance of the ALDS segmentation. Obs-2 repeated the same high performance achieved by Obs-3.

In the case of Obs-1, a comparable performance was achieved compared to all other observers.

The p values in Table 11.10 suggest and support the notion that Obs-2 and Obs-3 are very similar, with high p values of up to 0.98 and 0.99 for the right and the left lung, respectively. This suggests that another person can repeat a similar level of tracing, and that is very encouraging. When comparing Obs-1 versus Obs-2 and Obs-1 versus Obs-3, both yield values that are satisfactory and suggest that there is variability between observers. The p values for both the t test and the Mann-Whitney test increased significantly when the outliers from the BA plot are removed for Obs-1 versus Obs-2 and Obs-1 versus Obs-3 comparisons. The rise in p values indicates the ability of the tracings to be more similar with the omission of outliers. Thus, the observers have the ability to have less variability, which shows that the level of manual tracing can be repeated. The chi-square tests show that the p values for all relationships are higher than 0.05; thus, the observers are not independent from one another. We also show the CC and R^2 coefficient, which show the similarity between the observers. The relationship between Obs-2 and Obs-3 showed the highest CC of 0.999, which is slightly higher than 0.994 for both the Obs-1 versus Obs-2 and Obs-1 versus Obs-3 relationships, respectively, as seen in Table 11.9.

In addition to showing segmentation performance, introducing different observers could also affect the ability of the ALDS segmentation system to determine abnormal lungs. From the regression plots in Figure 11.12, we can see that all three observers produced visually very similar plots. The feature of abnormal lungs causing the most deviation from the GT is evident in all three observers' segmentations for both left and right lungs. BA plots for each observer for both abnormal and normal lungs are shown in Figures 11.13 and 11.14. For both left and right lungs, the abnormal plots were visually similar. For normal lungs, Obs-1 was noticeably different than Obs-2 and Obs-3 for both the left lung and the right lung. The 2SD ranges represented by dotted lines had a larger range in Obs-1. This represents the variability introduced when a different observer is enlisted. Although there was a difference between Obs-1 compared to Obs-2 and Obs-3, the 2SD ranges of normal lungs are smaller than abnormal lungs for all observers. This can be said to support the difference between normal and abnormal lungs.

There are a few possibilities of variability for this case of comparison. The first is the number of points done by an observer. More points used gives a more accurate and detailed tracing and vice versa. On average, the points traced by Obs-2 and Obs-3 are higher than that of Obs-1. Figure 11.15 shows an example of tracing. Obs-1 traced 49 points, Obs-2 traced 102 points, and Obs-3 traced 92 points. Due to the fewer number of points by Obs-1, details such as those indicated by the white arrows in Figure 11.15 are left out. From here, it can be said that since the fewer number of points decreases the detail of the tracing, it also causes the similarity coefficient to vary as well. From a randomly selected 10 images, the average points plotted were 43, 89, and 70 for Obs-1, Obs-2, and Obs-3, respectively. Obs-1 has significantly fewer points than Obs-2 and Obs-3 for these 10 images. Overall, Obs-1 also has the least DSC of all three observers

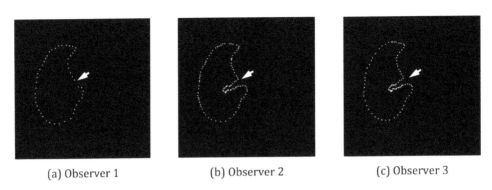

Figure 11.15   Sample of observers' tracing of the right lung (used with permission).

at 97.25% compared to that of 98.58% and 98.53% for Obs-2 and Obs-3, respectively. Thus, the fewer number of points traced results in a less detailed tracing and could lower the system's performance. However, the results still show an encouraging correlation between the system's output and all three observers' tracings. However, since the ODF was less than 10%, the tracings of Obs-1 are acceptable but can be improved with rigorous training.

Similar studies done for interobserver variability, such as a study by Hu et al. [14], proposed a segmentation algorithm that was tested on eight normal patients and compared between two observers. In this study, the distance between the segmentation and GT was calculated based on pixels and presented in the form of mean, max, and root mean square. Comparatively, our study had three observers and 96 patients consisting of 15 normal and 81 abnormal patients. Our study showed results visually as well as numerically using various methods.

Nery et al. [30] conducted an interobserver analysis compared with lung segmentation based on a watershed method. The study compared the performance of segmentation based on two observers who were physicians. The difference between the segmentation and the observers' segmentation was calculated with the DSC and Pratt's figure of merit. Observer analysis was done on two images. The study had two types of comparison. The first was done between observers only, and the second was done between the observers and the segmentation algorithm for two patients. This comparison is considered limited because of the low number of patients. In our study, we compared three observers to each other and compared the segmentation across 96 patient images. Another work by Nery et al. [31] evaluated the interobserver analysis based on Pratt's figure of merit and mean error compared to lung segmentation based on a watershed method [31]. The work also evaluated the BA plots of the difference of area and pixels of the lung segmentations from the observers and segmentation method. However, the work was also based on three observers alone on 41 CT slices, which is relatively small in terms of data.

Santos et al. [33] conducted an interobserver analysis compared with a lung segmentation method based on gray-level thresholding. The study did the analysis on

30 randomly selected images from eight patients. The observers were six radiologists. Although the number of observers was high, the number of randomly selected images to be evaluated was very low. Santos et al. [33] compared the observers' tracings based on Pratt's figure of merit, mean distance, and maximum distance. Kuhnigk et al. [32] also evaluated the interobserver variability compared with a lung segmentation method based on a watershed method, The study compared results from five observers on 24 patients. This again is relatively low in terms of number of patients compared to our study. Kuhnigk et al. [32] showed an incomplete difference between observers by showing the volume and mean distance for the right lung only.

The strength of this chapter is that it was able to demonstrate the variability and agreement between observers visually through various plots as well as numerically through various methods. In addition, the study also evaluated three observers for a relatively large database of 96 patients. The relatively high number of patients utilized offers diversity of data that consist of patients with normal lungs, ILD lungs, and non-ILD lungs. This allows validation to be done for the segmentation accuracy from all three observers. This chapter also investigates the characteristic of the segmentation system, which requires human interaction; thus, having diverse data would give a more holistic presentation of segmentation with different observers.

The limitation of this chapter is that it evaluates only interobserver variability and not intraobserver variability. This is due to the limited resources and time in this study. However, when more resources are made available, the authors would like to investigate intraobserver variability as well. For future work, the authors would like to evaluate the observer variability in a 3D perspective since this study was limited to 2D analysis.

11.5 Conclusion

This study performed the interobserver variability analysis of the manually traced lung borders by three observers compared against the automated segmentation system. The study presented the following statistical tests: (1) a test for normality using the D'Agostino-Pearson test, (2) an ANOVA test for studying the similarity between observers, and (3) significant difference tests using the t test, Mann-Whitney test, and chi-squared test. We showed that all three sets of tests were successful, which includes normality and ANOVA. The t test, Mann-Whitney test, and chi-square test showed that there is no significant difference for all three observers. The regression test showed a high degree of correlation between all observers. The performance indices DSC and Jaccard index between observers and the automated system for the right lung were 97.25% and 94.65%, respectively, for Obs-1; 98.58% and 97.24%, respectively, for Obs-2; and 98.53% and 97.15%, respectively, for Obs-3. For the left lung, the performance indices DSC and Jaccard index were 96.70% and 93.66%, respectively, for Obs-1; 98.21% and

96.52%, respectively, for Obs-2; and 98.26% and 96.62%, respectively, for Obs-3. Mean HD for Obs-2 and Obs-3 are less than 10 mm, while Obs-1 is less than 20 mm, which is consistent with the experience and assumptions of the three observers. Although Obs-1 has less experience compared to Obs-2 and Obs-3, the ODF shows that Obs-1 has less than a 10% difference compared to the other two, which is within the acceptable range as per our analysis.

Acknowledgments

This research was supported by the Research University Grant GUP QK130000.2540.06H35, Universiti Teknologi Malaysia, and Ministry of Higher Education, Malaysia. We would like to thank Dr. Amir Zeki, Pulmonary and Critical Care Medicine Division, University of California, Davis, School of Medicine, Davis, CA, USA, as well as all the clinicians and radiologists who contributed and made this study a success. We are grateful to AtheroPoint LLC, Roseville, CA, USA, for gracefully letting us use ImgTracer 1.0 software for tracing the manual borders of the lung. We would like to thank Springer Nature for allowing us to reuse, in part or in full, figures and text from previously published papers from the *Journal of Medical Systems* titled "Inter-Observer Variability Analysis of Automatic Lung Delineation in Normal and Disease Patients" (2016) and "Automatic Lung Segmentation Using Control Feedback System: Morphology and Texture Paradigm" (2015).

References

1. World Health Organization. *World Health Statistics 2011*. Geneva: World Health Organziation; 2011.
2. Centers for Disease Control and Prevention. Deaths: final fata for 2005. *Natl Center Health Stat Rep*. 2008:56.
3. Centers for Disease Control and Prevention. Deaths: final data for 2004. *Natl Vital Stat Rep*. 2007:55.
4. Sharman P, Wood-Baker R. Interstitial lung disease due to fumes from heat-cutting polymer rope. *Occup Med*. 2013;63:451–453. Available at: http://www.ncbi.nlm.nih.gov/pubmed/23881118.
5. O'Dwyer DN, Armstrong ME, Cooke G, Dodd JD, Veale DJ, Donnelly SC. Rheumatoid arthritis (RA) associated interstitial lung disease (ILD). *Eur J Intern Med*. 2013;24:597–603. Available at: http://www.ncbi.nlm.nih.gov/pubmed/23916467.
6. Schwarz MI, Matthay RA, Sahn SA, Stanford RM, L B, Scheinhorn DJ. Interstitial lung disease in polymyositis and dermatomyositis: analysis of six cases and review of the literature. *Medicine*. 1976;55:89–104.
7. Peroš-Golubičić T, Sharma O. *Clinical Atlas of Interstitial Lung Disease*. New York, NY: Springer; 2006.
8. Doi K. Computer-aided diagnosis in medical imaging: historical review, current status and future potential. *Comput Med Imaging Graph*. 2007;31:198–211. Available at: http://www.sciencedirect.com/science/article/pii/S0895611107000262.

9. Korfiatis P, Kalogeropoulou C, Karahaliou A, Kazantzi A, Skiadopoulos S, Costaridou L. Texture classification-based segmentation of lung affected by interstitial pneumonia in high-resolution CT. *Med Phys*. 2008;35:5290–5302.

10. Singh S, Maxwell J, Baker JA, Nicholas JL, Lo JY. Computer-aided classification of breast masses: performance and interobserver variability of expert radiologists versus residents 1. *Radiology*. 2011;258:73–80.

11. Nandy K. Interactive segmentation and tracking in optical microscopic images. *Cytometry Part A*. 2012;81:357–359.

12. Nagaraj S, Rao GN, Koteswararao K. The role of pattern recognition in computer-aided diagnosis and computer-aided detection in medical imaging: a clinical validation. *Int J Comput Appl*. 2010;8:18–22.

13. Noor NM, Than JCM, Rijal OM, Kassim RM, Yunus A, Zeki AA, et al. Automatic lung segmentation using control feedback system: morphology and texture paradigm. *J Med Syst*. 2015:1.

14. Hu S, Hoffman E a, Reinhardt JM. Automatic lung segmentation for accurate quantitation of volumetric X-ray CT images. *IEEE Trans Med Imaging*. 2001;20:490–498. Available at: http://www.ncbi.nlm.nih.gov/pubmed/11437109.

15. Wang A, Yan H. Delineating low-count defective-contour SPECT lung scans for PE diagnosis using adaptive dual exponential thresholding and active contours. *Int J Imaging Syst Technol*. 2010;20:149–54. Available at: http://doi.wiley.com/10.1002/ima.20222.

16. Dehmeshki J, Amin H, Valdivieso M, Ye X. Segmentation of pulmonary nodules in thoracic CT scans: a region growing approach. *IEEE Trans Med Imaging*. 2008;27:467–480.

17. Devan L, Santosham R, Hariharan R. Automated texture-based characterization of fibrosis and carcinoma using low-dose lung CT images. *Int J Imaging Syst Technol*. 2014;24:39–44. Available at: http://doi.wiley.com/10.1002/ima.22077.

18. van Rikxoort EM, van Ginneken B. Automated segmentation of pulmonary structures in thoracic computed tomography scans: a review. *Phys Med Biol*. 2013;187:R187.

19. Pope A. Reproducibility: intraobserver and interobserver variability. *Biostat Radiol*. 2009:125–140. Available at: http://www.springerlink.com/index/n51421559570263r.pdf.

20. Alberola-López C, Martín-Fernández M, Ruiz-Alzola J. Comments on: a methodology for evaluation of boundary detection algorithms on medical images. *IEEE Trans Med Imaging*. 2004;23:658–660. Available at: http://www.ncbi.nlm.nih.gov/pubmed/15147018.

21. Sheehan FH, Stewart DK, Dodge HT, Mitten S, Bolson EL, Brown BG. Variability in the measurement of regional left ventricular wall motion from contrast angiograms. *Circulation*. 1983;68:550–559. Available at: http://circ.ahajournals.org/cgi/doi/10.1161/01.CIR.68.3.550.

22. Saba L, Molinari F, Meiburger KM, Acharya UR, Nicolaides A, Suri JS. Inter-and intraobserver variability analysis of completely automated cIMT measurement software (AtheroEdge™) and its benchmarking against commercial ultrasound scanner and expert Readers. *Comput Biol Med*. 2013;43:1261–1272.

23. Wormanns D, Diederich S, Lentschig M. Spiral CT of pulmonary nodules: interobserver variation in assessment of lesion size. *Eur Radiol*. 2000;713:710–713. Available at: http://link.springer.com/article/10.1007/s003300050990.

24. Ko JP, Rusinek H, Jacobs EL, et al. Small pulmonary nodules: volume measurement at chest CT—phantom study 1. *Radiology.* 2003;228:864–870.

25. Abdullah N, Mesurolle B, El-Khoury M, Kao E. Breast imaging reporting and data system lexicon for US: interobserver agreement for assessment of breast masses. *Radiology.* 2009;252:665–672.

26. Watadani T, Sakai F, Johkoh T, Noma S. Interobserver variability in the CT assessment of honeycombing in the lungs. *Radiology.* 2013:266. Available at: http://pubs.rsna.org/doi/abs/10.1148/radiol.12112516.

27. van Rikxoort EM, de Hoop B, van de Vorst S, Prokop M, van Ginneken B. Automatic segmentation of pulmonary segments from volumetric chest CT scans. *IEEE Trans Med Imaging.* 2009;28:621–630. Available at: http://www.ncbi.nlm.nih.gov/pubmed/19211346.

28. Erasmus JJ, Gladish GW, Broemeling L, et al. Interobserver and intraobserver variability in measurement of non-small-cell carcinoma lung lesions: implications for assessment of tumor response. *J Clin Oncol.* [Internet]. 2003;21:2574–2582. Available at: http://www.ncbi.nlm.nih.gov/pubmed/12829678.

29. Hopper KD, Kasales CJ, van Slyke MA, et al. Analysis of interobserver and intraobserver variability in CT tumor measurements. *Am J Roentgenol.* 1996;167:851–854.

30. Nery F, Silva JS, Ferreira NC, Caramelo FJ, Faustino R. Automated identification of the lung contours in positron emission tomography. *J Instrum.* 2013;8:C03018.

31. Nery F, Silvestre J, Ferreira NC, Caramelo F, Silva JS, Faustino R. An algorithm for the pulmonary border extraction in PET images. *Procedia Technol.* 2012;5:876–884.

32. Kuhnigk JM, Hahn H, Hindennach M, Dicken V, Krass S, Peitgen HO. Lung lobe segmentation by anatomy-guided 3D watershed transform. *Med Imaging.* 2003:1482–1490. Available at: http://proceedings.spiedigitallibrary.org/proceeding.aspx?articleid=758286.

33. Santos BS, Ferreira C, Sousa Santos B, Silva JS, Silva A, Teixeira L. Quantitative evaluation of a pulmonary contour segmentation algorithm in x-ray computed tomography images. *Acad Radiol.* 2004;11:868–878.

34. Martin Bland J, Altman D. Statistical methods for assessing agreement between two methods of clinical measurement. *Lancet.* 1986;327:307–310.

35. Hollander M, Wolfe DA. *Nonparametric Statistical Methods.* New York, NY: John Wiley & Sons; 1999.

36. Jackson S. *Research Methods and Statistics: A Critical Thinking Approach.* Cengage Learning; 2011.

37. Otsu N. A threshold selection method from gray-level histograms. *Automatica.* 1975;11:23–27.

38. van Rikxoort EM, de Hoop B, Viergever MA, Prokop M, van Ginneken B. Automatic lung segmentation from thoracic computed tomography scans using a hybrid approach with error detection. *Med Phys.* [2009;36:2934. Available at: http://link.aip.org/link/MPHYA6/v36/i7/p2934/s1&Agg=doi.

39. Ali AM, Farag AA. Automatic lung segmentation of volumetric low-dose CT scans using graph cuts. In: Bebis G. et al. (eds) *Advances in Visual Computing.* ISVC 2008. Lecture Notes in Computer Science, vol 5358. Springer, Berlin, Heidelberg. DOI: https://doi.org/10.1007/978-3-540-89639-5_25.

40. Huttenlocher DP, Klanderman GA, Rucklidge WJ. Comparing images using the Hausdorff distance. *IEEE Trans Pattern Anal Mach Intell.* 1993;15:850–863.

41. Acharya UR, Vinitha Sree S, Mookiah MRK, et al. Diagnosis of Hashimoto's thyroiditis in ultrasound using tissue characterization and pixel classification. *Proc Inst Mech Eng Part H J Eng Med.* 2013;227:788–798.

42. Acharya UR, Sree SV, Krishnan MMR, et al. Atherosclerotic risk stratification strategy for carotid arteries using texture-based features. *Ultrasound Med. Biol.* 2012;38:899–915.

43. Churg A. *Thurlbeck's Pathology of the Lung.* New York, NY: Thieme; 2005.

12

Classification of Diseased Lungs Using a Combination of Riesz and Gabor Transforms and Machine Learning

Luca Saba, Joel C. M. Than, Norliza M. Noor,
Omar M. Rijal, Rosminah M. Kassim, Ashari Yunus,
Harman S. Suri, Michele Porcu, and Jasjit S. Suri

Contents

12.1 Introduction

Lung diseases make up the third-leading cause of death in the United States [1]. Deaths related to lung diseases were estimated to be 235,000 in 2010 alone. The main types of lung diseases that contribute to death are airway diseases (58.9%), influenza (21.4%), interstitial (12.3%), pulmonary circulation (5.9%), and neonatal (1.5%). In 2009, asthma, chronic obstructive pulmonary disease, and pneumonia had an economic burden that amounted to $106 billion [1]. In Malaysia, lung cancer is the third-highest occurring cancer and results in 10% patient death. Alarmingly, the majority of lung cancer cases (60%) are detected late in stage IV [2].

High-resolution computed tomography (HRCT) is a noninvasive solution for clinicians to view lung diseases, such as interstitial lung disease (ILD) [3]. There are common lung tissue patterns in ILD, such as ground glass opacities, reticular pattern, pleural thickening, honeycombing, and parenchymal consolidation [4]. A typical CT scan of a patient, as shown in Figure 12.1, may yield 30 to 300 slices, depending on

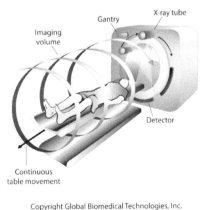

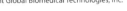
Copyright Global Biomedical Technologies, Inc.

(a) Scanning protocol.

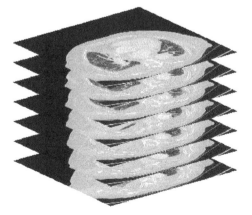

(b) Stack of CT lung slices as 3D display.

Figure 12.1   Scanning protocol for lung using CT scanner (used with permission).

the slice thickness and slice interval. This leads to fatigue in work flow and a drop in diagnostic accuracy [5]. Thus, this creates a further challenge for the radiologist in terms of decision making and risk stratification.

Computer-aided diagnosis (CADx) systems have shown indications of helping to improve diagnostic accuracy [6]. The main functions of CADx systems are to increase the specificity of lung disease detection and to decrease the false-negative rate that is caused by observational oversights. CADx systems are favorable compared to the usage of a second human observer since they do not require straining the demands of an already limited human personnel pool [7]. This study aims to contribute a system of morphological-based risk stratification that may benefit the development of a CADx system to stratify normal and diseased lungs. Such a study involves tissue-based characterization, which requires grayscale feature extraction using a variety of filters. A review of this topic is discussed in section 12.2 of this chapter.

This chapter presents a two-stage cascaded system consisting of (a) a semiautomated lung delineation subsystem (LDS) for lung region extraction (stage A) in CT slices, followed by (b) morphology-based lung tissue characterization (stage B) as shown in Figure 12.2.

We will show that directional transforms of Riesz and Gabor perform better than conventional textural features. We evaluate the accuracy of the machine learning (ML) system using the K-fold cross-validation protocol (K = 2, 3, 5, and 10). The lung database consisted of 96 patients: 15 normal and 81 diseased. We used five HRCT levels of the lung that represented different anatomy landmarks. The five levels of lung CT slices were chosen where disease is commonly seen [8]. Using various feature extraction techniques is important when devising a classification approach. We used five types of feature groups (Riesz transform [RT], Gabor transform [GT], gray-level co-occurrence matrix [GLCM], gray-level run length matrix [GLRLM], and fractal dimension [FD]) and their amalgamation. We used a support vector machine (SVM) classifier with a K-fold approach to split the global population into training data and testing data.

The layout of the study is as follows. Section 12.2 presents a background literature review and our current paradigm. Section 12.3 shows the materials and methods consisting of two subsections. Section 12.3.1 shows the acquisition of the CT lung volumes. The two-stage cascaded system is discussed in section 12.3.2. Experimental

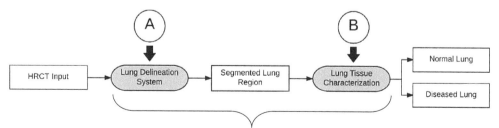

Lung risk stratification system depicted by cascaded two stage process: A and B.

Figure 12.2 Two-stage global system of lung delineation and lung disease stratification system (used with permission).

protocol is presented in section 12.4, while the results are discussed in section 12.5. The performance evaluation of the ML system is shown in section 12.6, followed by its discussion in section 12.7. Finally, the study presents the benchmarking strategies in section 12.8, followed by the conclusions in section 12.9.

12.2 Background Literature Review and Our Current Paradigm

Grayscale feature extraction for the ML paradigm has shown promising results. The GT is a commonly used method for feature extraction. It allows for directional analysis that is also scalable. The GT has a wide application in different classifications for the lung [9], brain [10], liver [11], and carotid [12]. A big advantage of using the GT is that its properties are invariant to illumination, rotation, scale, and translation [13]. The RT is an emerging technique that has a growing application in the medical imaging field [14–16]. Previous studies have shown that it is useful for classification in the lung, liver, and brain. It has shown promising results for classification and tissue characterization. The RT is an effective feature extraction paradigm due to its steerable filter bank. This property allows it to find textural information in various directions that can be used for morphological-based tissue characterization. Further, the RT's property of scalability adds more features and in turn increases the information detected [14–16].

Several authors have tried the GT and RT with limited success in morphological-based tissue characterization without a hybridization paradigm. This study is motivated by recent work by Suri in breast cancer and vascular areas [17–19]. In this study, we take advantage of the directional and scale properties of the RT (24 features) and GT (60 features) by combining them in the ML framework. Along with these, we compute low-level features, such as the GLCM (four features), the GLRLM (11 features), and FD (one feature), thus totaling 100 grayscale features. The understanding of tissue characteristics segregation was introduced using the lung feature segregation index (LFSI) concept, leading to the strategy for dominant feature extraction. Since this system is a two-stage cascaded system, we studied the effect of LDS on tissue characterization models. Finally, another effective contribution is the understanding of the stability and reliability of the system in such an ML paradigm.

12.3 Materials and Methods

12.3.1 Data Acquisition

The data used in this study were in the form of HRCT thorax images that were retrieved retrospectively from the Department of Diagnostic Imaging at the Kuala Lumpur Hospital for 96 patients. These images were taken using a Siemens Somatom Plus4 CT scanner at 10–30-mm intervals of patients in supine position at full inspiration.

Images were in DICOM format and sized at 512×512 pixels. The five levels of each lung were selected by a senior radiologist. The 96 patients were determined by a clinician to be of 15 healthy (normal cases) and 81 diseased cases. The diseased cases consisted of ILD patients and non-ILD patients. Relevant consent was obtained from the ethics board for the use of these anonymized data.

12.3.2 Methodology: Two-Stage Cascaded System

Our cascaded model was developed while keeping in mind that the transmission of information from stage A to stage B has the highest impedance match to maximize the error that is lost. This requires a global system for regional lung extraction followed by a local-based approach for tissue characterization. Further, it is a requirement that the local approach adapting morphological-based feature extraction be less sensitive to the lung regional extraction in the global space, and this is important to have low changes in sensitivity in stage B due to variations in stage A. Keeping these fundamental requirements, we developed a two-stage cascaded model for lung risk stratification. This study was inspired by Suri's work that showed risk stratification for breast and vascular areas [17–19]. In our study, we address the risk stratification problem for lungs by designing a two-stage cascaded (back-to-back) system that works hand in hand to stratify normal and diseased lungs as discussed in Figure 12.2.

The scope of this study is focused primarily on discovering the best amalgamation of the grayscale features for lung risk stratification (so-called stage B), while stage A of the cascaded two-stage system was adapted using our prior study labeled as LDS [20]. Having identified the lung region using the global extraction system, the majority of this study is focused on understanding different directional transforms and combining them with texture features to segregate the diseased lung against controls. Further, we deeply study the feature analysis using a special segregation index, both with and without amalgamation. Since LDS was our previous study, we only briefly discuss stage A as follows.

12.3.2.1 LDS (Stage A)

The LDS consists of a two-stage process that allows automated delineation paired with human interaction from the radiologist to ensure optimal regional lung segmentation [20]. The first stage of delineation, called intermediate segmentation, involves an empirical threshold process and morphology operations. The morphology operations use a structure element ("square") sized at 3×3 pixels for erosion and dilation. The output of the first segmentation is called the intermediate segmented lung, which is compared against the ground truth. If an error criterion is reached, the lung is delineated again by the final segmentation. The second stage of segmentation also uses morphology operations coupled with an entropy filter. The flowchart of this system is shown in Figure 12.3. The output of the final segmentation is a mask of the lung region that is adapted for tissue risk stratification. For reference, samples of the

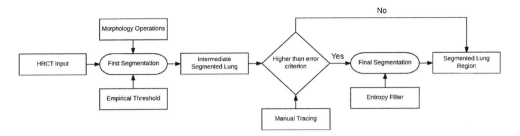

Figure 12.3   Lung delineation system (stage A) (used with permission).

segmented normal lungs and diseased lungs are shown in Figures 12.4 and 12.5. Note that our objective in this study was not to explore segmentation-based systems for lung delineation but rather to explore the different directional transforms while combining them with texture features for lung risk assessment system.

12.3.2.2 Lung Tissue Characterization System (Stage B)

The lung tissue characterization at the heart of the system in stage B is driven mainly by the power to extract the grayscale features by amalgamating the optimized set of transforms. The amalgamation is driven by the motivation that certain sets of features, when adapted in a classification framework during the cross-validation protocol, yield an optimal performance. This is considered a class of hybridization

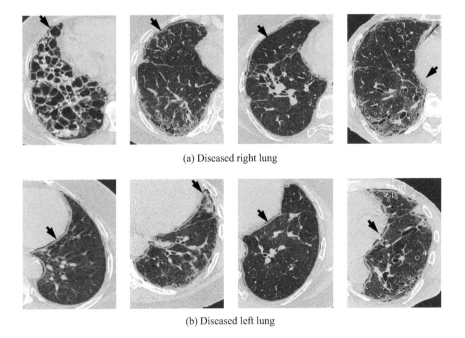

Figure 12.4   Diseased lungs with segmentation boundary (green) and ground truth (red) (used with permission).

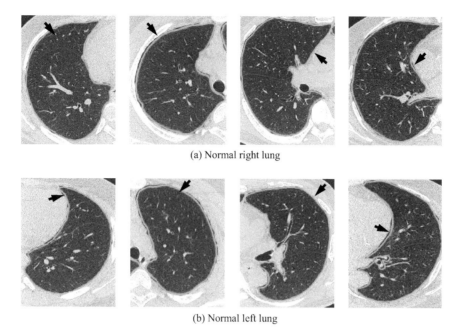

(a) Normal right lung

(b) Normal left lung

Figure 12.5 Normal lung with segmentation boundary (green) and ground truth (red) (used with permission).

procedure. Thus, we need grayscale feature extraction systems or combination of systems that, when amalgamated, yield the highest classification accuracy.

A grayscale feature extraction method that has the ability to both capture the dynamic changes in the tissue characteristics and traverse in a 360° direction is being considered as one of the significant contributions of our study. High-frequency components of an image need to be picked up best in the frequency domain framework. This must be done while ensuring that all the directions are traversed. Thus, we adapted the best-fitting transform, which is named after its property, the RT [21–23]. A second grayscale feature that has the ability to scale while keeping the direction in mind comes from the well-proven filter named the GT [24, 25]. Taking different scales of the lung helps in adapting the fineness and coarseness of the cancerous region in all directions. We take this one step further by picking up the texture components that have chaotic or nonchaotic patterns.

Under the class of texture components, we used the famous Haralick texture using the gray-level co-occurrence framework in conjunction with the run length–based texture paradigm. Even though these features have been applied by our group in some way or another, the novelty of this study is that it combines them for CT-based lung images by formulating a paradigm for tissue characterization and risk stratification. This is depicted by the dotted block (shown by the arrows) in Figure 12.6 while using the cross-validation protocol in the ML framework. The cross-validation protocol depends on the number of patients adapted during the training phase, and we used the conventional four sets of K-fold protocols: (K = 2, 3, 5, and 10). We used the SVM-based classifier, which has been a well-proven and adapted strategy for training

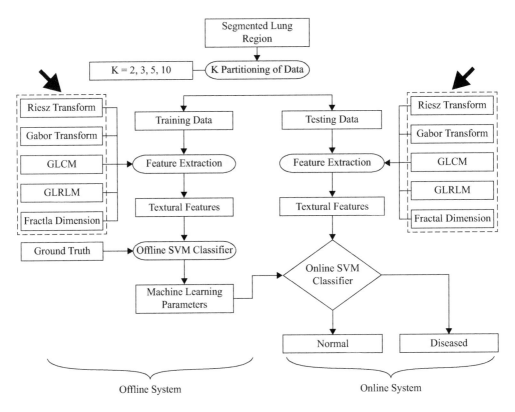

Figure 12.6 Overview of stage B: lung tissue characterization system (used with permission).

and testing phases, as shown in Figure 12.6. Note that the predicted class label for the test patient is estimated by transforming the online grayscale test features (from test patients' lung regional images) using the offline training parameters. Having discussed the global and local systems, we now explore the mathematical formulations of these grayscale features in more detail.

12.4 Grayscale Feature Extraction and Selection

The mathematical formulation of the feature extraction and its amalgamation for best combination selection is presented in this section. The group of five features are RT, GT, GLCM, GLRLM, and FD, resulting in a total of 100 features.

12.4.1 2D RT

The RT is an extension of the Hilbert transform [26]. The function of the RT follows a filter bank strategy. The two main parameters that provide the richness to the RT are "order" and "scale." The RT maps any function $f(x)$ to its harmonic conjugate. For a

Filter 1	Filter 2	Filter 3	Filter 4	Filter 5	Filter 6

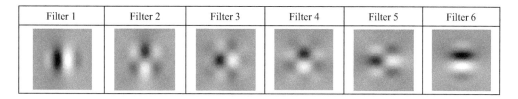

Figure 12.7 Directional filters for the RT using fifth order.

2D function of $f(x)$, the different components of the nth-order RT R are defined in the Fourier domain as equation 1 [26]:

$$\overline{R^{(o_1,o_2)}f(x)} = \sqrt{\frac{o_1+o_2}{o_1!o_2!}}\frac{(-j\omega_1)^{o_1}(-j\omega_2)^{o_2}}{\|\omega\|^{o_1+o_2}}\hat{f}(\omega) \tag{1}$$

where $\hat{f}(x)$ is the Fourier transform of $f(x)$, N is the order of transform where $O = o_1 + o_2$. ω represents the frequency, and ω_1 represents the x-axis and ω_2 the y-axis.

We used the fifth order and four scales using RT. Using the fifth order provides six directional filters or channels, as shown in Figure 12.7. This order adapted is suitable to detect the directional change in texture features.

The application of RT is constrained in a region of interest of 64×64 squared pixels. Since there are six channels (directions) and four scales (resolution), one can obtain a set of 24 images for every input lung region of interest (ROI) image. Since the texture information is represented by the variation in the patterns, one can characterize this variation by computing the variance of these RT images. It is likely that the higher-variance images will represent the chaotic behavior, that is, the disease. This information can then be used for training the SVM classifier for risk stratification.

12.4.2 2D GT

The GT is a powerful application to extract textural information. It has properties of both scalability and steerability. It has an impulse response that can be represented by a sinusoidal wave (a plane wave for 2D Gabor filters with a particular frequency and orientation). The 2D Gabor function, $\psi_{(\alpha,s)}$, can be represented as equation 2 [21]:

$$\psi_{(\alpha,s)}(x,y) = \frac{1}{2\pi\sigma_m\sigma_n}\exp\left\{-\frac{1}{2}\left[\left(\frac{x}{\sigma_x}\right)^2+\left(\frac{y}{\sigma_y}\right)^2\right]\right\} + 2\pi j\omega x \tag{2}$$

where (x,y) are the rectilinear coordinates in the spatial domain, ω is the frequency of the sinusoid, and σ_x and σ_y are the standard deviations of the Gaussian envelopes.

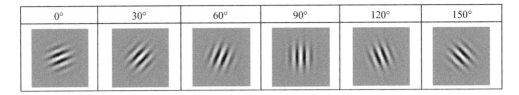

0°	30°	60°	90°	120°	150°

Figure 12.8 Gabor filter representation for different orientations (used with permission).

The 2D Gabor wavelets are obtained by dilation and rotation of the mother wavelet using the Gabor function in equation 3:

$$\psi_{(\alpha,s)}(x,y) = a^{-1}\psi\left[a^{-1}\left(x\cos\theta + y\sin\theta\right), a^{-1}\left(-x\sin\theta + y\cos\theta\right)\right], a>1 \quad (3)$$

where a^{-1} is a scale factor, (α,s) are integers, the orientation θ is given by $\theta = \alpha\pi/\Theta$, and Θ is the number of orientations. Thus, the GT of an image $I(x, y)$ is given by equation 4:

$$G_{(s,\alpha)}(x,y) = I(x,y) * \psi_{(s,\alpha)}(x,y) \quad (4)$$

where $*$ represents convolution operation, α values are such that $\alpha =1, 2, 3 \dots, \Theta$ and Θ is the total number of orientations available, and s represents the scale and takes the values $s = 1, 2, 3 \dots, S$, where S is the total number of scales available. The GT directional filters used are shown in Figure 12.8.

12.4.3 GLCM Texture Features

GLCM is a widely known method of texture extraction. GLCM shows the spatial relationship of neighboring pixels and calculates the occurrence of a pixel with a specific gray level or intensity compared to its neighbors in a number of directions. Textural information is contained in that spatial relationship.

The matrices are designed to measure the spatial relationships between pixels. The method is based on the belief that texture information is contained in such relationships. Using GLCM, the main features observed are energy, correlation, contrast, and homogeneity [27]. A GLCM is denoted here as $c(m, n)$, which is normalized by dividing each element in the matrix by the total number of pixel pairs. These features are represented in equations 5 to 8:

$$\text{Energy (E)} = \sum_m\sum_n\left[c(m,n)\right]^2 \quad (5)$$

$$\text{Correlation (Corr)} = \frac{\sum_m\sum_n(m,n)c(m,n) - \mu_m\mu_n}{\sigma_m\sigma_n} \quad (6)$$

$$\text{Contrast (Co)} = \sum_m \sum_n (m-n)^2 \, c(m,n) \tag{7}$$

$$\text{Homogeneity (Ho)} = \sum_m \sum_n \left[\frac{c(m,n)}{1+(m,n)^2} \right] \tag{8}$$

When disease is present in an image, the probability of having higher textural information increases. This is because lung disease affects the radiologic and morphologic properties of lung tissue. GLCM represents the spatial relationship between neighboring pixels, and within this relationship, we can detect the textural information regarding those pixels. Thus, more information represented by a higher energy, correlation, and contrast may indicate disease. When an image has a high homogeneity, it means that the image does not have much change in textural information, suggesting normality of the image.

12.4.4 GLRLM Texture Features

GLRLM gives a holistic representation of an image. It represents the frequency (j) of pixels that have the same gray-level intensity (i) in specific directions (0°, 45°, 90°, or 135°). GLRLMs are based on a run length matrix (RLM) that can be defined as a set of consecutive, collinear pixels having the same gray level. For this study, we used GLRLM features such as short-run emphasis (SRE), long-run emphasis (LRE), low gray-level run emphasis (LGRE), high gray-level run emphasis (HGRE), short-run low gray-level emphasis (SRLGE), short-run high gray-level emphasis (SRHGE), long-run low gray-level emphasis (LRLGE), long-run high gray-level emphasis (LRHGE), gray-level nonuniformity (GLN), run length nonuniformity (RLN), and run percentage (RP) [28].

The presence of disease may cause fluctuations in grayscale values. This is because lung diseases cause changes to lung tissue that affect their radiologic properties, thus affecting their grayscale values compared to normal patients. These variations cause the RLMs to decrease because of the inconsistency in grayscale values. This feature enables the stratification of diseased and normal patients.

12.4.5 FD Feature

FD can be defined as a ratio that demonstrates the degree of complexity in an image. It analyzes the roughness of a pattern in an image [29, 30]. These details can be also termed a fractal pattern. FD pattern is the measure of the space-filling capacity of a pattern. This gives information of how a fractal scales differently from the space it is embedded in. When disease is present, it can cause lung tissue to have scarring and changes in morphologic properties. This introduces roughness and causes FD to be higher. This is a feature that enables the distinguishability between normal and diseased patients. For this study, the Minkowski method is used to calculate FD [31]. FD can be calculated as D_F in equation 9:

$$D_F = -\frac{\log N(\epsilon)}{\log \epsilon} \qquad (9)$$

where $N(\epsilon)$ represents the total boxes of size and ϵ required to fill the entire area of an image.

12.4.6 LFSI

One of the key aspects in our study is the design of the LFSI, which helps in understanding the segregation power of features. This index is mathematically expressed as equation 10:

$$\text{LFSI}(\%) = \left(\left| \frac{F_N - F_D}{F_N} \right| \right) \times 100 \qquad (10)$$

where F_N represents the mean feature value for normal patients and F_D is the mean feature value for the diseased patients. LFSI has the ability to distinguish the features of normal and diseased lungs. Note that this index shows the normalized percentage difference between the mean diseased lung feature values and mean normal lung feature value.

12.4.7 Feature Selection

Feature selection allows the system to avoid redundant features and features that may contribute in lowering classification accuracies. It allows the optimal number of features to be used. This is particularly important when a large set of features is available. For this study, we used a straightforward feature selection technique that relies on feature dominance. The dominance of each feature is calculated using LFSI. The dominance level is directly proportional to the difference between the mean values of each feature from the two classes. The features are arranged from the most dominant feature to the least dominant feature. In this way, a total of 100 feature combinations are arranged, beginning with the most dominant feature, and are gradually combined with each lesser dominant feature until reaching the least dominant feature. The combination that produced the highest accuracy is used.

12.5 Experimental Protocols

Since the heart of the ML system consists of the grayscale features, we focused on the individual features or combination or hybridization of the features and their roles in the ML system. Since both RT and GT are directional-based filters, we studied the individual power of these features and how they are related to the stratification accuracy. In the second set of experiments, we used a hybridization protocol where we combined the directional-based features with textural-based features to generate the hybrid set of features. Finally, since the data size helps in knowing the diversity of the training parameters, we studied the effect of the size of the data on the stratification accuracy. These are divided into three fundamental experimental protocols.

12.5.1 Experiment 1: Comparing Individual Feature Sets

This study focuses on five types of feature extraction techniques (RT, GT, GLCM, GLRLM, and FD). We compared these five techniques under the same protocol. We used two-, three-, four-, five-, and 10-fold classification protocols using T = 20 trials to ensure generalization and reproducibility. In our study, we use several metrics to evaluate the performance in stratification of the lung disease into normal and abnormal. The 2×2 confusion matrix, consisting of true positive (TP), false positive (FP), true negative (TN), and false negative (FN), was evaluated for all combinations in each fold, where TP is the rate of occurrences that the system was able to classify diseased lungs that were actually diseased lungs, FP is the rate at which normal lungs were identified as diseased lungs, TN is the rate of normal lungs being correctly identified as normal lungs, and FN is the rate at which diseased lungs were identified as normal lungs. Using these, the metrics are as follows: sensitivity (SEN), equation 11; specificity (SP), equation 11; positive predictive value (PPV), equation 12; accuracy (ACC), equation 12; and area under the curve (AUC). AUC is the area under the ROC curve. The ROC curve's vertical axis represents sensitivity, and its horizontal axis represents (100% specificity) [28]:

$$SEN(\%) = \left(\frac{TP}{TP+FN} \right) \times 100 \quad \& \quad SP(\%) = \left(\frac{TN}{FP+TN} \right) \times 100 \tag{11}$$

$$PPV(\%) = \left(\frac{TP}{TP+FP} \right) \times 100 \quad \& \quad ACC(\%) = \left(\frac{TP+TN}{TP+FN+TN+FP} \right) \times 100 \tag{12}$$

12.5.2 Experiment 2: Hybridization of Feature and Its Effect on Accuracy

We hybridized the techniques of RT with other features to form three kinds of feature sets. We used RT, (RT + GLCM), (RT + GT), and (RT + GLCM, + GT + FD + GLRLM). This study used a feature selection technique based on the dominance of each feature. We showed the ability of RT to improve based on the combination of different features. Thus, we are able to combine features based on their ability to stratify diseased and normal lungs. Again, we used all four sets of K-fold classification protocol combinations—two-, three-, four-, five-, and 10-fold—using T = 20 trials to ensure generalization and reproducibility.

12.5.3 Experiment 3: Effect of Training Data on Classification Accuracy

In this experiment, we varied the number of total patients used (N) from 10 patients to 96 patients. A set of possible values were considered: 10, 20, 30, 40, 50, 60, 70, 80, and 96. This gave us nine possible values of total patient size (N). When N changes, the amount of training data changes, but the ratio of normal and diseased patients is set to be the same throughout all possible N values. This is in order to see the effectiveness of classification with different numbers of patients. Again we used two-, five-, and 10-fold classification protocols under trials of T = 20 to ensure generalization and reproducibility. This relationship will also evaluate the memorization versus generalization paradigm [32].

12.6 Results

We demonstrate here the abilities of our risk stratification system in many shapes and forms. First, we show the power of individual features when used in the ML framework. Here, we will see how the ROC curves get increasing AUC values for an increasing feature power set. In the second set of results, we will show how the different combinations of fusions of these features behave in the ML paradigm. This includes the following combinations: (RT + GLCM), (RT + GT), and (RT + GLCM + GT + FD + GLRLM). The third set of results consisted of studying the effect of increasing the population size using different partition protocols. One of the most important innovations of this study lies in understanding which features contribute the most to LFSI when arranged in ascending order of the LFSI values. The last part of the data analysis and results consisted of how the classification accuracy reaches the point of diminishing returns when features are added as per the LFSI. All these results are well covered using the plots and supporting tables.

12.6.1 Classification Accuracy Using Individual Features

Individual features considered in this experiment were GT, RT, GLCM, GLRLM, and FD under different K-fold protocols. Since there are four cross validation (CV) protocols, we show these four tables (Tables 12.1–12.4) corresponding to K = 2 to

TABLE 12.1 Classification Performance with Individual Features Using the K = 2 Protocol (T = 20, N = 96, L = 5) (Used with Permission)

Individual Features	SEN (%)	SP (%)	PPV (%)	ACC (%)	AUC
FD	54.09	52.67	84.96	53.85	0.53
GLCM	75.47	70.37	92.65	74.61	0.73
GT	99.01	95.44	99.08	98.41	0.97
RT	99.18	87.40	97.50	97.20	0.93
GLRLM	63.84	68.67	90.89	64.66	0.66

TABLE 12.2   Classification Performance with Individual Features Using K = 3 Protocol (T = 20, N = 96, L = 5) (Used with Permission)

Individual Features	SEN (%)	SP (%)	PPV (%)	ACC (%)	AUC
FD	54.02	52.80	84.97	53.85	0.53
GLCM	75.61	70.23	92.63	74.71	0.73
Gabor	99.22	96.13	99.22	98.70	0.98
Riesz	99.30	87.75	97.57	97.36	0.94
GLRLM	63.80	69.25	91.04	64.73	0.67

TABLE 12.3   Classification Performance with Individual Features Using K = 5 Protocol (T = 20, N = 96, L = 5) (Used with Permission)

Individual Features	SEN (%)	SP (%)	PPV (%)	ACC (%)	AUC
FD	54.54	52.22	84.96	54.15	0.53
GLCM	75.60	70.23	92.63	74.70	0.73
Gabor	99.36	96.48	99.29	98.87	0.98
Riesz	99.38	87.88	97.60	97.45	0.94
GLRLM	63.83	69.35	91.07	64.77	0.67

K = 10. As can be seen, FD and GLCM showed accuracies below 80% for all K-fold approaches. The highest accuracy was achieved using GT (98.87%) followed by RT (97.45%). This observation suggests the power of GT and RT in stratifying normal and diseased patients. The scalability and directional properties of these two transforms allow them to perform better than others. The highest accuracies were obtained using the 10-fold approach followed by the five-, three-, and two-fold approaches. This happened since the higher the K-fold, the more data are used for training. We also present the ROC curves for the five feature extraction methods (Figure 12.9). The ROC curves concur with the earlier observation that RT and GT perform better compared to the rest of the feature extraction methods.

TABLE 12.4   Classification Performance with Individual Features Using K=10 Protocol (T = 20, N = 96, L =5) (Used with Permission)

Individual Features	SEN (%)	SP (%)	PPV (%)	ACC (%)	AUC
FD	53.61	53.24	85.01	53.55	0.53
GLCM	75.66	70.22	92.64	74.75	0.73
Gabor	99.42	96.74	99.34	98.97	0.98
Riesz	99.43	88.03	97.63	97.52	0.94
GLRLM	63.86	69.35	91.07	64.79	0.67

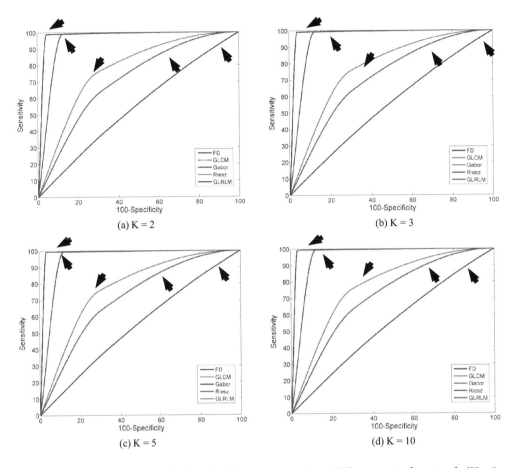

Figure 12.9 ROC curves of individual features using four different sets of protocols (K = 2, 3, 5, 10; T = 20; N = 96; L = 5) (used with permission).

12.6.2 Hybridization of RT and GT Features

Since there are different features available, it is beneficial to hybridize RT and other separate features to form three types of feature hybridization configurations to be compared with the RT alone and in feature combination sets (RT + GLCM, RT + GT, RT + GLCM + GT + FD + GLRLM). The highest accuracy was observed when all five features were used (99.53%). This shows that all features are contributing to improving the segregation index. The RT + GT combination showed the second-highest accuracy results (98.73%), followed by RT + GLCM (98.43%), for all the K-folds, as seen in Table 12.5 (K = 2), Table 12.6 (K = 3), Table 12.7 (K = 5), and Table 12.8 (K = 10). The improvement in accuracy by the combinational feature set against the solo RT feature is intuitive; however, it is important to see the use of RT + GT and RT + GLCM in offering close results that may take less computational time, especially since fewer features were used. This is an encouraging observation that RT is beneficial in stratifying normal and diseased patients. The ROC curves for the features

TABLE 12.5   Classification Performance by Combining Different Features Using K = 2 Protocol (T = 20, N = 96, L = 5) (Used with Permission)

Hybridization Feature Set	SEN (%)	SP (%)	PPV (%)	ACC (%)	AUC
Riesz	99.18	87.40	97.50	97.20	0.93
RT + GLCM	99.13	92.21	98.44	97.97	0.96
RT + GT	99.76	93.05	98.61	98.63	0.96
RT + GLCM + GT + FD + GLRLM	99.35	97.32	99.46	99.01	0.98

TABLE 12.6   Classification Results by Combining Different Features Using K = 3 Protocol (T = 20, N = 96, L = 5) (Used with Permission)

Hybridization Feature Set	SEN (%)	SP (%)	PPV (%)	ACC (%)	AUC
RT	99.30	87.75	97.57	97.36	0.94
RT + GLCM	99.33	92.76	98.55	98.23	0.96
RT + GT	99.78	93.40	98.68	98.71	0.97
RT + GLCM + GT + FD + GLRLM	99.65	98.06	99.61	99.39	0.99

TABLE 12.7   Classification Results by Combining Different Features Using K = 5 Protocol (T = 20, N = 96, L = 5) (Used with Permission)

Hybridization Feature Set	SEN (%)	SP (%)	PPV (%)	ACC (%)	AUC
RT	99.30	87.75	97.57	97.36	0.94
RT + GLCM	99.33	92.76	98.55	98.23	0.96
RT + GT	99.78	93.40	98.68	98.71	0.97
RT + GLCM + GT + FD + GLRLM	99.65	98.06	99.61	99.39	0.99

TABLE 12.8   Classification Performance by Combining Different Features Using K = 10 Protocol (T = 20, N = 96, L = 5) (Used with Permission)

Hybridization Feature Set	SEN (%)	SP (%)	PPV (%)	ACC (%)	AUC
RT	99.38	87.88	97.60	97.45	0.94
RT + GLCM	99.39	92.93	98.58	98.30	0.96
RT + GT	99.77	93.46	98.69	98.71	0.97
RT + GLCM + GT + FD + GLRLM	99.75	98.16	99.63	99.48	0.99

combination can be seen in Figure 12.10. The ROC curves also concur with the accuracies in Tables 12.5–12.8, suggesting that features performed better followed closely by RT + GT and RT + GLCM.

12.6.3 Effect of Increasing the Training Data Size on Classification Accuracy

We also show the accuracies from varying the number of patients, N, for all four folds in Table 12.9. The classification accuracy increases when the number of patients, N, is increased. The classification of the most patients yields the highest accuracy for all

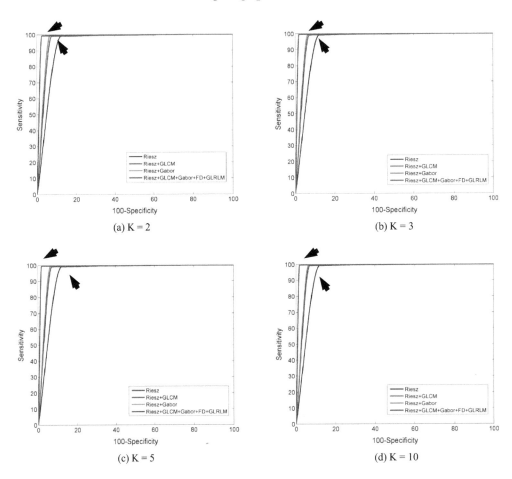

Figure 12.10   ROC curve by combining different features using four different sets of hybrid-ization feature set protocols (K = 2, 3, 5, 10; T = 20; N = 96; L = 5) (used with permission).

TABLE 12.9   Effect of Changing Population on Classification Accuracies for Four Protocols (K = 2, 3, 5, 10; T = 20, N = 96, L = 5) (Used with Permission)

	Accuracy (%)			
N	K = 2	K = 3	K = 5	K = 10
10	94.65	95.28	95.79	95.90
20	95.91	96.66	97.05	97.29
30	97.19	97.76	98.11	98.34
40	97.84	98.43	98.78	98.97
50	98.28	98.77	99.04	99.13
60	98.45	98.93	99.11	99.24
70	98.77	99.17	99.27	99.36
80	99.00	99.33	99.45	99.50
96	99.10	99.40	99.48	99.54

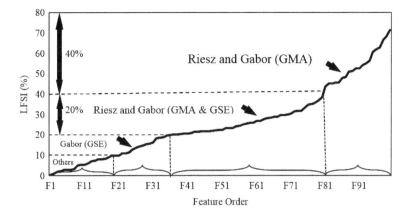

Figure 12.11   LFSI percentages of each feature in ascending order from 1 to 100 (used with permission).

four folds, whereas the classification using the least patients yielded the lowest accuracy for all four folds. It is encouraging that the maximum difference of accuracy is 4.45%, which is less than 5%. This gives an indication of the applicability of the classification system using different data sizes.

12.6.4 Demonstration of Segregation Index for Understanding the Feature Strength

Figure 12.11 shows the distribution of all features and their LFSI values in ascending order. Each feature is arranged in a feature order and represented as F_O. The feature for each F_O is given in Table 12.10. The highest contributions in feature capability to stratify normal and diseased lungs are GMA and RT features. This means that the top 40% of the feature list consists of features that belong to GMA and RT. Further, the LSFI, which covers 20% to 40% of the segregation, is contributed mainly by features such as GSE, GMA, and RT (Figure 12.11).

This is an indication of the effectiveness of the RT and GT methods to offer meaningful textural information for stratifying lung diseases. As shown by the dotted lines in Figure 12.11, the features that range from 10% to 20% of LFSI consists of GT features only. Above that LFSI mark, features consist of RT and GT. Features that contribute below 10% LFSI consist of other sets of features that include FD and GLCM and GLRLM. This observation suggests that directional transforms of RT and GT are stronger compared to general textural features.

12.6.5 Evidence for Optimal Feature Selection and Point of Stable Accuracy

An example of the feature selection used is seen in Figure 12.12. The classification accuracy starts to peak and stabilize when a feature combination of 50 was used. The features that contribute to the peak consist mainly of R and GT (GMA and GSE).

TABLE 12.10   Feature Labels and Feature Order (F$_O$) in Ascending from 1 to 100 (Used with Permission)

F$_O$	Feature Name	F$_O$	Feature Name	F$_O$	Feature Name	F$_O$	Feature Name
F1	H	F26	GSE, F6, S2	F51	GSE, F6, S4	F76	GMA, F1, S2
F2	SRLGE	F27	GSE, F2, S2	F52	GMA, F3, S2	F77	GMA, F6, S3
F3	Co	F28	GSE, F4, S3	F53	GSE, F2, S4	F78	R, F1, S2
F4	SRHGE	F29	GSE, F3, S3	F54	GSE, F1, S4	F79	R, F2, S3
F5	FD	F30	GSE, F1, S2	F55	R, F4, S2	F80	GMA, F2, S3
F6	SRE	F31	GSE, F5, S3	F56	R, F3, S1	F81	GMA, F1, S3
F7	RP	F32	GSE, F6, S3	F57	GMA, F6, S1	F82	GMA, F4, S4
F8	E	F33	GSE, F4, S4	F58	GSE, F6, S5	F83	GMA, F3, S4
F9	LGRE	F34	GSE, F2, S3	F59	GSE, F2, S5	F84	R, F1, S3
F10	HGRE	F35	GSE, F4, S5	F60	R, F2, S1	F85	R, F6, S4
F11	LRLGE	F36	R, F5, S1	F61	GSE, F1, S5	F86	GMA, F5, S4
F12	GLN	F37	GSE, F3, S4	F62	R, F3, S2	F87	R, F5, S4
F13	GSE F4 S1	F38	GSE, F1, S3	F63	GMA, F2, S1	F88	R, F4, S4
F14	GSE F5 S1	F39	R, F6, S1	F64	GMA, F6, S2	F89	GMA, F6, S4
F15	Corr	F40	GMA, F4, S1	F65	GMA, F4, S3	F90	R, F1, S4
F16	GSE F3 S1	F41	GMA, F5, S1	F66	GMA, F3, S3	F91	GMA, F2, S4
F17	LRHGE	F42	GSE, F5, S4	F67	R, F5, S3	F92	R, F3, S4
F18	LRE	F43	GSE, F3, S5	F68	R, F2, S2	F93	GMA, F1, S4
F19	RLN	F44	R, F6, S2	F69	GMA, F5, S3	F94	R, F2, S4
F20	GSE, F6, S1	F45	R, F5, S2	F70	R, F6, S3	F95	GMA, F3, S5
F21	GSE, F4, S2	F46	GMA, F4, S2	F71	GMA, F2, S2	F96	GMA, F4, S5
F22	GSE, F5, S2	F47	GMA, F3, S1	F72	R, F1, S1	F97	GMA, F5, S5
F23	GSE, F3, S2	F48	GSE, F5, S5	F73	GMA, F1, S1	F98	GMA, F2, S5
F24	GSE, F2, S1	F49	R, F4, S1	F74	R, F4, S3	F99	GMA, F6, S5
F25	GSE, F1, S1	F50	GMA, F5, S2	F75	R, F3, S3	F100	GMA, F1, S5

Abbreviations: GSE, Gabor square energy; GMA, Gabor mean amplitude; R, Riesz; F$_O$, feature order; FX, feature orientation, X from 1 to 6; SY, scale order, Y from 1 to 5.

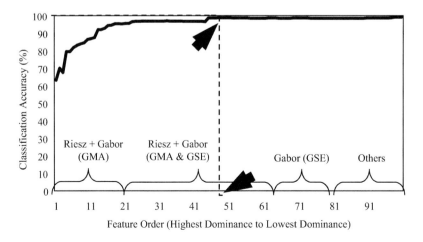

Figure 12.12 Feature selection based on feature combination (used with permission).

Note that GT (GSE) does have some features past this peak that are slightly less effective. Any addition of other features does not cause a change in the accuracy, as seen in Figure 12.12. Thus, it can be said that the classification accuracy starts to be constant at a certain feature number being used. This observation shows the effectiveness of RT and GT in stratifying normal and diseased lungs as compared to the other features used. These features show superiority due to their inherent characteristics of scalability and steerability. Again, this indicates to us that directional transforms of R and GT perform better compared to general textural features.

12.7 Performance Evaluation

The objective of this section is to demonstrate the evaluation of the ML system due to variabilities in stages A and B of the entire pipeline. Furthermore, it ensures the repeatability in the design and control of the error reduction propagation, if any. We present two kinds of performance evaluation (PE) paradigms. In the first design of PE, our focus was to evaluate the system's stability and reliability, while in the second framework, we evaluated the effect of the stage A on stage B.

12.7.1 Stability and Reliability Analysis

A crucial analysis of a classification system's performance is the assessment of stability and reliability. This assessment is crucial because it gives an indication of how the system performs under repeated conditions and under different conditions. This affirms that the results are consistent and repeatable. The definition of reliability is the ability to maintain a specific performance level under specific conditions. Reliability of the system is computed while running a 20-trials approach. Reliability is represented by a reliability index (ξ_N), as shown in equation 12:

$$\xi_N(\%) = \left(1 - \frac{\partial_N}{\mu_N}\right) \times 100 \qquad (13)$$

where ∂_N is the standard deviation of the accuracy when using a particular set of patients (N) for the experiment and μ_N is the mean of accuracy.

Stability assessment analyses show the system changes across repeated conditions. We do this by using a similar approach to dynamics of the control theory [33]. First, a maximum stability criterion of 5% variation is defined. When a system varies more than 5%, it is said that the system is not stable. Next, we calculate the standard deviation (SD) for each computation of different N. If the SD is less than 5%, we give a stable rating [33]. We present the performance of the system based on the results of the reliability tests for four different protocols in Table 12.11. The reliability indices for all four K-fold protocols are above 0.95, indicating a strong reliability of the classification system when running each set of patient population size ranging from 10 to 95. Note that for each N selected, 20 random trials are executed. As can be seen

TABLE 12.11   Reliability Index ξ_N When Changing Population for Four Protocols (K = 2, 3, 5, 10; T = 20; N = 96; L = 5) (Used with Permission)

	Reliability Index (ξ_N) for Different Set of Data Sizes (N)								
K-Fold	10	20	30	40	50	60	70	80	95
K = 2	0.993	0.995	0.998	0.998	0.999	0.998	0.999	0.999	0.999
K = 3	0.994	0.997	0.998	0.999	0.999	0.999	0.999	0.999	0.999
K = 5	0.996	0.998	0.998	0.999	0.999	0.999	0.999	0.999	0.999
K =10	0.996	0.998	0.999	0.999	0.999	0.999	0.999	0.999	0.999

in the Table 12.11, down the row and across the columns, the reliability index either remains constant or increases, indicating the effect of data size N or increase in the number of patients during the CV training protocol.

12.7.2 Effects of Over- and Undersegmentation on Classification

In this study, we also investigated the effects of over- and undersegmentation that may happen during the segmentation phase. We wanted to see the effects of inaccuracies in segmentation on classification. We intentionally introduced these inaccuracies by using dilation operations for oversegmentation and erosion operations for undersegmentation. We use a "square" structure element (SE) that ranges in size from 3×3 to 5×5 to 10×10 to 15×15 to 20×20). The reason we use the maximum of 20 pixels is because some of the lungs become totally eroded at sizes above 20×20 pixels. Examples of the morphology operations are shown in Figure 12.13.

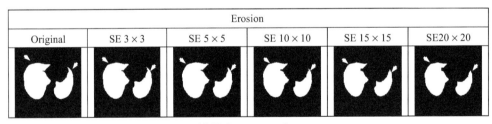

(a) Under-segmentation

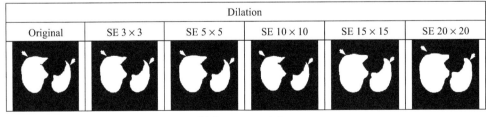

(b) Over-segmentation

Figure 12.13   Examples of over- and undersegmentation (used with permission).

TABLE 12.12   Effect of Lung Undersegmentation on Classification Accuracy While Adopting Four CV Protocols (K = 2, 3, 5, 10; T = 20; *N* = 96; L = 5) (Used with Permission)

K-Fold	Accuracy (%)				
	SE* 3×3	SE 5×5	SE 10×10	SE 15×15	SE 20×20
K = 2	99.21	98.64	98.40	98.30	97.96
K = 3	99.01	99.52	98.87	98.23	95.54
K = 5	99.26	99.21	99.06	98.79	99.05
K = 10	99.32	99.37	99.26	98.95	99.20

TABLE 12.13   Effect of Lung Oversegmentation on Classification Accuracy While Adopting Four CV Protocols (K = 2, 3, 5, 10; T = 20; *N* = 96; L = 5) (Used with Permission)

K-Fold	Accuracy (%)				
	SE 3×3	SE 5×5	SE 10×10	SE 15×15	SE 20×20
K = 2	99.56	99.83	99.84	99.85	99.90
K = 3	99.70	99.92	99.90	99.92	99.95
K = 5	99.75	99.95	99.93	99.95	99.96
K = 10	99.81	99.96	99.94	99.96	99.97

Tables 12.12 and 12.13 show the change in accuracy after stage B due to the change in lung segmented region (stage A). This mimics the process of under- and oversegmentation in stage A. The application of erosion generally shows a trend of decreasing accuracies when the level of erosion increases. The application of dilation, on the other hand, shows an increase in accuracy as dilation increases. Note that the accuracy does not change more than 5%. This suggests that the classification stage is not considerably affected due to changes in the segmentation stage A.

12.8 Discussion

The main objective of this study was to understand the role of the directional-based transforms (RT and GT) tissue characterization approach for risk stratification and to understand the amalgamation of directional transforms such as RT and GT with GLCM, GLRLM, and FD, which led to 100 grayscale features. Another subobjective of the study was to understand the lung segregation index between normal and abnormal subjects using the attribute of feature strengths. We further show a complete system that connects in tandem the stages for segmentation and tissue characterization and that studies the effect of the segmentation phase on the tissue characterization phase. As part of the comprehensive data analysis, we established the validity of our results by computing the behavior of the accuracy curves with respect to changes in data size and change in cross-validation partition protocol. Further, our analysis shows that directional transforms are more powerful compared to textural feature extractions.

12.8.1 Feature Hybridization

Our hybridization protocol showed encouraging results when fusing GT, FD, GLRM, and GLCM with RT (Tables 12.5–12.8). The classification accuracies for K = 10 and RT alone versus three types of amalgamated features using Riesz are RT alone (97.52%), RT + GLCM (98.43%), RT + GT (98.73%), and RT + FD + GLCM + GT + GLRLM (99.53%). Note that as the amalgamation of features increases, so do the accuracies. RT is a powerful feature extraction technique because of its steerability and scalability factors. Similarly, the combination of GT and GLRLM possesses similar properties of steerability. GLRLM, on the other hand, offers textural information covering spatial distribution. Thus, combining directional and spatial information helps improve the segregation index, thereby boosting the accuracies. The combination of different features, especially based on their ability to segregate between normal and diseased lungs, creates a robust approach.

12.8.2 A Short Note on the Effect of Training Data Size on Stratification Accuracy

Even though it is intuitive, with an increase in the population size, the accuracy should increase (nearly ~5% in our case; Table 12.10). The key point to understand is that the accuracy will eventually start becoming constant, or there will be a slight dip justifying the change from memorization to generalization. When we change the population size (N) from 10 patients to 96 patients, our accuracies gradually increased for all CV partition protocols, and there was no dip or drop. This shows that the learning was still happening and memorization still active. This further means that the system is capable of picking larger population sizes. One solution would be to subsample this data set into quadrants for increasing the data size for a better test to see when generalization can be triggered. One can say with assurance that the RT's behavior to lead to higher accuracy in all protocols with an increase in N was consistent, ensuring a direct relationship between the directional information during tissue characterization and cross validation.

12.8.3 Influence of Under- and Oversegmentation on Stratification Accuracy

We simulated the effect of error propagation from stage A (segmentation phase) to stage B (tissue characterization along with ML phase) in two different ways: (1) undersegmentation (Table 12.12) and (2) oversegmentation in stage A (Table 12.13).

During the undersegmentation, there is a loss of lung regional area, causing textural loss, penalizing the directional filters (RT and GT) and textural filters (GLCM and GLRLM), and thereby compromising the accuracy. The reverse pattern was observed during the oversegmentation. Although the pattern showed consistency in behavior, there was no special cutoff observed to obtain a certain level of accuracy. A larger data size could improve the statistical means and standard deviations, which could be our next plausible approach, but the current results were encouraging and consistent.

12.8.4 Benchmark Against the Current Literature

We compared our algorithm against the existing algorithms available in the literature over one decade (Table 12.14). The comparison includes type of classifiers used, types of features extracted, and performance measures such as sensitivity, specificity, accuracy, and AUC. It is important to note that although a direct comparison cannot be done between our work and other studies due to nonavailability of data sets and exact replicas of methods available in the literature, we have done our best to show the mappings for the same set of parameters. At the outset, we would like to share that, using the conventional classifiers, our system performs exceedingly well, showing a maximum of a 17% (serial #4, column 7: 82.5% when compared against our proposed method; serials #6 and #7, column 7: 98.73% and 99.53%) improvement in accuracy. Further, most of the techniques in the literature do not show full data, such as sensitivity, specificity and AUC (Table 12.14). Seeing all the above challenges, we will share the key algorithmic differences and performances below.

Zrimec et al. [34] used rudimentary features that are first-order spectra, such as variance, skewness, and kurtosis. They used a Naive Bayes (NB) classifier and yielded an accuracy of 87.2%. Our current work used features that offer more detailed information because of the RT's and GT's attributes of steerability and scalability. This detailed information can prove effective in classifying normal and diseased lungs, which is indicated by its higher performance.

Sørensen et al. [35] stratified normal and diseased lungs using features such as local binary patterns and intensity histograms coupled with a k-nearest neighbor (k-NN) classifier. Their work yielded a classification accuracy of 95.2%. Their work has an encouraging accuracy but does not show the amalgamation that is an innovation in our current study and that includes five feature groups and 100 grayscale features leading to higher accuracy behavior. Further, Sørensen et al. [35] also did not show other classification performance, such as sensitivity, specificity, and AUC.

Kim et al. [36] used elementary features of texture—GLCM and histogram coupled with the circularity of the lung—to detect diseases with an overall best accuracy of 86.47%. Their work showed an interesting approach using various ROI image sizes, such as 16×16, 32×32, and 64×64. Our work used only 64×64 ROIs since the resolution of RT and GT approaches required a minimum size of ROI to be

TABLE 12.14   Comparison with the Existing Literature (Used with Permission)

SN	Authors	CADx system	Feature Type	Total No. of Features	Feature Hybridization	Classifier Type	Data Size	Data Analysis	Performance	SEN	SP	ACC	AUC
1	Zrimec et al. [34] (2007)	Seg + TC*	First order and GLCM	63	✓	NB	16	—	✗	97.40	85.50	87.20	✗
2	Sørensen et al. [35] (2008)	TC	Local binary patterns and intensity histogram	6	✗	k-NN	25	Optimal ROI size analysis	✗	✗	✗	95.20	✗
3	Kim et al. [36] (2009)	Seg + TC	Texture and shape (circularity)	24	✓	SVM	92	Optimal ROI size analysis	✗	93.5	97.85	86.47	✗
4	Arzhaeva et al. [37] (2010)	Seg + TC	General purpose filter banks	25	✓	LDA, k-NN, SVM	75	Interobserver analysis	✗	—	—	82.50	✗
5	Park et al. [38] (2011)	Seg + TC	Histogram and RLM	26	✓	ANN	30	Optimal ROI size analysis	✗	80.00	85.70	86.70	0.88
6	**Proposed Work (2017)**		**RT + GT**	**84**	✓			**Data size analysis**	**Stability & reliability evaluation**	**99.78**	**93.53**	**98.73**	**0.97**
7	**Proposed Work (2017)**	**Seg + TC**	**RT + GT + GLRLM + FD + GLCM**	**100**	✓	**SVM**	**96**	**Feature power analysis** LFSI analysis	**Effect of Stage A on Stage B**	**99.76**	**98.39**	**99.53**	**0.99**

Abbreviations: Seg, segmentation; TC, tissue characterization.

able to produce higher performance. Kim et al. [36] concur with our reasoning of using 64×64 image sizes, showing that it returns a higher accuracy, sensitivity, and specificity.

Arzhaeva et al. [37] showed classification work of stratifying lungs to their disease based on two subsequent scans (in an interval) for 75 patients. Their work used lower levels of features, such as first-order statistics and texture. As a contrast, our study used five sets of features (low and high level) that collectively offered richer and more diversified information. However, their study's advantage compared to our work is the use of two observers in identifying the disease in the patient. This offers interobserver information that can be helpful. Arzhaeva et al. [37] used accuracy only as a classification performance measure. On the other hand, our work used more classification measures, allowing for a holistic and in-depth view of the data analysis and classifcation performance of different features (sensitivity, specificity, accuracy, AUC, and PPV).

Park et al. [38] aimed to classify early ILD using low-dose CT images using RLM and histogram features on 30 patients. Their work managed to achieve an accuracy of 86.70%. A weakness of their study was that the amount of features used was limited and therefore may not offer a wide depth of textural information for classification. In addition, the amount of patients used was relatively small compared to our work with 96 patients. Comparing all the works listed, our work showed an approach of using feature amalgamation of high-level and low-level features. This extensive approach focused on the characteristics of RT and GT, ensuring a robust approach to classification. As compared to the other studies, we showed data analysis when using different population sizes. In addition, the introduction of segmentation errors in stage A had not been done in the other studies.

12.8.5 Strengths and Weaknesses of This Study

The major advantage of this study is that it used 20-trial and four K-fold approaches. These measures helped to ensure repeatability and consistency of the results. This study also measured the feature strength using the LFSI, which helps in understanding the feature's ability to segregate between normal and diseased lungs. Another advantage of this study was the analysis of the stability and reliability of the classification system. The stability and reliability studies helped to validate the classification accuracy provided under different conditions. Understanding the stability and reliability fluctuations is useful in learning and making predictions about diseased lungs.

However, there are several components that could be improved. First, this study was done only on 2D data and can be extended into 3D classification with extensive feature sets. Second, a multicenter evaluation needs to be conducted to evaluate robust performance of our risk stratification system. Third, studies need to be conducted that evaluate the risk labels on the blind test patients instead of using CV protocols. In addition the above extensions, the current prototype design is very encouraging and has unique contributions to make.

12.9 Conclusion

In conclusion, we have shown different features and their combinations and the ability to classify normal and diseased lungs. The highest accuracy was achieved using all the features. RT was able to perform well when combined with other features as well. The addition of other features showed an increase to 98.73% using RT and GT, when only 23 subfeatures were used when 84 were available. This study has also showed that the classification system used is not heavily influenced by over- and undersegmentation, where changes in classification accuracy varied less than 5%. We also have shown that our system is reliable, with a RI of 0.98–0.99 when changing the number of patients.

Acknowledgments

We would like to thank Springer Nature for allowing us to reuse, in part or in full, figures and text from a previously published paper from *Computers in Biology and Medicine* titled "Lung Disease Stratification Using Amalgamation of Riesz and Gabor Transforms in Machine Learning Framework."

References

1. National Heart, Blood, and Lung Institute. *Disease Statistics, NHLBI Fact Book, Fiscal Year 2012*. Bethesda, MD: National Heart, Blood, and Lung Institute; 2012:35.
2. Azizah AM, Nor Saleha I, Noor Hashimah A. et al. *Malaysia National Cancer Registry Report 2007-2011*. Kuala Lumpur: Malaysia Ministry of Health; 2011.
3. Saba L, Suri JS. *Multi-Detector CT Imaging: Abdomen, Pelvis, and CAD Applications*. Boca Raton, FL: CRC Press;2013.
4. Collins J. CT signs and patterns of lung disease. *Radiol Clin North Am*. 2001;39:1115–1135.
5. Krupinski EA, Berbaum KS. Does reader visual fatigue impact interpretation accuracy? *Proc SPIE*. 2010;7627:76270M–76270M.
6. El-Baz A, Suri JS. *Lung Imaging and Computer Aided Diagnosis*. Boca Raton, FL: CRC Press; 2011.
7. Castellino RA. Computer aided detection (CAD): an overview. *Cancer Imaging*. 2005;5:17–19.
8. Kazerooni EA, Martinez FJ, Flint A, et al. Thin-section CT obtained at 10-mm increments versus limited three-level thin-section CT for idiopathic pulmonary fibrosis: correlation with pathologic scoring. *Am J Roentgenol*. 1997;169:977–983.
9. Cirujeda P, Müller H, Rubin D, et al. 3D Riesz-wavelet based covariance descriptors for texture classification of lung nodule tissue in CT. In: *37th Annual International Conference of the Engineering in Medicine and Biolgy Society*. 2015:7909–7912.
10. Barker J, Hoogi A, Depeursinge A, Rubin DL. Automated classification of brain tumor type in whole-slide digital pathology images using local representative tiles. *Med Image Anal*. 2016;30:60–71.
11. Depeursinge A, Kurtz C, Beaulieu C, Napel S, Rubin D. Predicting visual semantic descriptive terms from radiological image data: preliminary results with liver lesions in CT. *IEEE Trans Med Imaging*. 2014;33:1669–1676.

12. Sharma AM, Gupta A, Kumar PK, et al. A review on carotid ultrasound atherosclerotic tissue characterization and stroke risk stratification in machine learning framework. *Curr Atheroscler Rep.* 2015;17:1–13.

13. Kyrki V, Kamarainen JK, Kälviäinen H. Simple Gabor feature space for invariant object recognition. *Pattern Recognit Lett.* 2004;25:311–318.

14. Depeursinge A, Foncubierta-Rodriguez A, Van De Ville D, Müller H. Lung texture classification using locally-oriented Riesz components. In: *Lecture Notes in Computer Science.* New York, NY: Springer; 2011:231–238.

15. Unser M, Van De Ville D. Higher-order Riesz transforms and steerable wavelet frames. In: *16th IEEE International Conference on Image Processing.* 2009:3801–3804.

16. Depeursinge A, Chin AS, Leung AN, et al. Automated classification of usual interstitial pneumonia using regional volumetric texture analysis in high-resolution computed tomography. *Invest Radiol.* 2015;50:261–267.

17. Singh BK, Verma K, Thoke AS, Suri JS. Risk stratification of 2D ultrasound-based breast lesions using hybrid feature selection in machine learning paradigm. *Measurement.* 2017;105:146–157.

18. Acharya UR, Krishnan MMR, Sree SV, et al. Plaque tissue characterization and classification in ultrasound carotid scans: a paradigm for vascular feature amalgamation. *IEEE Trans Instrum Meas.* 2013;62:392–400.

19. Acharya UR, Sree SV, Krishnan MMR, et al. Atherosclerotic risk stratification strategy for carotid arteries using texture-based features. *Ultrasound Med Biol.* 2012;38:899–915.

20. Noor NM, Than JCM, Rijal OM, et al. Automatic lung segmentation using control feedback system: morphology and texture paradigm. *J Med Syst.* 2015;1:22.

21. Lee C-J, Wang S-D. Fingerprint feature extraction using Gabor filters. *Electron Lett.* 1999;35:288–290.

22. Depeursinge A, Rodriguez AF. Lung texture classification using locally-oriented Riesz components. *Components.* 2011;1:231–238.

23. Cirujeda P, Cid YD, Müller H, et al. A 3-D Riesz-covariance texture model for prediction of nodule recurrence in lung CT. *IEEE Trans Med Imaging.* 2016;35:2620–2630.

24. Acharya UR, Sree SV, Mookiah MRK, et al. Diagnosis of Hashimoto's thyroiditis in ultrasound using tissue characterization and pixel classification. *Proc Inst Mech Eng Part H J Eng Med.* 2013;227:788–798.

25. Acharya UR, Mookiah MRK, Sree SV, et al. Evolutionary algorithm-based classifier parameter tuning for automatic ovarian cancer tissue characterization and classification. *Ultraschall Med Eur J Ultrasound.* 2014;35:237–245.

26. Unser M, Chenouard N, Van De Ville D. Steerable pyramids and tight wavelet frames. *IEEE Trans Image Process.* 2011;20:2705–2721.

27. Haralick RM, Shanmugam K, Dinstein LH. Textural features for image classification. *IEEE Trans Syst Man Cybern.* 1973;6:610–621.

28. Shrivastava VK, Londhe ND, Sonawane RS, Suri JS. Computer-aided diagnosis of psoriasis skin images with HOS, Texture and color features: a first comparative study of its kind. *Comput. Methods Programs Biomed.* 2016;126:98–108.

29. Chaudhuri BB, Sarkar N. Texture segmentation using fractal dimension. *IEEE Trans Pattern Anal Mach Intell.* 1995;17:72–77.

30. Sarkar N, Chaudhuri BB. An efficient approach to estimate fractal dimension of textural images. *Pattern Recognit.* 1992;25:1035–1041.

31. Lewandowski Z, Beyenal H. Fundamentals of Biofilm Research. Boca Raton, FL: CRC Press; 2013.

32. Araki T, Jain PK, Suri HS, et al. Stroke risk stratification and its validation using ultrasonic echolucent carotid wall plaque morphology: a machine learning paradigm. *Comput Biol Med*. 2017;80:77–96.

33. Shrivastava VK, Londhe ND, Sonawane RS, Suri JS. Reliable and accurate psoriasis disease classification in dermatology images using comprehensive feature space in machine learning paradigm. *Expert Syst Appl*. 2015;42:6184–6195.

34. Zrimec T, Wong JS. Improving computer aided disease detection using knowledge of disease appearance. *Stud Health Technol Inform*. 2007;129:1324–1328.

35. Sørensen L, Shaker SB, de Bruijne M. Texture classification in lung CT using local binary patterns. In: *Proceedings of the 11th International Conference on Medical Image Computing and Computer-Assisted Intervention*. 2008:941.

36. Kim N, Seo JB, Lee Y, Lee JG, Kim SS, Kang SH. Development of an automatic classification system for differentiation of obstructive lung disease using HRCT. *J Digit Imaging*. 2009;22:136–148.

37. Arzhaeva Y, Prokop M, Murphy K, et al. Automated estimation of progression of interstitial lung disease in CT images. *Med Phys*. 2010;37:63–73.

38. Park SC, Tan T, Wang X, et al. Computer-aided detection of early interstitial lung diseases using low-dose CT images. *Phys Med Biol*. 2011;56:1139–1153.

Appendix A: Symbols for Equations

Symbol	Meaning	Equation
$f(x)$	2D function	1
$\overline{R^{(o_1,o_2)}f(\omega)}$	Riesz transform of $f(x)$	1
O	Order where $O = o_1 + o_2$	1
$\hat{f}(\omega)$	Fourier transform of $f(x)$	1
ω_1	Frequency of x-axis	1
ω_2	Frequency of y-axis	1
ω	Frequency	1, 2
$\psi_{(\alpha,s)}$	2D Gabor function	2–4
(x,y)	Rectilinear coordinates in spatial domain	2
σ_x, σ_y	Standard deviations of the Gaussian envelopes	2
θ	Angle where $\theta = \alpha\pi/\Theta$	3
a^{-1}	Scale factor	3
α	Orientation	2–4
Θ	Total number of orientations	4
s	Scale	2–4
S	Total number of scales	4
$I(x,y)$	Image	
$G_{(s,\alpha)}$	Gabor of an image	4
$*$	Convolution	4
$c(m,n)$	Co-occurrence matrix	5–8
i	Gray level	Section 12.4.4
j	Frequency of pixel with i	Section 12.4.4
$p(i,j)$	Number of runs of pixels that have gray level i and length group j having a specific direction	Section 12.4.4
DF	Fractal dimension	9
ϵ	Boxes of size, ϵ	9
$N(\epsilon)$	Total boxes of size, ϵ	9
LFSI	Lung feature segregation index	10
FD	Mean feature value for diseased patients	10
FN	Mean feature value for normal patients	10

(*continued*)

Symbol	Meaning	Equation
SEN	Sensitivity	11
SP	Specificity	11
PPV	Positive predictive value	12
ACC	Accuracy	12
TP	True positive	11, 12
TN	True negative	11, 12
FN	False negative	11, 12
FP	False positive	11, 12
ξ_N	Reliability index	
∂_N	Standard deviation of the accuracy when using a particular number of patients (N)	12
μ_N	Mean of accuracy when using N	12

13

An Unsupervised Parametric Mixture Model for Automatic Three-Dimensional Lung Segmentation

Mohammed Ghazal, Samr Ali, Mohanad AlKhodari, and Ayman El-Baz

Contents

13.1 Introduction

Computer-aided diagnosis (CAD) systems have made a large impact in the medical field, for they significantly aid in supporting the decisions of radiologists and medical doctors. This is due to the continuous improvements made in the various different subfields of medical image analysis and imaging techniques. One such important subfield is the segmentation of the lungs. Lung segmentation is the process that refers to the accurate identification of lung tissue and its separation from the chest background. This may be applied to the various imaging modalities used for the lungs, such as computed tomography (CT). Accurate segmentation of lung tissue allows radiologists and medical doctors to investigate abnormalities in a clearer manner and as such make better-informed decisions that may save a person's life. Consequently, lung segmentation plays a major role in CAD system development and is still heavily researched.

Image features, such as quantitative visual appearance, aid in the discrimination between object structures and image background and are hence used for accurate medical segmentation. Such available prior information in terms of an appearance or spatial model is extracted from a set of training images that have been manually segmented by medical experts. Appearance features are associated with the visual appearance or gray-level intensity of a single pixel in two-dimensional (2D) images or a voxel in 3D ones. It is often refined with association of a spatial interaction model between the aforementioned intensities whether in a pairwise iteration or higher-order neighborhood definition as per the requirements of the chosen or developed model. Such combined features are usually used to better guide the segmentation procedure and lead to improved accuracies and enhanced segmentation results. On successful application of these models, most of the voxels in a 3D image or of pixels in a 2D one of an object can be correctly classified as per the derived threshold from the model.

In this chapter, we discuss a novel methodology for 3D automatic lung segmentation and present our experimental results and findings. The chapter is organized as follows. Section 13.2 provides background of the anatomy and key functions of the lung; Section 13.3 expands on related work on lung segmentation. Section 13.4 discusses the proposed method and algorithms. Section 13.5 presents the experimental results of the proposed method. Section 13.6 provides concluding remarks for the chapter.

13.2 Anatomy and Key Functions of the Lung

Lungs are pyramid-shaped major organs in the respiratory system. They weight around 300–500 g each in adults, and their volume ranges between 3.5 and 8.5 L each [1, 2]. The left lung has a smaller volume than the right lung, which is wider and shorter. Lungs are placed on both sides of the thorax, and they are sealed and protected by the rigid thoracic cage. Lungs are connected by the diaphragm from the inferior side and are linked to the trachea by right and left bronchias, as shown in Figure 13.1. On the

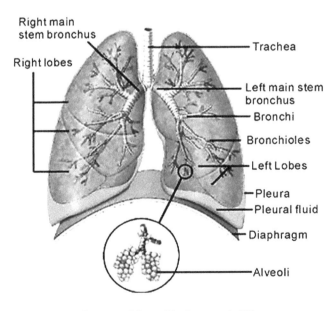

Figure 13.1   Lung anatomy (retrieved from Hashim et al. [4]).

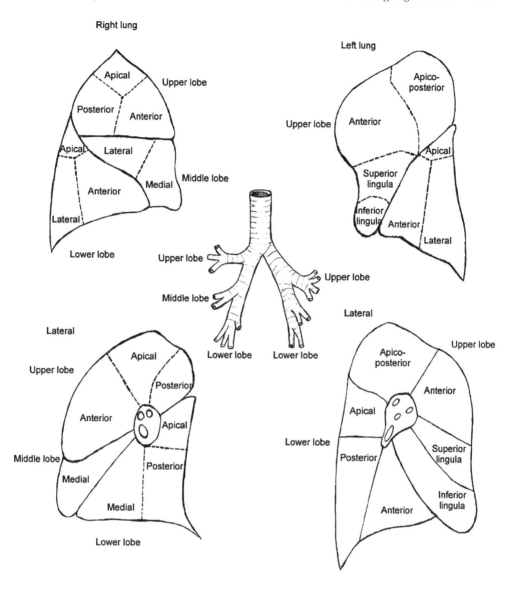

Figure 13.2   Lung lobes and fissures (retrieved from Celis et al. [6]).

surface of the left lung, there is a cardiac notch where the heart is located [3] between the left and right lungs. The air passes through the throat and nose toward the larynx, which is the voice box, reaching into the trachea. The trachea is separated into two parts, the bronchi tubes, and air flows through them into each lung. The absorbed air reaches the alveoli air sacs that allow the oxygen and carbon dioxide to move between the lungs and blood [4].

Both lungs are likely to be symmetrical and are divided into different lobes, as shown in Figure 13.2. The right lung consists of three lobes, while the left lung has only two lobes [5]. Lobes are separated from one another by diagonal and horizontal

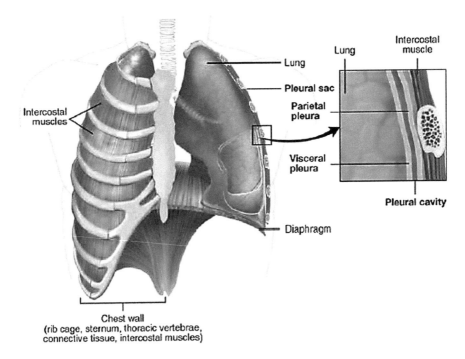

Figure 13.3   Cross-sectional view of lungs showing the pleura (retrieved from Betts et al. [3]).

fissures to form segments [1]. In the right lung, there are 10 different segments. The apical, anterior, and medial are in the right upper lobe. The medial and lateral are in the right middle lobe. The superior, medial, anterior, lateral, and posterior are in the right lower lobe. On the other side, the left lung lobes include eight segments. In the left upper lobe, there are the apicoposterior, anterior, superior lingula, and inferior lingula, while in the left lower lobe; there are the superior, anteromedial, lateral, and posterior [6].

Figure 13.3 shows a cross-sectional view for the lungs. Each lung is covered with glistening visceral pleura, which has a translucent nature. This pleura looks pink, and it may accumulate black pigment due to age because of the exposure to environment particulates [5]. The pleura that covers each lung is a membrane consisting of two main layers: the visceral pleura and the parietal pleura. The visceral pleura extends into the lung fissures and forms invaginations into both lungs, while the parietal pleura connects the diaphragm and the mediastinum by the thoracic wall. The main function of the lung pleura is to reduce the friction between lung layers during the breathing process, to maintain the position of the lungs within the chest wall [3], and to produce the pulmonary ligament that holds the lungs over the diaphragm [6].

Lungs are the essential organs for the respiration process. Breathing in (aspiration) and out (inhalation) is done mainly by the lungs. The diaphragm plays a critical role in this process by increasing or decreasing the air pressure within the lungs and therefore allows them to absorb or eject air. In the inhalation process, the diaphragm muscle gets tighter, which increases the size of lungs, allowing air to pump through them. In exhalation, the size of the lungs decreases as a result of the relaxation process of the diaphragm muscle; therefore, air is pushed out of the lungs [7, 8]. Moreover, as a respiratory function, the lungs are considered to be the gas exchange organs in the respiratory system. The main function of the lungs is to provide the blood with filtered oxygen and to take the carbon dioxide away from it. Through the process of ventilation, the exchange of oxygen and carbon dioxide takes place between the airways of the lungs and the blood. Oxygen (O_2) is absorbed from the air by inspiration, while in expiration, carbon dioxide (CO_2) is expelled from the respiratory system [4]. In external respiration, gases do exchange within the tissues and blood of the body. Oxygen and carbon dioxide switch between the air in the alveoli and the blood in the pulmonary capillaries. The oxygen concentration in the lung alveoli is higher than that in the lung capillaries. Thus, the oxygen diffuses from the alveoli toward the blood. On the other side, the carbon dioxide concentration in blood is higher than in the air sacs, so the process is done on the opposite side [8]. This oxygen and carbon dioxide gradient results in having a successful exchange of gases between air sacs and blood in the body. In addition, most of carbon dioxide reaches the lungs in plasma as bicarbonate ions (HCO_3-). These ions, along with the hydrogen ions, are converted into carbonic acid (H_2CO_3) once the blood reaches the pulmonary capillaries. Then they return into carbon dioxide and water by the enzyme carbonic anhydrase. The removal of these ions allows hemoglobin to build more oxygen in the blood by providing more neutral pH levels and therefore relieve the blood of its burden of waste and return refreshed blood to heart. If breathing occurs at a high rate, this interaction will result in high pH levels in the blood, and therefore dizziness symptoms might appear along with tetanic contractions of muscles [9].

A nonrespiratory function of lungs is done through the respiratory epithelium, which is a barrier that filters the inspired air from fibrin clumps and chemicals before it reaches the respiratory system, mainly alveoli. In the physical filtration process, lungs act as filters for blood-borne substances. The pulmonary capillaries are around 7 μm in diameter. This size is considered small for the pulmonary circulation to act as filters. However, after coughing, the pressure increases in the right atrium, which produces demonstrable blood flow between both the left and the right atria. Thus, gas emboli pass through the pulmonary capillary or bypass the lung entirely through the foramen ovale [10]. Without providing such filtering processes within lungs, the risk of increased emboli in the arterial system increases. In addition, emboli may pass the alveoli through precapillary anastomoses that exist in the pulmonary circulation. However, microcirculation maintains alveolar perfusion in front of a large degree of embolization by its ability to dilate pulmonary capillaries. This helps minimize dangerous hypertension following pulmonary embolus, and therefore the lungs succeed in maintaining their physical filtering functionality [11]. The lungs are considered the main defensive organs that provide protection from any substances that might be absorbed through the breathing process. Moreover, they provide a metabolic function, as they include a fiberinolytic system that undergoes clots in the pulmonary vessels [4, 10].

13.3 Related Work on Lung Segmentation

Images obtained from radiography (X-ray) or CT go through CAD techniques and are analyzed to provide data about the volume, shape, and movement of organs or even any occurrence of diseases, such as lung cancer or pulmonary edema [13]. Researchers have been trying to segment lungs efficiently through the years. However, the lung segmentation process suffers from accuracy and robustness problems because of the variations in the anatomical lung shape [14]. Various techniques have been followed, such as thresholding-based and deformable boundary model-based lung segmentation. In threshold-based segmentation, the main objective lies in separating the background from the foreground based on the intensity of the object (lungs and chest). If the object intensity is above this certain threshold, it is valued at 1, and the resulting image is a binary one that represents this object. Such a technique suffers from a drawback in that in most CT images, the intensity-based segmentation process may be affected by the variation in brightness between the foreground and background. Therefore, if the lung segment is dark and close to the background brightness, the accuracy of the segmentation process may be affected [15]. In deformable boundary model–based segmentation, boundaries of the lung are determined through using specific internal and external guiding forces to fit the shape of lung. In this model, a snake algorithm initiates manual seed points deformed iteratively by choosing neighboring pixels with minimal energy to guide the segmentation process, while level sets segment the image by extracting all the gray-level values and assign it in one label set [16]. Moreover, lung segmentation could be possible based on the appearance and shape techniques. Lung segmentation can be classified into three main categories: appearance model, shape model, and appearance-shape model techniques. Below, we review the related work on lung segmentation following these three main categories.

In appearance model techniques, the segmentation process is considered successful for medical imaging analysis. However, routine clinical setting, caused by pathological changes or medical interventions, results in gross disturbances of objects. Considering such disturbances, a number of relevant works have been cited in the literature. Beichel et al. [17] introduced a novel Robust Active Appearance Model (RAAM) that consists of two main stages. The first stage of RAAM analyzes initial residuals using the mean-shift–based mode detection, while the second stage uses an objective function to select a mode combination that does not represent the gross outliers. This RAAM resulted in up to 50% object area covered by the gross gray-level disturbances. Another technique was proposed by Wang et al. [18], providing a 3D tensor-based active appearance model (AAM), which overcame the problem of accuracy caused by transforming 3D appearance matrices into 1D vectors for CT slices. In this technique, the AAM was applied on 3D scans rather than on 1D scans, and a Higher Order Singular Value Decomposition (HOSVD) was proposed as a tensor-based model that is built with a block-based Kronecker. In fact, HOSVD was introduced mainly to represent and process the lung in tensor space. For lung CT scans, the model was designed to determine the optimal scheme for a low-rank representation of appearance tensors. It is worth mentioning here that most AAM segmentation processes operate on patterns represented by vectors. Thus, before applying the AAM on CT images, it has to be vectored first through concatenation methods, which leads to the loss of some implicit structural or local contextual information. Therefore, as an update to this technique, Wang et al. [19] introduced new methods for HOSVD used for the segmentation of 3D CT images in tensor space while reducing the computer memory usage at the same time. The technique was applied on images for 310 diseased lungs, and the evaluation resulted in an average Dice coefficient of 97.0 ± 0.59 and a mean absolute surface distance error of 1.0403 ± 0.5716 mm. In Beichel et al. [20], a new 3D AAM was performed to segment the diaphragm from CT data sets. It consists of a 2D closed curve, an elevation image that forms the 3D shape information, and texture layers representing the image intensity as well as the surrounding layers. The reference curve was generated from the CT images by a parallel projection of the diaphragm dome outline in the axial direction. The landmark point placement, which is the bounding curve of the elevation image, was applied only on the 2D curve. Matching was then performed based on a gradient-descent optimization process that used image intensity appearance around the actual dome shape. Results from 60 CT data sets generated as phantom data by computer showed a positioning error of 0.16 ± 2.95 mm. The validation using real CT data sets resulted in a positioning error of 0.16 ± 2.95 mm.

In shape model techniques, researchers have implemented various approaches to segment lungs, which can be atlas-based or model-based methods. From its name, atlas-based methods make use of preobtained information about the lungs used for recognition and delineation in order to create a human lung atlas. This preobtained image is treated as a sample image with labels for the thoracic regions. It is then registered to a new target image so that the labels are transformed into the target [21]. Li et al. [22] acquired quantitative CT-based measurements of lung structure and function to create a computerized human lung atlas. Those measurements were then linked to six target CT images using the 3D intensity-based image registration. In the atlas-based approach, researchers register a template image volume to the rest of the CT image (target) volumes in order to reconstruct the atlas by deforming the template with average transformation. As a result, the reconstructed computerized human lung atlas would provide a basis for establishing regional ranges of normative values for structural and functional measures of the human lung to be segmented. The technique used in this work reduced landmark registration error from 10.5 to 0.4 mm and the average volume overlap error from 0.7 to 0.11 for the six images acquired for testing. Gill et al. [14] introduced another approach for constructing a human lung atlas using the Active Shape Model (ASM) to represent lung features and average shape, which was applied on 190 3D lung CT images. The proposed technique creates an atlas for the human lung by calculating the average lung shape from a set of lung features through affine transform. These features can be matched to new images through mapping that transforms the average lung shape to the new image space. This technique of segmentation uses local features identified in CT volume rather than a small set of specific salient points. The result of this work was an average dice coefficient of 0.746 ± 0.068 for initialization and 0.974 ± 0.017 for segmentation. The mean absolute surface distance error was 0.948 ± 1.537.

Model-based methods take into account the variations in shape and texture of lung images, where the gray level of the lungs derives the segmentation process by coping with the variability of the target image. The process is finalized when the model finds its best match for the CT data to be segmented [21]. Sun et al. [23] provided a model-based segmentation technique of pathological lung CT data sets by adopting a novel 3D Robust Active Shape Model (RASM) for the segmentation of the lungs. As a first step of the procedure, the rib cage of the chest was detected to determine the initial position of the RASM. After that, a global optimal surface-finding method was used to identify human lungs in CT scans. The left and right lungs were then extracted separately. The objective was to segment 40 CT scans of abnormal lungs and 20 CT scans of normal right/left lungs in order to extract data of high-density lung diseases, such as cancer, fibrosis, and pneumonias. Extracted data were compared to an independent reference of 11 CT images for diseased lungs and nine CT images for healthy lungs. For this shape-model segmentation, two steps were followed. The first step was the generation of a lung model to present lung shapes through the means and variations of lungs. The second step was to perform a RASM matching to segment lungs by matching the model to the target structures. In this work, the standard matching process was extended to include another step for outlier detection. The goal of this extra step was to find normal shape patterns of landmark subsets to be utilized through ASM matching in order to identify or reject outliers. As a result, 116 seconds was needed for the segmentation process with an average Dice coefficient of 0.975 ± 0.006 and a mean absolute surface distance error of 0.84 ± 0.23 mm. Gill et al. [24] introduced a technique for 4D segmentation of lungs through RASM matching. It manually utilizes the CT data sets volumes in order to provide an accurate segmentation for each data set. In 3D, the ASM is applied and then extended to the 4D volume. This technique was applied on 152 CT data sets and results in a Dice coefficient of 0.9773 ± 0.0254, which was better than the 3D technique results of 0.9659 ± 0.0517. This technique opens the space for more research work on lung segmentation based on shape models through 4D data sets.

In appearance-shape model segmentation techniques, Shao et al. [25] proposed a joint shape and appearance sparse learning method for the process of lung segmentation. Images were acquired from posterior-anterior (PA) chest radiography. Using a robust initialization method, the initial shape was created to look close at the lung boundaries. To overcome the differences in lung shape through images, a set of shape composition models was built based on local lung shape segments. Thus, the accuracy of the process can be improved. Local appearance models of lungs were used by a sparse representation that captures the local lung appearance and therefore determines the lung boundaries. In order to integrate the shape/appearance information, a hierarchical deformable framework was used at the end of the segmentation process. The result from 247 PA radiographs showed that it outperformed the normal model and appearance techniques. Tan et al. [26] combined techniques of marker-controlled watershed, geometric active contours, and Markov random fields (MRF) as an active shape and appearance model. This method is used to segment one object in each process. It selects a region of interest (ROI) that covers any lesion on the slice. A marker-controlled watershed is then used to generate 3D initial surface for the lesion. Moreover, MRF was used as an improvement in the extraction of ground glass opacity parts of part-solid lesions. However, the technique would be difficult to use if tumors occur, which are small lesion regions. This is because of the lack of training examples used to generalize the model of objects. The results of Lung Image Database Consortium data set, which contains 23 lung nodules with six radiologists' delineated contours, had mean overlap ratios of lesion of 69% (for the computer algorithm) and 65% (for the radiologists). The intraclass correlation coefficient was 0.998. Shen et al. [27] introduced a novel predictive model for objects boundary which includes deformable surface (shape), volumetric interior statistics (appearance), and an embedded classifier to separate object from background based on current feature information. This model only focuses on the foreground object rather than analyzing the background methods such as Snakes, Level Sets, and MRF. As an elastic 3D model, the shape used in the process provides thousands of vertices within the surface, which is a simplex-mesh surface. Through liner systems, the model deformations are generated after encoding the ROI boundaries. This technique can be called active volume models because it does not require offline training data and it is self-contained generative object. This technique was applied on human thorax to extract the right lung segment and resulted in having 93.6 sensitivity and 99.8 specificity with Dice Similarity Coefficient of 95.2 in only 1,000s.

In recent work on lung segmentation, El-Baz et al. [28] introduced Markov-Gibbs random fields (MGRF)–based segmentation for lung regions obtained from CT scans. A linear combination of discrete Gaussian (LCDG) model with positive and negative components of the distribution was applied. Voxel classification using a Bayesian maximum a posteriori (MAP) classifier and an iterative conditional model (ICM) were used in the segmentation process. A total of 487 radiograph images were used, and the segmentation accuracy was 94.37%. Kockelkorn et al. [29] introduced a segmentation process that contains the volumes of interest (VOIs) from chest CT images. The textural features of each VOI are then extracted and trained using k-nearest neighbors classifier. In this research work, 22 CT scans were used and resulted in having an overlap measure of 0.96 and mean absolute surface distance error of 1.68 mm. Mendonca et al. [30] segmented lungs from chest radiograph images through a spatial edge detector. By observing the rectangular ROIs (right and left lungs), the lung boundary is then accurately extracted based on these regions. This technique eliminates the outlying edges and detects mediastinal pixels, costal edges, and bottom and top edges. They used 47 data sets and achieved a sensitivity (P) of 0.9225 and 0.968 as positive predictive value. Table 13.1 summarizes lung segmentation techniques using CT/radiography.

13.4 Methods

Let the finite arithmetic grid $R = (i, j, z): 1 \leq i \leq I, 1 \leq j \leq J, 1 \leq z \leq Z$ where i, j, and z correspond to the Cartesian coordinates of the supported grayscale CT image $g: R \mapsto Q$, of size $I \times J \times Z$ and its corresponding region maps $m: R \mapsto X$.

$Q = \{0,...,Q-1\}$ refers to the set of gray levels, where Q denotes the number of gray levels in g and $X = \{1,...,X\}$ is the set of region labels with X as the total number of classes to be separated during segmentation of the respective image. That is, the segmentation divides an image g into X connected objects or subimages such that $g_x : R_x \mapsto Q; x \in X; R_x \subset R$, $\bigcup_{x \in X} R_x = R$ with no overlaps $(R_x \cap R_{x'} = \phi \mid x \neq x', \forall (x,x') \in X)$.

The MGRF image segmentation model is given by the CT image joint probability distribution and the desired region maps:

$$P(g,m) = P(m)P(g \mid m) \tag{1}$$

Here, $P(m)$ is an unconditional distribution of maps, and $P(g \mid m)$ is a conditional distribution of images, given a map. $P(m)$ may also be referred to as the spatial model, while $P(g \mid m)$ represents the appearance model of the image and is often used as an initialization for the approximation of $P(m)$. The Bayesian MAP estimate of the map, given the image $g, m^* = argmax_m L(g,m)$, maximizes the log-likelihood function:

$$L(g,m) = logP(m) + logP(g \mid m) \tag{2}$$

13.4.1 Intensity Model of CT Lung Images

We approximate an unsupervised parametric intensity model of the CT images with a mixture of discrete Gaussians. That is, let $q; q \in Q = \{0,...,Q-1\}$ denote the Q-ary gray level. Then as seen in Figure 13.4

$$P(g \mid m) = \Psi(q) = \sum_{r=1}^{K} w_r \varphi(q \mid \theta_r) \tag{3}$$

where $\Psi(q)$ is the approximated unsupervised parametric intensity model, K is the number of the distributions, w_r is the prior probability or mixing weight, and $\varphi(q \mid \theta_r)$ is the probability density function model for the Gaussian distribution r such that $\varphi(q \mid \theta) = \Phi_\theta(q+0.5) - \Phi_\theta(q-0.5)$ for $q = 1,...,Q-2, \varphi(0 \mid \theta) = \Phi_\theta(0.5)$, $\varphi(Q-1 \mid \theta) = 1 - \Phi_\theta(Q-1.5)$, where $\Phi_\theta(q)$ is the cumulative Gaussian probability function with $\theta = (\mu, \sigma^2)$ as the shorthand notation for the respective mean μ and variance σ^2. Note that

$$\sum_{r=1}^{K} w_r = 1 \tag{4}$$

TABLE 13.1   Summary of Lung Segmentation Techniques Using CT/Radiography

Study	Database	Dim	Approach	Performance
Beichel et al. [17]	45 data sets	3D	Active Appearance Model	50% object area covered by the gross gray-level disturbances
Wang et al. [18]	310 data sets	3D	Active Appearance Model Higher Order Singular Value Decomposition (HOSVD)	Average Dice Similarity Coefficient (DSC) of 97.0 ± 0.59 mm. Mean absolute surface distance error of 1.0403 ± 0.5716
Beichel et al. [20]	60 data sets (phantom data)	3D	Active Appearance Model	Positioning error of −0.16 ± 2.95 mm
Li et al. [22]	6 data sets	3D	Atlas-Based Segmentation	Reduced landmark registration error from 10.5 to 0.4 mm Average volume overlap error reduced from 0.7 to 0.11
Sun et al. [23]	40 diseased 20 normal data sets	3D	Model-Based Segmentation Active Shape Model	116 seconds was needed for the segmentation process. Average DSC of 0.975 ± 0.006 mm. Mean absolute surface distance error of 0.84 ± 0.23
Gill et al. [14]	190 data sets	3D	Atlas-Based Segmentation Active Shape Model Affine Transform	Average DSC was 0.746 ± 0.068 initialization and 0.974 ± 0.017 for segmentation. Mean absolute surface distance error was 0.948 ± 1.537
Gill et al. [24]	152 data sets	3D/4D	Robust Active Shape Model (RASM)	DSC of 0.9773 ± 0.0254
Shao et al. [25]	247 data sets	2D	Joint Shape and Appearance Model	NA
Tan et al. [26]	23 lung nodules with six radiologists contours	3D	Marker-Controlled Watershed Geometric Active Contours Markov Random Fields (MRF)	The intraclass correlation coefficient (ICC) is 0.998
Shen et al. [27]	NA	3D	Joint Shape and Appearance Model Active Volume Model	93.6 sensitivity and 99.8 specificity DSC of 95.2
El-Baz et al. [28]	487 radiograph images	3D	Markov-Gibbs Random Fields (MGRF)	Segmentation accuracy was 94.37%
Kockelkorn et al. [29]	22 CT data sets	3D	Volumes of Interest (VOIs) Segmentation	Overlap measure of 0.96 Mean absolute surface distance error of 1.68 mm
Mendonca et al. [30]	47 data sets	3D	Spatial Edge Detector	Sensitivity (P) of 0.9225 Positive predictive value of 0.968

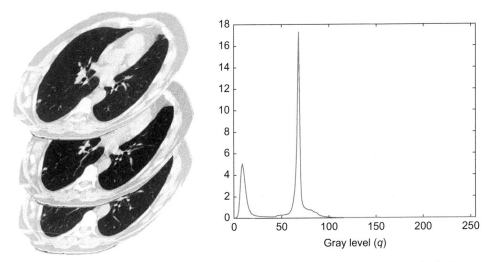

(a) Typical chest slices from a spiral CT scan.   (b) Normalized histogram for the intensity distribution.

Figure 13.4   Illustration of joint Markov-Gibbs model of CT lung images.

The objective is to maximize the log likelihood of the empirical data by the model parameters assuming statistically independent signals:

$$L_{app}(w,\theta) = \sum_{q \in Q} f(q)\log \Psi_{w,\theta}(q) \tag{5}$$

As such, the local log likelihood is given by the expectation maximization (EM) technique to find out the parameters w_r and θ_r. That is, the relative contributions of each signal $q \in Q$ to each Guassian at iteration m are specified by the respective conditional weights,

$$\Pi_r^{[o]}(w_r \mid g(i,j,z)=q) = \frac{w_r^{[o]}\varphi\left(q \mid \theta_r^{[o]}\right)}{\sum_{l=1}^{K} w_l^{[o]}\varphi\left(q \mid \theta_l^{[o]}\right)}, 1 \le i \le I, 1 \le j \le J, 1 \le z \le Z, 1 \le r \le K \tag{6}$$

such that

$$\sum_{l=1}^{K} \Pi_r^{[o]}\left(w_r \mid g(i,j,z)=q\right) = 1 \tag{7}$$

$$\varphi_r\left(g(i,j,z)=q \mid \mu_r, \sigma_r^2\right) = \frac{1}{\sqrt{2\pi\sigma_r^2}} e^{-\frac{(q-\mu_r)^2}{2\sigma_r^2}} \tag{8}$$

That is the following two steps iterate until the log likelihood $L_{app}(w,\theta)$ no longer changes or becomes as small as a preset Δ_{EM}:

- E step $[o + 1]$: Find the conditional weights or the responsibility $\Pi^{[o]}$ of equation 6 under the fixed parameters $w^{[o]}$ and $\theta^{[o]}$ from the previous iteration o.
- M step $[o + 1]$: Find conditional maximum likelihood estimates $w^{[o+1]}$ and $\theta^{[o+1]}$ by maximizing $L(w,\theta)$ under the fixed weights of equation 6.

$$w_r^{[o+1]} = \frac{\sum_{i=1}^{I}\sum_{j=1}^{J}\sum_{z=1}^{Z} \Pi_r^{[o]}\left(w_r \mid g(i,j,z) = q\right)}{\sum_{l=1}^{K}\sum_{i=1}^{I}\sum_{j=1}^{J}\sum_{z=1}^{Z} \Pi_l^{[o]}\left(w_r \mid g(i,j,z) = q\right)}, 1 \le r \le K \tag{9}$$

$$\mu_r^{[o+1]} = \frac{\sum_{i=1}^{I}\sum_{j=1}^{J}\sum_{z=1}^{Z} \Pi_r^{[o]} g(i,j,z)}{\sum_{i=1}^{I}\sum_{j=1}^{J}\sum_{z=1}^{Z} \Pi_r^{[o]}} \tag{10}$$

$$\left(\sigma_r^{[o+1]}\right)^2 = \frac{\sum_{i=1}^{I}\sum_{j=1}^{J}\sum_{z=1}^{Z} \Pi_r^{[o]}\left((i,j,z) - \mu_r^{[o]}\right)^2}{\sum_{i=1}^{I}\sum_{j=1}^{J}\sum_{z=1}^{Z} \Pi_r^{[o]}} \tag{11}$$

13.4.2 Spatial Interaction Model of CT Images

Pairwise interactions between each region label and its neighbors are taken account of in the Markov-Gibbs model of region maps whereby we assume relative region orientation-independent interactions due to symmetry considerations only up to a 26-neighborhood system, that is, the nearest voxel, as shown in Figure 13.5 for the arbitrary Gibbs potentials identified from image data. These are dependent only on whether the labels of the voxel pair considered are matching, that is, interregion or intraregion locations of each of the voxel pairs. Consequently, the developed model differs from an autobinomial one in just having analytical estimates and Gibbs potentials that are unrelated to a particular function.

The discussed symmetric label interactions are fourfold, whereby we consider the following: the closest two horizontal in the current slice (h), the closest two vertical in the current slice (v), the closest four diagonal in the current slice (d), and the closest in the upper slice with the closest in the lower slice (ul). The potentials of each type are bivalued because only whether the labels match (coincide or are similar) or do not (different) is taken into consideration. As such, let

$$V_a = \begin{cases} V_a(\rho,\chi) = V_{a,eq}, & \text{if } \rho = \chi \\ V_a(\rho,\chi) = V_{a,ne}, & \text{if } \rho \ne \chi \end{cases}$$

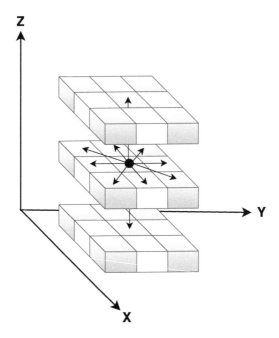

Figure 13.5   Spatial interaction model.

denote the bivalued Gibbs potentials to describe the symmetric pairwise interactions of type $a \in A = \{h, v, d, ul\}$ between the region labels. Let $N_h = \{(-1,0,0),(1,0,0)\}$, $N_v = \{(0,-1,0),(0,1,0)\}, N_d = \{(-1,-1,0),(1,1,0),(1,-1,0),(1,1,0)\}$, and $N_{ul} = \{(0,0,-1),(0,0,1)\}$ be subsets of intervoxel offsets for the 26-neighborhood system. Then the Gibbs probability distribution of region maps is as follows:

$$P(m) \propto exp \sum_{(i,j,z) \in R} \sum_{a \in A} \sum_{(\zeta, \eta, \kappa) \in N_a} V_a(m_{i,j,z}, m_{i+\zeta, j+\eta, z+\kappa}) \tag{12}$$

To identify the MGRF model described in equation 12, we have to estimate the Gibbs potentials V. In this chapter, we apply the analytical maximum likelihood estimation for the Gibbs potentials defined as

$$V_{a,eq} = \frac{X^2}{2(X-1)}\left(f_{eq} - \frac{1}{X}\right)$$
$$V_{a,ne} = \frac{X^2}{2(X-1)}\left(f_{ne} - \frac{1}{X}\right) \tag{13}$$

where f_{eq} and f_{ne} denote the relative frequency of the equal or matched and nonequal or mismatched equivalent voxel pairs of the labels as in $\{[(i,j,z),(i+\zeta, j+\eta, z+\kappa)] : (i,j,z) \in R; (i+\zeta, j+\eta, z+\kappa) \in R; (\zeta, \eta, \kappa) \in N_a\}$, respectively.

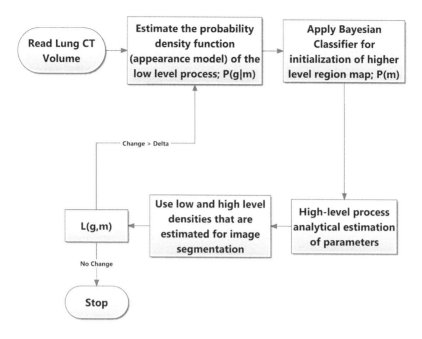

Figure 13.6   Segmentation approach proposed.

To further improve the segmentation, we then train with global features to handle any homogeneity in the lung structure. This is achieved with extracted scale-space features at multiple scales of image smoothing. This follows the same principle that allows humans to extract appearances and shapes as well as fine details of an image along with larger features, hence better guiding the medical image segmentation [31–34]. As such, we repeatedly apply spatial or frequency domain filters to the resulting scaled images on computation of the different levels of smoothing [35]. We also note that since the Gaussian distribution, that is, the mixture of which the appearance model is made of, is symmetric, such features are rotation independent. Moreover, we apply 3D region analysis for the computation of 3D connectivity for further segmentation enhancement. Finally, we use majority voting for the final segmentation result.

The complete iterative segmentation procedure is as follows:

1. Estimate X from the appearance model developed $\Psi(q)$ for each of the classes in X (lung or chest).
2. Use the resultant Bayesian MAP classification $\Psi(q)$ as initialization of the MGRF region map.
3. Refine iteratively the map:
   a. Potential values estimation for region map model using equation 13.
   b. Current regions' empirical gray-level densities recollection followed by their reapproximation in order to update the region map. This is performed by the Bayesian pixel-wise classification as shown in Figure 13.6.

     c. Perform the ICM algorithm. That is, for each site $(i, j, z) \in R$:

         i. Compute $P(m)_x = P(g_{(i,j,z)} = x \mid g_a) \forall X$.

         ii. Set $g_{(i,j,z)}$ to the label x which has the maximum probability.

     d. Repeat step 3c until there is no further change or it is less than predefined Δ.

4. Image smoothing at different scale spaces and repeat previous steps for each scale space.

5. 3D connectivity analysis.

6. Majority voting for final segmentation generation. Note that in step 4, we choose an odd total number in order to have a final decision by majority.

13.5 Experimental Results

Figure 13.7 illustrates a sample of our intensity model, which we also use as an initialization for the MGRF model. On approximation of the distributions that make up the signal, we find the threshold of the intensity model dynamically following this algorithm:

1. Initialize threshold value $T = T_{old} = T_{new}$ at the first distribution's μ. That corresponds to the peak of the lung probability distribution.

2. Increment threshold T_{old} by 1 for the updated value of the threshold $\left(T_{new} = T_{old} + 1\right)$.

3. If the probability density function value at $T_{new} < T_{old}$, then repeat step 2; otherwise, set the final threshold value $T = T_{old}$.

Figure 13.8 shows the results of the lung segmentation based only on the intensity model, while Figure 13.9 depicts the improvement of the segmentation on combining the spatial model with refinement with the appearance model. On the other hand, the final segmentation result to be fed to our 3D connectivity and region analysis is shown in Figure 13.10 after incorporation of two additional generated scale space volumes.

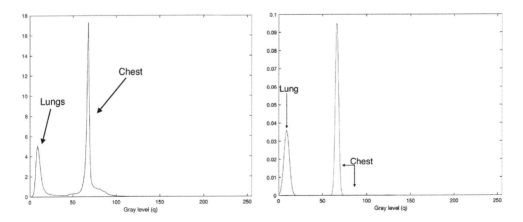

Figure 13.7   Illustration of approximated appearance model of CT lung images.

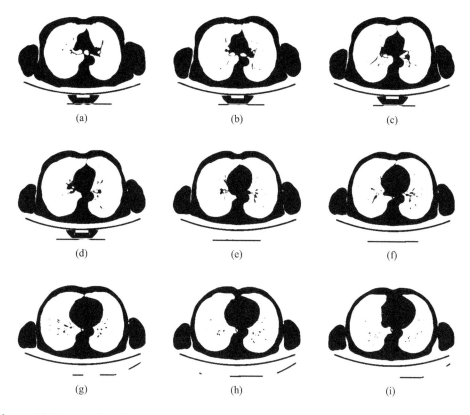

Figure 13.8   Results of lung segmentation with only intensity model applied.

Last but not least, Figure 13.11 shows a 3D visualization of the final segmentation results of our approach.

We validate the proposed segmentation approach on CT images through the analysis of the performance metrics of dice α, precision β, and recall γ: α is a local volumetric measure that allows us to measure the accuracy of the segmentation approach in comparison with the ground truth generated by a radiologist or a medical doctor; β, which is otherwise known as the positive predictive value, is the measure of how accurate a certain class prediction is. We define it as

$$\beta = TP / (TP + FP) \tag{14}$$

where TP is the number of true positives and FP is the number of false positives.

Next, sensitivity or the true positive rate γ is the capability of the model to select occurrences of a particular class given a data set. It is denoted as

$$\gamma = TP / P = TP / (TP + FN) \tag{15}$$

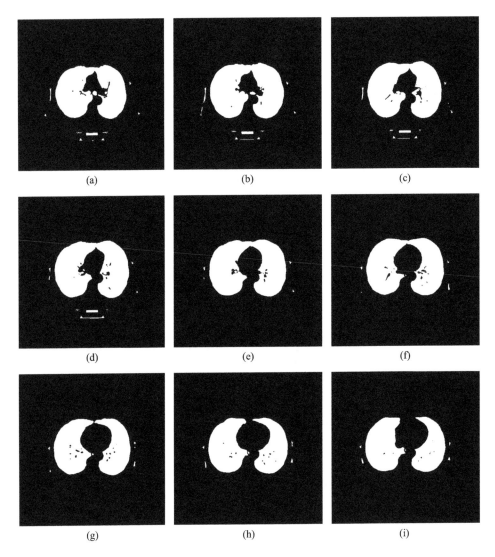

Figure 13.9 Results of lung segmentation with combined intensity and refined spatial models applied.

where P are all the positive or correct occurrences and FN is the number of false negatives.

13.6 Conclusion

In conclusion, the experimental results indicate that the proposed segmentation algorithm for lung tissue in CT images shows promising results. Our algorithm is based on an unsupervised parametric MGRF model that includes accurate

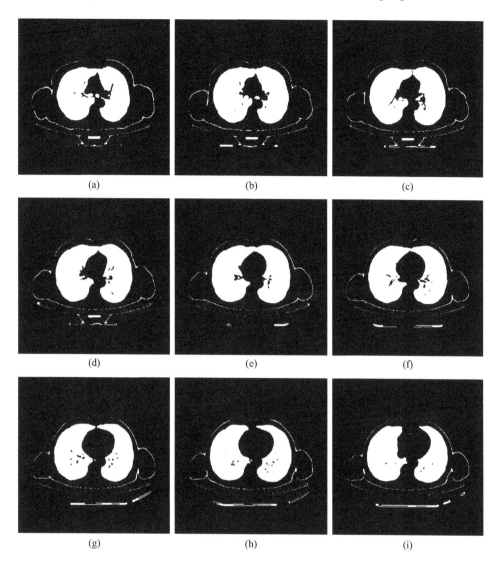

Figure 13.10   Results of lung segmentation with combined intensity and spatial models after different scale space incorporation.

appearance model formation that is also used as an initialization map for the conditional MGRF model. In addition, we also form and use a spatial interaction model and iteratively refine the map accordingly. Advantages of the proposed approach include the absence of any requirement of postprocessing steps for construction of a 3D visualization of the segmented lung. With our current implementation of the algorithm, processing of the – CT testing images took around seconds. Each of these images was 512 by 512 pixels with 126 slices per CT test subject.

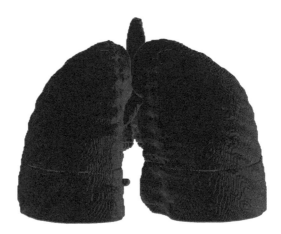

Figure 13.11   Segmented lung visualization using the proposed approach.

References

1. Tomashefski J, Farver C. Anatomy and histology of the lung. In: *Dail and Hammar's Pulmonary Pathology*. New York, NY: Springer; 2009:20–48.
2. Prakash C, Deopa D, Thakkar HK. Study of internal organ weight and its correlation to body weight in Kumaon region of Uttarakhand. *J Indian Acad Forensic Med.* 2013;35(1):29–32.
3. Betts JG, Desaix P, Johnson JE, et al. *Anatomy and Physiology*. Vol. 3. 2013.
4. Hashim A, Hashim ZH, El-Ahmady O, Khaled HM, Elmazar M. Serum VEGF165 and HGF in Egyptian patients with lung and pleural cancers. *Int J Adv Phram Biol Chem.* 2015;3(4):1048–1059.
5. Johnson R, Hsia C. Anatomy and physiology of the human respiratory system. *WIT Trans State Art Sci Eng.* 2006;24:1–29.
6. Celis E, Diaz-Mendoza J, Mosenifar Z. Medscape lung anatomy 2016. Available at: https://emedicine.medscape.com/article/1884995-overview. Date accessed June 29, 2016.
7. Robson R, Tidy C. The lungs and respiratory tract. Patient. https://www.wyevalleysurgery.co.uk/health-information. Date accessed November 13, 2015.
8. Suddarth B. Gas Exchange and Respiratory Function. Medical-Surgical Nursing http://downloads.lww.com/wolterskluwer_vitalstream_com/sample-content/9780781785891_Smeltzer/samples/Chapter021.pdf. Unit 5, Chapter 25. 2009.
9. Sylvia S. Mader Dr, Windelspecht M. The respiratory system. In: *Human Biology*, 15e. New York, NY: McGraw-Hill Education; 2017.
10. Joseph D, Puttaswamy R, Krowidi H. Non-respiratory functions of the lung. *Br J Anesth.* 2013;3(3):98–102.
11. Lumb A, Walwyn S. Non-respiratory functions of the lung. In: *Anaesthesia Science*. London: Wiley Online Library; 2006:257–264.
12. Magdy E, Zayed N, Fakhr M. Automatic classification of normal and cancer lung CT images using multiscale AM-FM features. *Int J Biomed Imaging.* 2015. doi: org/10.1155/2015/230830.

13. Dhalia J, Nehemiah H, Kannan A. Patient-specific model based segmentation of lung computed tomography images. *J Inf Sci Eng*. 2006;32(5):1373–1394.
14. Gill G, Toews M, Beichel R. Robust initialization of active shape models for lung segmentation in CT scans: a feature-based atlas approach. *Int J Biomed Imaging*. 2014. doi: 10.1155/2014/479154.
15. Karthikeyan A, Valliammai M. Lungs segmentation using multi-level thresholding in CT images. *Int J Electron Comput Sci Eng*. 2012;1(3)1509–1513.
16. Huidrom R, Chanu Y, Singh K. A study on lung segmentation for the detection and diagnosis of lung cancer. *Int J Adv Res Comput Sci Softw Eng*. 2016;6(11):55–66.
17. Beichel R, Bischof H, Leberl F, Sonka M. Robust active appearance models and their application to medical image analysis. *IEEE Trans Med Imaging*. 2005;24(9):1151–1169.
18. Wang Q, Na S, Wang B. Three-dimensional active appearance model based on tensor mode and its application in lung field segmentation from CT images. *Pattern Recognit Artif Intell*. 2015;28(8):750–759.
19. Wang Q, Kang W, Hu H, Wang B. HOSVD-Based 3D Active Appearance Model: Segmentation of Lung Fields in CT Images. Springer. 2016;40(7):176.
20. Beichel R, Gotschuli G, Sorantin E, Leberl F, Sonka M. Diaphragm dome surface segmentation in CT data sets: a 3D active appearance model approach. In: *Proceedings of SPIE: Medical Imaging Image Processing*. 2002(4684):475–485.
21. Mansoor A, Bagci U, Foster B, et al. Segmentation and image analysis of abnormal lungs at CT: current approaches, challenges, and future trends. *RadioGraphics*. 2015;35(4):1056–1076.
22. Li B, Christensen G, Hoffman E, McLennan G, Reinhardt J. Establishing a normative atlas of the human lungs: intersubject warping and registration of volumetric CT images. *Acad Radiol*. 2003;10(3):255–265.
23. Sun S, McLennan G, Hoffman E, Beichel R. Model-based segmentation of pathological lungs in volumetric CT data. In: *Proceedings of Third International Workshop on Pulmonary Image Analysis*. 2010(1):31–40.
24. Gill G, Beichel R. Lung segmentation in 4D CT volumes based on robust active shape model matching. *Int J Biomed Imaging*. 2015. doi: 10.1155/2015/125648.
25. Shao Y, Gao Y, Guo Y, Shi Y, Yang X, Shen D. Hierarchical lung field segmentation with joint shape and appearance sparse learning. *IEEE Trans Med Imaging*. 2014;33(9):1761–1780.
26. Tan Y, Schwartz LH, Zhao B. Segmentation of lung lesions on CT scans using watershed, active contours, and Markov random field. *Med Phys*. 2013;40(4):043502.
27. Shen T, Li H, Qian Z, Huang X. Active volume models for 3D medical image segmentation. *IEEE Trans Med Imaging*. 2011;30(3):774–791.
28. El-Baz A, Gimelfarb G, Falk R, Holland T, Shaffer T. A framework for unsupervised segmentation of lung tissues from low dose computed tomography images. In: *Proceedings of the British Machine Vision Conference*. 2008:855–865.
29. Kockelkorn T, Van Rikxoort E, Grutters J, Van Ginneken B. Interactive lung segmentation in CT scans with severe abnormalities. In: *Proceedings of the 7th IEEE International Symposium on Biomedical Imaging*. 2010:564–567.
30. Mendonca A, da Silva J, Campilho A. Automatic delimitation of lung fields on chest radiographs. In: *Proceedings of the International Symposium on Biomedical Imaging*. 2004;2:128790.
31. Vincken KL, Koster ASE, Viergever MA. Probabilistic multiscale image segmentation. *IEEE Trans Pattern Anal Mach Intell*. 1997;19(2):109–120.

32. Snel JG, Venema HW, Grimbergen CA. Detection of the carpal bone contours from 3-D MR images of the wrist using a planar radial scale-space snake. *IEEE Trans Med Imaging.* 1998;17(6):1063–1072.
33. Gauch JM. Image segmentation and analysis via multiscale gradient watershed hierarchies. *IEEE Trans Image Process.* 1999;8(1):69–79.
34. Petrovic A, Divorra Escoda O, Vandergheynst P. Multiresolution segmentation of natural images: from linear to nonlinear scale-space representations. *IEEE Trans Image Process.* 2004;13(8):1104–1114.
35. El-Baz A. *Multi Modality State-of-the-Art Medical Image Segmentation and Registration Methodologies.* New York, NY: Springer; 2011.

14

How Deep Learning Is Changing the Landscape of Lung Cancer Diagnosis

Sarfaraz Hussein and Ulas Bagci

Contents

14.1 Introduction

One of the leading causes of death in the world is cancer. Out of 8.2 million deaths due to cancer worldwide, lung cancer accounts for the highest number of mortalities at 1.59 million [1]. The diagnosis of lung nodules as benign or malignant can help identify cancer stage, leading to better treatment and improved survival rates. In this regard, the development of an automated system to automatically stratify lung nodules can save radiologists a lot of tedious work and precious time.

Early diagnosis of nodules can aid in reducing deaths related to lung cancer [2]. Large-scale lung screening programs can help in early diagnosis. For lung cancer detection and diagnosis, the most common imaging modality is low-dose computed tomography (CT). Although CT imaging remains the gold standard for lung cancer detection and diagnosis, computer-aided diagnosis (CAD) and quantification tools are often necessary. An additional advantage of developing highly accurate CAD systems comes from the exploration of imaging features and biomarkers that can be then incorporated by radiologists to improve clinical decisions.

14.1.1 Challenges to Lung Nodule Diagnosis

It is vital to have fast, accurate, and robust CAD systems for the diagnosis of lung nodules. The research in the detection and diagnosis of lung nodules has been accelerated with the accessibility to large publicly available data set, such as LIDC-IDRI from the Lung Image Database Consortium (LIDC) [3]. The task of accurate diagnosis of lung cancer, however, remains challenging due to the significant variance in the shape, intensity, extent, and position of lung nodules. Moreover, the difference between the malignancy and attribute scores from different radiologists increases the challenge. Given these variations of lung nodules, it may be important to have a significantly large number of labeled training examples in order to develop a highly accurate system. Recent advances in machine learning, particularly deep learning, have boosted the diagnostic performance of CAD systems. Traditionally, the CAD frameworks for the diagnosis of lung nodules relied on handcrafted feature extraction and cumbersome feature selection and engineering. However, with the advancements in deep learning, approaches have moved the CAD-based decision making toward accurate and robust (image) feature learning.

14.1.2 Approaches to Lung Nodule Analysis

Conventionally, the detection and categorization/classification (i.e., diagnosis) tasks in medical imaging were performed mainly with handcrafted features and off-the-shelf classifiers, such as support vector machines (SVM) and random forests (RF) [6, 9]. Between feature extraction and classification, feature selection or engineering approaches were usually applied to obtain the most discriminative set of features for classification. With the success of deep learning in all other tasks of visual domains, the research in medical image analysis transitioned from feature engineering to feature learning. In this chapter, we first provide an overview of conventionally used different feature extraction and selection approaches. We then discuss various feature learning and classification schemes, including deep learning–based strategies. We analyze a combination of deep features and handcrafted features for the diagnosis of lung nodules. End-to-end training of a two-dimensional (2D) deep neural network is studied for improved diagnosis followed by a 3D CNN–based approach that incorporates high-level lung nodule attributes. This chapter is based mainly on works of lung nodule diagnosis [9, 28, 29] from our lab and discusses potential future developments of lung cancer diagnosis with deep

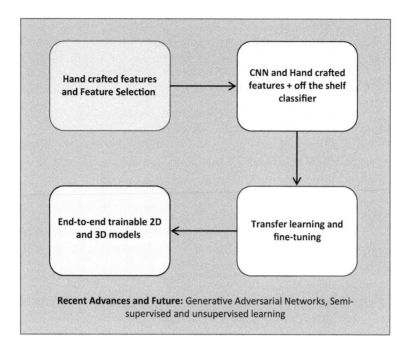

Figure 14.1   A broad overview of different machine learning techniques used for the automatic diagnosis of lung nodules. A transition from feature engineering to feature learning as well as future research directions are indicated.

learning methodologies. Figure 14.1 shows a transition from feature engineering to feature learning (deep learning), which affected almost all fields, including CAD designs for lung cancer diagnosis. While initial works in this field were in the intersection of feature extraction and feature learning jointly (due to a lack of hardware and other limitations of deep learning), more recent works focus solely on deep learning methods; a complete shift from feature extraction to feature learning is observed.

14.1.2.1 Feature Extraction and Selection

The usual methods of characterization of lung nodules included nodule segmentation and extraction of handcrafted imaging features, followed by the use of a stand-alone classifier/regressor. Uchiyama et al. [4] extracted various physical measures, such as intensity statistics, and performed classification with artificial neural networks. The method by El-Baz et al. [5] relied on segmentation of lung nodules using appearance-based models followed by shape analysis with spherical harmonics (SH). Finally, the classification was performed with k-nearest neighbor. The approach by Han et al. [6] extracted 2D texture features, such as Gabor, Haralick, and local binary patterns, along with their extension to 3D. The final class labels were obtained using SVM. In a classical work by Way et al. [7], segmentation is performed using 3D active contours, and a rubber band straightening transform was applied to the surrounding voxels to obtain the texture features. Linear discriminant analysis (LDA) was employed as a classifier. In an effort to incorporate the complementary information from both imaging and clinical data, Lee et al. [8] presented a feature selection–based approach. An ensemble classifier was used to combine genetic algorithm and random subspace method and applied to measure feature relevance and information content. The reduced feature was classified with an LDA classifier.

14.1.2.2 Feature Learning with Classification/Diagnosis

Recently, deep learning has successfully tackled the challenging problems of detection, segmentation, and classification in images and videos. Following up with that success, efforts had been made to transit from feature selection and engineering toward feature learning. However, taking into account a scarcity of labeled data in medical images, convolutional neural network (CNN) pretrained on nonmedical data sets were used to extract discriminative features followed by a separate classification stage [9, 10]. These approaches still relied on handcrafted features, such as SH. The goal is to incorporate both handcrafted and machine learning features to improve the classification performance. Most of these approaches are based on 2D image analysis [11], thus potentially ignoring important anatomical and contextual cues.

14.2 CNNs and Handcrafted Features

In the earlier lung cancer CAD works deep learning have been used to learn more discriminative features, but due to hardware, memory, and other limitations (e.g., the 3D nature of the images) of the deep learning methods, architectures were not so deep. Therefore, scientists were interested in fusing not-so-deep features (often appearance was dominant in such features) with the known feature extraction methods. One such example was to encode shape information from the nodules, as the not-so-deep networks were not as good in encoding the shape of the nodules [9]. In order to fuse information from both shape and appearance features, a combination of SH and CNN can be used. In order to model the variations in nodule shape, a surface parameterization scheme based on SH conformal mapping was employed. In parallel, image patches were passed through a pretrained CNN in order to obtain texture and intensity features. The features from SH and CNN were fused, and an RF classifier was trained to yield final malignancy outputs. The approach was evaluated on the LIDC-IDRI data set [3]. In the following, as an example of earlier deep learning methods for lung cancer diagnosis, we present details of the fusion of SH- and CNN-based features for lung cancer diagnosis.

14.2.1 Spherical Harmonics (SH)

SH comprises of a basis series that represent functions over a unit sphere S^2. The use of SH is meant to transform a 3D Euclidean shape into an SH space. The first step in this regard is to map the shape onto a unit sphere using conformal mapping. Conformal mapping is based on one-to-one surface transformations that maintain local angles. This transformation is important for surfaces with large differences, including cortical surfaces of the brain [12].

Consider M and N be two Riemannian manifolds such that a mapping $\varphi : M \rightarrow N$ remains conformal (local angles are preserved). A spherical parameterization of the surface can be obtained by mapping this simple surface to a unit sphere S^2. For genus zero closed surfaces, conformal mapping remains equivalent to a harmonic mapping and satisfies the Laplace equation, $\Delta f = 0$. Here, it is important to note that lung nodules are spherical in shape with limited local variations. In this regard, the spherical mapping of lung nodules to a unit sphere remains a natural option. The variations in the shapes of nodules can be modeled by conformal mapping to a unit sphere. In order to discriminate the differences of mapping to a unit sphere, SH are used. SH map S^2 to real space R.

With SH, a given function $f \in S^2$ can be decomposed into a direct sum of irreducible subexpressions given as

$$f = \sum_{l \geq 0} \sum_{|m| \leq l} \hat{f}(l,m) Y_l^m$$

where Y_l^m is the mth harmonic basis of degree l and $\hat{f}(l,m)$ is the corresponding SH coefficient. This decomposition yields representations that are invariant to scale, rotation, and transformation [12]. Moreover, it is comparatively easier to compute a correlation between vectors than surfaces. As the malignancy classification of lung nodules is influenced by determining the shape characteristics, the obtained decomposition is important for representing varying shapes of lung nodules.

The steps for obtaining SH representations are depicted in Figure 14.2. SH coefficients of segmented nodules with varying levels of malignancy are shown, along with the segmentations of the same nodules from different radiologists. First, a 3D mesh is generated from the segmented nodule. The mesh is then conformally mapped to a unit sphere and is decomposed into SH coefficients. It can be observed that SH coefficients are more discriminative for malignant and benign nodules compared to the segmentations for the same nodule. This qualitatively establishes that SH coefficients can be used for the characterization of malignancy. For smaller nodules, however, segmentation variations could yield different SH coefficients, motivating the use of appearance features using CNN.

14.2.2 CNN Features

In order to complement shape features, appearance features are extracted from CNN, and this can possibly improve the determination of malignancy. Features are extracted from the same network architecture as done by Krizhevsky et al. [13], which consists of five convolutional and three fully connected layers. The trained network provides different levels of image representation useful for training a discriminative classifier.

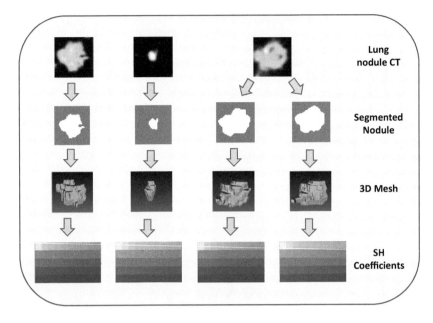

Figure 14.2 Example of SH coefficients for different nodules and segmentations. The top two rows show CT and segmented lung nodules, respectively. The third row depicts their 3D mesh followed by their SH coefficients. The first two columns show malignant and benign nodules, respectively, and the last column shows a lung nodule with different segmentation masks.

As the CNN takes a 2D RGB image, the local 3D CT image is transformed to have two dimensions and three channels. For each segmentation center of mass, a fixed-size cubic region of interest is fitted with the dimensions of the largest nodule in the data set. The data set is processed to have isotropic dimensions via interpolation.

For each nodule, three orthogonal axes, x', y', z', are identified within the conventional x, y, z space of axial, coronal, and sagittal planes. These axes are obtained using principal components analysis (PCA) on the binary segmentation. In the transformed space, three planes, $x'y'$, $x'z'$, and $y'z'$, are extracted that correspond to the three RGB channels of the image used as an input to the CNN. In order to avoid training the network from scratch, the pretrained model is used, and the features from the first fully connected layer of the network are used as appearance descriptor. This is inspired by the use of transfer learning from natural images to the medical imaging domain [14, 15].

14.2.3 Classification with RF

SH and CNN yield shape and appearance features that are used to determine malignancy. These features serve as an input to a classifier where the goal is to learn a discriminative model that returns accurate malignancy scores. Inspired by the approach in Sampaio et al. [16], here the SH and CNN features are combined to train a classifier. In this case, RF is employed for classification. RF-based classifiers are found to be accurate and efficient for similar problems [17]. The classifier comprises of a set of trees that are built by random sampling in feature and sample space so as to maximize the discriminativity at each node. A testing sample traverses through the trees, and a final classification label is obtained by a majority vote. For this particular application and data set, a set of 200 trees is found to have accurate and efficient classification performance.

14.2.4 Experiments and Results

The method is trained and tested on the LIDC image collection [3], which consists of 1,018 helical thoracic CT scans. Each scan was processed by four blinded radiologists who provided segmentations as well as malignancy ratings. Inclusion criteria consisted of scans with a collimation and reconstruction interval less than or equal to 3 mm and those with between approximately one and six lung nodules, with the longest dimensions between 3 and 30 mm. In total, 2,054 nodules were extracted with 5,155 segmentations, whereas 1,432 nodules were marked by at least two annotators.

To evaluate the performance of the proposed framework, "off-by-one" accuracy is used, which means that a malignancy rating with ±1 is considered as acceptable. For evaluation, 10-fold cross validation is performed (see Table 14.1). The results show that deep CNN and SHs provide complementary appearance and feature information, which help improve the malignancy characterization of lung nodules.

14.3 End-to-End 2D CNN for Lung Cancer Diagnosis

Another approach for the diagnosis of lung nodules is based on end-to-end training of CNN. Bearing a similarity with the previous approach, this method is also based on a 2D CNN, where multiple views of the lung nodules are fused as different channels of an RGB image. However, in sharp contrast to the previous method, here end-to-end training of CNN from scratch is performed in order to realize the full potential of the neural network, that is, to learn discriminative features. In addition,

TABLE 14.1 Off-by-One Accuracy for SH Only, DCNN Only, and Hybrid Models for Different Sets of Numbers of Annotators and Numbers of SH Coefficients

Minimum Annotations	No. of SH Coefficients	DCNN Only	SH Only	SH + DCNN
	100		0.772	0.812
1	150	0.791	0.783	0.824
	400		0.774	0.807
	100		0.761	0.803
2	150	0.759	0.779	0.793
	400		0.761	0.824

the complementary significance of high-level nodule attributes such as calcification, lobulation, sphericity, and others is analyzed so as to improve the determination of malignancy.

14.3.1 Architecture

The trained CNN model used for the characterization of lung nodules is named TumorNET, which was inspired by the architecture of Krizhevsky et al. [13], which consists of five convolutional layers, three fully connected layers, and a softmax classification layer. The first, second, and fifth convolutional layers are followed by a max-pooling layer. The input to the network is a three-channel image where the CT image patches from lung nodules are 3D. In an effort to combine information across all three views, median intensity projection of the image across each view is calculated. For each dimension of the image patch I, the median projected image ϕ can be represented as

$$\phi(y,z) = \underset{x}{med}\left[I(x,y,z)\right]$$

$$\phi(x,z) = \underset{y}{med}\left[I(x,y,z)\right]$$

$$\phi(x,y) = \underset{z}{med}\left[I(x,y,z)\right]$$

where *med* is the median operator. These projections corresponding to each axes (plane) of the image are concatenated to yield a 3D tensor, $\Phi = \left[\phi(y,z), \phi(x,z), \phi(x,y)\right]$. The CNN is trained end to end by considering this tensor Φ as a 2D image with three channels. An overview of the network is shown in Figure 14.3.

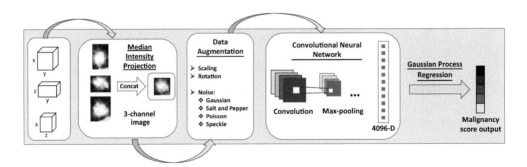

Figure 14.3 An overview of an end-to-end 2D CNN–based approach. First, the median intensity projection is performed across each axis, which are then concatenated as three channels of an image. Data augmentation is performed using scaling and rotation and adding Gaussian, Poisson, salt-and-pepper, and speckle noise. The CNN comprising five convolution and three fully connected layers is trained from scratch. While testing, the three-channel image is fed to the trained network to obtain a 4,096-dimensional feature. Gaussian process regression is employed to get the final malignancy score.

14.3.2 Data Augmentation

A deeper network such as TumorNET comprises a large number of parameters that need a large data set to perform full training. Here, obtaining features from the last layers of a pretrained network can provide suboptimal solutions, thus failing to realize the full potential of a deep network. In order to deal with the absence of a large number of examples to train a network from scratch, data augmentation is performed. Data augmentation gives extra samples corresponding to a single sample from the training data. The data augmentation is performed with rotation and scaling of the original examples. The input patch is randomly rotated along with scaling (upscaling and downscaling). Moreover, Gaussian noise with random mean, Poisson, salt-and-pepper, and speckle noise further adds new examples. Rotation, scaling, and noise add sufficient positive and negative examples to train the network.

14.3.3 Gaussian Process Regression

The next step is to train the deep network with the augmented examples until the loss converges. The first fully connected layer of the network denotes the high-dimensional feature representation of the input data consisting of $d = 4{,}096$ dimensions. With a large number of examples to train a discriminative regression model, $n = 2{,}000$ examples from the training data are sampled. Consider $X = [X_1, X_2 \ldots X_n]$ as the feature matrix, where $X \in R^{n \times d}$ and the regression labels are represented as $Y = [Y_1, Y_2 \ldots Y_n]$, where $Y \in R^{n \times 1}$. As each nodule has different malignancy scores from different radiologists, Y is the average score of these malignancy scores. Here, the target is to learn the regression estimator from the training data, which can be used to regress the malignancy scores of the testing examples.

Here, it's important to model the interobserver variation in the malignancy scores of different radiologists. The Gaussian process (GP) models this variation in which the prediction for each input also consists of an uncertainty measure.

In the GP formulation, each feature vector X_i is modeled by a latent function f_i with $f = (f_1, f_2 \ldots f_n)$ which is represented as

$$f \mid X \sim N\big(m(X), K(X, X)\big),$$

where $m(X)$ is the mean function and K is the covariance matrix such that $K_{ij} = k(X_i, X_j)$.

The GP regression, corresponding to a single observation Y, is constructed by a latent function and Gaussian noise ϵ:

$$Y = f(X) + \epsilon, \epsilon \sim N\big(0, \sigma_n^2\big).$$

Let f and $\tilde{f}$ be training and testing outputs, so their joint distribution is represented as

$$
\begin{bmatrix} f \\ \tilde{f} \end{bmatrix} \sim N\left(0, \begin{bmatrix} K(X,X) & K(X,\tilde{X}) \\ K(\tilde{X},X) & K(\tilde{X},\tilde{X}) \end{bmatrix}\right)
$$

where $K(\tilde{X},X)$ are the covariances, which are computed between all pairs of training and testing sets. The mean of this distribution is the best estimator for $\tilde{f}$.

14.3.4 Experiments and Results

The evaluation data set is the LIDC-IDRI data set [3]. The data set comprises 1,018 scans with slice thickness varying from 0.45 to 5.0 mm. Four expert radiologists annotated lung nodules with diameters greater than or equal to 3 mm. In the training and evaluation set, nodules annotated by at least three radiologists were used. There were 1,340 nodules satisfying this criterion. The nodules have a malignancy rating from 1 to 5, where 1 represents low malignancy and 5 is for highly malignant nodules. In order to account for the indecision among radiologists, nodules with an average score equal to 3 are excluded. The final data set consists of 635 benign and 510 malignant nodules for classification. All images were resampled to have 0.5-mm spacing in each dimension.

The evaluation consisted of 10-fold cross validation over 1,145 nodules. The data augmentation generated 50 extra samples corresponding to each example in the training data. An equal number of positive and negative examples are used to perform balanced training of the network. As the validation set, 10% of the examples from the training data were sampled. The network was trained for approximately 10,000 iterations as the loss function converged around it.

After training the network, features were extracted from randomly sampled 2,000 examples from the training data. The features were from the first fully connected layer of the network. The GP regression was then applied to those features. For testing, the images from the testing set were fed through the network to produce the feature representation followed by GP regression.

The success criterion is defined to have the malignancy predicted within a ±1 margin of the true score. Support vector regression, elastic net, and the least absolute shrinkage and selection operator (lasso) serve as other methods for comparison. All methods used CNN features from training and testing. As it can be inferred from Table 14.2 that TumorNET with GP regression outperforms popular classification and regression methods by a significant margin.

We also explored the significance of high-level nodule attributes, such as calcification, sphericity, texture, and others, for the determination of nodule malignancy. Fortunately, for the LIDC-IDRI data set, the radiologists have also provided the

TABLE 14.2 Comparison of the Proposed Approach with Support Vector Regression, Elastic Net, and Lasso Using Accuracy Measure and Standard Error of the Mean (SEM)

Methods	Regression Accuracy % (SEM %)
Support vector machine	79.91 (1.36)
Elastic net	79.74 (0.94)
Lasso	79.56 (1.14)
GP regression (TumorNET)	**82.47 (0.62)**

TABLE 14.3 Regression Accuracy and Standard Error of the Mean (SEM) Using a Combination of High-Level Attributes and CNN Features

Methods	Regression Accuracy % (SEM %)
High-level attributes	86.58 (0.59)
High-level attributes + CNN	**92.31 (1.59)**

scores corresponding to each of these attributes for nodules larger than 3 mm. We aim to analyze how these high-level attributes can aid classification of a nodule in conjunction with the appearance features obtained using the TumorNET framework. Another reason for our interest in these high-level attributes is that they can be easier to detect and annotate compared to malignancy. In this regard, crowdsourcing can be employed to get these attributes with high efficiency and efficacy.

For this particular experiment, we used six attributes: calcification, spiculation, lobulation, margin, sphericity, and texture. We computed the average scores in cases where scores from multiple radiologists were available. We performed two sets of experiments. For the first, we used GP regression over the set of these six features, and for the second, we concatenated them with a 4,096-dimension feature vector from TumorNET. We found that the combination of the high-level attributes and CNN features notably improves the regression accuracy (Table 14.3).

14.4 3D CNN with Multitask Learning

Capitalizing on the significant progress of deep learning technologies for image classification and their potential applications in radiology [15], we propose a 3D CNN–based approach for rich feature representation of lung nodules. We argue that the use of 3D CNN is paramount in the classification of lung nodules in low-dose CT scans, which are 3D by nature. By using the conventional CNN methods, however, we implicitly lose the important volumetric information, which can be very significant for accurate risk stratification. The superior performance of 3D CNN over 2D networks has been well studied by Tran et al. [18]. We also avoid handcrafted feature extraction, painstaking feature engineering, and parameter tuning. Moreover, any information about six high-level nodule attributes, such as calcification, sphericity, margin, lobulation, spiculation, and texture (Figure 14.4), can help improve the benign–malignant risk assessment of the nodules. Taking forward this idea, we

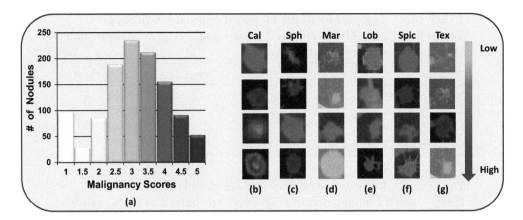

Figure 14.4 Graph showing the number of nodules with different malignancy scores (a) and lung nodule attributes with different scores. As we move from the top (attribute missing) to the bottom (attribute with the highest prominence), the prominence of the attributes increases. (b) and (c) show calcified and spherical nodules; (d) represents the margin, where the top row is for poorly defined nodules and the bottom row shows well-defined nodules. (e) and (f) show lobulated and spiculated nodules, whereas (g) represents nodules with different textures. The top row in (g) represents nonsolid nodule, and the bottom row shows solid nodule.

identify features corresponding to these high-level nodule attributes and fuse them in a multitask learning framework to obtain the final risk assessment scores. An overview of the proposed approach is presented in Figure 14.5. Overall, our main contributions in this work can be summarized as follows:

- We propose a 3D CNN–based method to utilize the volumetric information from a CT scan that would be otherwise lost in the conventional 2D CNN–based approaches. Moreover, we also circumvent the need for a large amount of volumetric training data to train the 3D network by transfer learning. We use the CT data to fine-tune a network that is trained on 1 million videos. To the best of our knowledge, our work is the first to empirically validate the success of transfer learning of a 3D network for lung nodules.
- We perform experimental evaluations on one of the largest publicly available datasets comprising lung nodules from more than 1,000 low-dose CT scans.
- We employ graph-regularized sparse multitask learning to fuse the complementary feature information from high-level nodule attributes for the determination of malignancy. We also propose a scoring function to measure the inconsistency in risk assessment among different experts (radiologists).

14.4.1 Problem Formulation

Let $X = [x_1, x_2 \ldots x_n] \in R^{n \times d}$ be the data matrix comprising features from n data points in R^d. Each sample corresponds with a regression score given by $Y = [y_1, y_2 \ldots y_n]$, where $Y \in R^{n \times 1}$. Here, the objective is to learn the coefficient vector or the regression

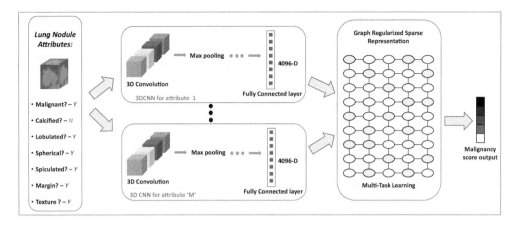

Figure 14.5   An overview of the 3D CNN–based approach. First, the 3D CNNs are fine-tuned using labels for malignancy and six attributes. The input volume is then passed through different 3D CNNs, each corresponding to an attribute (task). The 3D CNN architecture consists of five sets of convolutions, max poolings, and two fully connected layers. The output from the first fully connected layer is utilized as the feature representation. The features from different CNNs are fused together using graph-regularized sparse least-squares optimization function to obtain coefficient vectors corresponding to each task. While testing, the feature representations of the testing image are multiplied with the coefficient vector to obtain the malignancy score.

estimator W from the training data. In this case, the l_1-regularized least-squares regressor is defined as

$$\min_{W} \| XW - Y \|_2^2 + \lambda \| W \|_1$$

where λ controls the sparsity level for coefficient vector $W = [w_1, w_2 \ldots w_d]$. The problem in the above equation is an *unconstrained convex optimization* problem, and it remains nondifferentiable when $w_i = 0$. Hence, the closed-form solution corresponding to the global minimum is not possible. Thus, the above equation is represented in the following way as a *constrained optimization* function:

$$\min_{W} \| XW - Y \|_2^2 \; s.t. \| W \|_1 \leq t$$

where t is inversely proportional to λ. In the representation given in the above equation, both optimization function and the constraint are convex.

14.4.2 Network Architecture and Transfer Learning

We use the lung nodules data set to fine-tune a 3D CNN trained on the Sports-1M data set [19]. The sports data set comprises 1 million videos with 487 classes. In the absence of a large number of training examples from lung nodules, we use a transfer learning strategy to obtain rich feature representation from a larger data set

(Sports-1M) for lung nodule characterization. The Sports-1M data set is used to train a 3D CNN [18]. The 3D architecture consists of five sets of convolutions, two fully connected classification layers, and one soft-max classification layer. Each convolution set is followed by a max-pooling layer. The input consists of 16 nonoverlapping slices with a total dimension of $3 \times 16 \times 128 \times 171$. The numbers of filters in the first three convolution layers are 64, 128, and 256, respectively, whereas there are 512 filters in the last two layers. The fully-connected layers have a dimension 4096 which is also the length of feature vectors used as an input to the MTL framework.

14.4.3 Multitask Learning

Consider a problem with M tasks representing different attributes corresponding to a given data set D. These tasks may be related and share some feature representation, both of which are unknown. The goal in multitask learning (MTL) is to perform joint learning of these tasks while exploiting dependencies in feature space so as to improve regressing one task using the others. In contrast to multilabel learning, tasks may have different features in MTL. Each task has model parameters denoted by W_m, used to regress the corresponding task m. Moreover, when $W = [W_1, W_2 \ldots W_M] \in R^{M \times d}$ represents a rectangular matrix, rank is considered an extension to the cardinality. In that case, trace norm, which is the sum of singular values, is a replacement to the l_1 norm. Trace norm, also known as nuclear norm, is the convex envelope of the rank of a matrix (which is nonconvex), where the matrices are considered on a unit ball. By replacing l_1 norm with trace norm, the trace norm–regularized least-squares loss function is given by

$$\min_{W} \sum_{i=1}^{M} \| X_i W_i - Y_i \|_2^2 + \rho \| W \|_*$$

where ρ tunes the rank of the matrix W and trace norm is defined as $\| W \|_* = \sum_{i=1} \sigma_i (W)$ with σ representing singular values.

Another regularizer, pertinent to MTL, is the regularization on the graph representing the relationship between the tasks [20, 21]. Consider a complete graph $G = (V, E)$ such that nodes V represent the tasks and the edges E encode any relativity between the tasks. The complete graph can be represented as a structure matrix $S = [e^1, e^2 \ldots e^{\|E\|}]$, and the difference between all the pairs connected in the graph is penalized by the following regularizer:

$$\| WS \|_F^2 = \sum_{i=1}^{\|E\|} \| We^i \|_2^2 = \sum_{i=1}^{\|E\|} \| W_{e_a^i} - W_{e_b^i} \|_2^2$$

where e_a^i, e_b^i are the edges between the nodes a and b. The above regularizer can also be written as

$$\| WS \|_F^2 = tr((WS)^T (WS)) = tr(WSS^T W^T) = tr(WLW^T)$$

where *tr* represents the trace of a matrix and $L = SS^T$ is the Laplacian matrix. Since there may exist disagreements among the scores from different experts (radiologists), we propose a scoring function to measure potential inconsistencies:

$$\Psi(j) = (e^{\frac{-\Sigma_i (x_i^j - \mu^j)^2}{2\sigma^j}})^{-1}$$

The inconsistency measure corresponding to a particular example j is represented by $\Psi(j)$. The term x_i^j is the score given by the expert (radiologist) i, and μ^j and σ^j denote mean and standard deviation of the scores, respectively. Here, for simplicity, we have dropped the index for the task; however, note that the inconsistency measure is computed for all the tasks. The final proposed graph-regularized sparse least-squares optimization function with the inconsistency measure can then be written as

$$\min_{W} \sum_{i=1}^{M} \|(X_i + \Psi_i)W_i - Y_i\|_2^2 + \rho_1 \|WS\|_F^2 + \rho_2 \|W\|_1$$

where ρ_1 controls the level of penalty for graph structure and ρ_2 controls the sparsity. In the above optimization, the least-squares loss function the first part considers tasks to be decoupled, whereas the second and third consider the interdependencies between different tasks.

The optimization function in the above equation cannot be solved through standard gradient descent because the l_1 norm is not differentiable at $W = 0$. Since the optimization function has both smooth and nonsmooth convex parts, estimating the nonsmooth part can help solve the optimization function. Therefore, an *accelerated proximal gradient method* [22, 23] is employed to solve the above equation. The accelerated proximal method is the first-order gradient method with a convergence rate of $O(1/k^2)$, where k is the iteration counter. Note that in the above equation, the l_1 norm comprises the nonsmooth part and the proximal operator is used for its estimation.

14.4.4 Results

We used the 3D CNN trained on the Sports-1M data set [19], which had 487 classes. We fine-tuned the network using samples from lung nodule data set. In order to generate the binary labels for the six attributes and the malignancy, we used the center point and gave positive (or negative) labels to samples having scores greater (or lesser) than the center point. In the context of our work, tasks represented six attributes and malignancy. We fine-tuned the network with these seven tasks and performed 10-fold cross validation. By fine-tuning the network, we circumvented the need to have a large amount of training data. Since the 3D network was trained on image sequences with three channels and with at least 16 frames, we replicated the same gray-level axial channel for the other two. Moreover, we also ensured that all input volumes

TABLE 14.4   Classification Accuracy and Mean Absolute Score Difference of the Proposed Multitask Learning Method in Comparison with the Other Methods

Methods	Accuracy	Mean Score Difference
GIST + lasso	76.83%	0.675
3D CNN + lasso (pretrained)	86.02%	0.530
3D CNN + lasso (transfer learning)	88.04%	0.497
3D CNN MTL + trace norm	80.08%	0.625
Graph-regularized MTL	**91.26%**	**0.459**

have 16 slices by interpolation when necessary. We used the 4,096-dimension output from the first fully connected layer of the 3D CNN as a feature representation.

To find the structure matrix S, we computed the correlation between tasks by finding an initial normalized coefficient matrix W using lasso with the least-squares loss function followed by computing the correlation coefficient matrix [21]. We then applied a threshold on the correlation coefficient matrix to obtain a binary graph structure matrix. For testing, we multiplied the features from network trained on malignancy with the corresponding coefficient vector W to obtain the score.

For evaluation, we used metrics for both classification and regression. We calculated classification accuracy by considering classification to be successful if the predicted score lies in ± 1 of the true score. We also reported the average absolute score difference between the predicted score and the true score. Table 14.4 shows the comparison of our proposed multitask learning method with GIST features [24] + lasso and 3D CNN multitask learning with trace norm. Our proposed graph-regularized MTL outperforms the other methods by a significant margin. Our approach improves the classification accuracy over GIST features by about 15% and over trace norm regularization by 11%. Moreover, the average absolute score difference reduces by 32% and 27% when compared with GIST and trace norm, respectively. Figure 14.6 shows the qualitative results from the 3D CNN–based approach.

In order to evaluate the significance of transfer learning via fine-tuning, we project the features onto a low-dimensional space. This is done by computing the proximity between boundary points using t-distributed stochastic neighborhood embedding (t-SNE) [25]. As our feature space is high dimensional (4,096 dimensions), t-SNE is useful in revealing the structure of data at different scales. It can be seen in Figure 14.7 that fine-tuning the network on the lung nodule data set distinctively improves the separation between benign and malignant classes.

14.5 Discussion and Conclusion

In this chapter, we focused on different deep learning techniques for the risk stratification of lung nodules. An overview of handcrafted feature engineering and deep learning–based feature learning is provided. Moreover, a transition from 2D to 3D

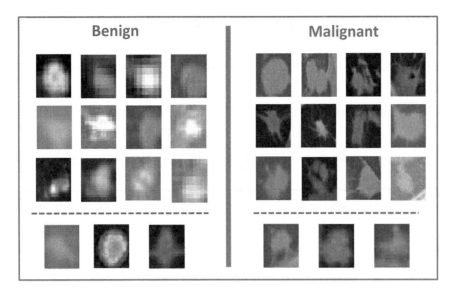

Figure 14.6 Qualitative results using our proposed approach. Left and right show axial views of benign and malignant nodules, respectively, where the top three rows consist of successful cases (where the prediction was within ±1 of the expert score) and the last row (below the dotted line) shows failure cases.

CNN is discussed along with techniques to incorporate the high-level nodule attributes within the risk stratification framework.

Risk stratification of lung nodules can be extended by training a 3D CNN end to end. Moreover, a single architecture can be employed to perform joint detection, segmentation, and diagnosis of lung nodules. A more pertinent clinical application

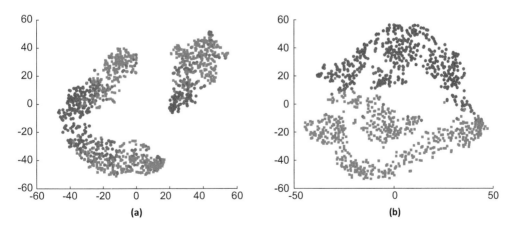

Figure 14.7 Effect of fine-tuning on 3D CNN features. *t*-SNE visualization for features obtained from (a) pretrained network and (b) network after fine-tuning. The separation between features belonging to two classes, that is, benign nodules (represented in blue) and malignant nodules (shown in red), can be readily observed in (b).

would be to use sequential CT scans for automatic lung cancer diagnosis. A possible research direction is to use recurrent neural networks and Long Short Term Memory Networks to perform prediction on sequential data. Incorporation of other imaging modalities, such as positron emission tomography, can also be useful, especially to compute the metabolic tumor volume.

There still remains critical challenges to incorporate deep learning–based strategies in clinical practice for the diagnosis of lung nodules. Until fairly recently, deep learning has remained a black box for clinicians and researchers that has made it difficult to gain acceptance for clinical use cases. However, the discussion and research about the interpretability of deep learning are paving the path toward identifying new imaging biomarkers that are important for radiologists. In this regard, the use of class activation maps is of significant value [26, 27]. More research is needed in this area to avoid mistrust of artificial intelligence in health care in general and in lung cancer diagnosis specifically.

Training a deep neural network generally requires a large number of labeled training examples, which may not be easier to obtain, especially pertaining to medical images. In this regard, there is a lot of potential for research in developing unsupervised approaches for medical imaging applications. Moreover, there usually exists a large variability in labels provided by different radiologists. As discussed in this chapter, transfer learning has helped to address the lack of annotated examples. However, the efficacy of transfer learning is limited by the large differences that exist between the domains of medical and natural images. Additionally, it is comparatively easier to obtain scan-level labels than slice-level labels. For this purpose, weakly supervised approaches, such as multiple instance learning, can help perform learning on scan-level labels. In the future, these research directions, along with unsupervised learning, can be pursued to address challenges in lung nodule diagnosis and to incorporate deep learning approaches in routine clinics.

References

1. Stewart BW and Wild CP, 2014. *World Cancer Report 2014*. Lyon, France: International Agency for Research on Cancer. *World Health Organization*.
2. van Beek EJ, Mirsadraee S, Murchison JT. Lung cancer screening: computed tomography or chest radiographs? *World J Radiol*. 2015;7(8):189.
3. Armato SG, McLennan G, Bidaut L, et al. The Lung Image Database Consortium (LIDC) and Image Database Resource Initiative (IDRI): a completed reference database of lung nodules on CT scans. *Med Phys*. 2011;38(2):915–931.
4. Uchiyama Y, Katsuragawa S, Abe H, et al Quantitative computerized analysis of diffuse lung disease in high-resolution computed tomography. *Med Phys*. 2003;30(9):2440–2454.
5. El-Baz A, Nitzken M, Khalifa F, Elnakib A, Gimel'farb G, Falk R, El-Ghar MA. 3D shape analysis for early diagnosis of malignant lung nodules. In: *Biennial International Conference on Information Processing in Medical Imaging*. Berlin, Heidelberg: Springer; 2011;772–783.
6. Han F, Wang H, Zhang G, et al. Texture feature analysis for computer-aided diagnosis on pulmonary nodules. *J Digit Imaging* 2015;28(1):99–115.

7. Way TW, Hadjiiski LM, Sahiner B, et al. Computer-aided diagnosis of pulmonary nodules on CT scans: segmentation and classification using 3D active contours. *Med Phys.* 2006;33(7, pt1):2323–2337.

8. Lee MC, Boroczky L, Sungur-Stasik K, et al. Computer-aided diagnosis of pulmonary nodules using a two-step approach for feature selection and classifier ensemble construction. *Artif Intell Med.* 2010;50(1):43–53.

9. Buty M, Xu Z, Gao M, Bagci U, Wu A, Mollura DJ. Characterization of lung nodule malignancy using hybrid shape and appearance features. In: *International Conference on Medical Image Computing and Computer-Assisted Intervention.* Springer, Cham.: 2016;662–667.

10. Kumar D, Wong A, Clausi DA. *Lung nodule classification using deep features in CT images.* In: New York, NY: Institute of Electrical and Electronics Engineers; 2015:133–138.

11. Chen S, Ni D, Qin J, Lei B, Wang T, Cheng JZ. Bridging computational features toward multiple semantic features with multi-task regression: A study of CT pulmonary nodules. In: *International Conference on Medical Image Computing and Computer-Assisted Intervention.* Springer, Cham.: 2016;53–60.

12. Gu X, Wang Y, Chan TF, Thompson PM, Yau S-T. Genus zero surface conformal mapping and its application to brain surface mapping. *IEEE Trans Med Imaging.* 2004;23(8):949–958.

13. Krizhevsky A, Sutskever I, Hinton GE. Imagenet classification with deep convolutional neural networks. In: *Advances in neural information processing systems.* 2012;1097–1105.

14. Bar Y, Diamant I, Wolf L, Lieberman S, Konen E, Greenspan H. Chest pathology detection using deep learning with non-medical training. In: *IEEE International Symposium on Biomedical Imaging. ISBI.* 2015;294–297.

15. Shin H-C, Roth HR, Gao M, et al. Deep convolutional neural networks for computer-aided detection: CNN architectures, dataset characteristics and transfer learning. *IEEE Trans Med Imaging.* 2016;35(5):1285–1298.

16. Sampaio WB, Diniz EM, Silva AC, De Paiva AC, Gattass M. Detection of masses in mammogram images using CNN, geostatistic functions and SVM. *Comput Biol Med.* 2011;41(8):653–664.

17. Breiman L. Random forests. *Mach Learn.* 2001;45(1):5–32.

18. Tran D, Bourdev L, Fergus R, Torresani L, Paluri M. Learning spatiotemporal features with 3d convolutional networks. In: *Proceedings of the IEEE international conference on computer vision.* 2015;4489–4497.

19. Karpathy A, Toderici G, Shetty S, Leung, T., Sukthankar, R. and Fei-Fei, L. Large-scale video classification with convolutional neural networks. In: *Proceedings of the IEEE conference on Computer Vision and Pattern Recognition.* 2014;1725–1732.

20. Evgeniou T, Pontil M. *Regularized multi-task learning.* In: New York, NY: Association for Computing Machinery; 2004:109–117.

21. Zhou J, Chen J, Ye J. *Malsar: Multi-Task Learning via Structural Regularization.* Tempe, AZ: Arizona State University; 2011:21.

22. Nesterov Y. *Introductory Lectures on Convex Optimization: A Basic Course.* New York, NY: Springer Science and Business Media; 2013.

23. Parikh N, Boyd S. Proximal algorithms. *Found Trends Optim.* 2014;1(3):127–239.

24. Oliva A, Torralba A. Modeling the shape of the scene: a holistic representation of the spatial envelope. *Int J Comput Vis.* 2001;42(3):145–175.

25. Maaten LVD, Hinton G. Visualizing data using t-SNE. *J Mach Learn Res.* 2008;9: 2579–2605.

26. Zhou B, Khosla A, Lapedriza A, Oliva A, Torralba A. Learning deep features for discriminative localization. In: *Proceedings of the IEEE Conference on Computer Vision and Pattern Recognition.* 2016:2921–2929.

27. Selvaraju RR, Cogswell M, Das A, Vedantam R, Parikh D, Batra D., 2017, October. Grad-CAM: visual explanations from deep networks via gradient-based localization. In: *International Conference on Computer Vision (ICCV)* 2017:618–626.

28. Hussein S, Gillies R, Cao K, Song Q, Bagci U. Tumornet: lung nodule characterization using multi-view convolutional neural network with Gaussian process. In: *IEEE 14th International Symposium on Biomedical Imaging.* 2017:1007–1010.

29. Hussein S, Cao K, Song Q, Bagci U. Risk stratification of lung nodules using 3D CNN-based multi-task learning. In: *International Conference on Information Processing in Medical Imaging.* 2017:249–260.

15

Early Assessment of Radiation-Induced Lung Injury

Ahmed Soliman, Fahmi Khalifa, Ahmed Shaffie,
Ali Mahmoud, Neal Dunlap, Brian Wang, Adel Elmaghraby,
Georgy Gimel'farb, Robert Keynton, Mohammed Ghazal,
Jasjit S. Suri, and Ayman El-Baz

Contents

15.1 Introduction

The main side effect of radiation therapy (RT) for lung cancer patients is the development of lung radiation–induced lung injury (RILI). Almost 40% of patients who undergo RT develop lung injuries following treatment [1]. Lung injury can be acute radiation pneumonitis (RP), which always happens in less than 6 months, or lung fibrosis, which happens after 6 months [2]. Early detection of lung injury will help to improve management of the treatment and reverse the injury progression (see Figure 15.1). Currently, global pulmonary function tests (PFT), such as spirometry, measure an airflow obstruction/restriction without providing regional lung function information. Alternatively, the lung functionality can be locally evaluated using nuclear imaging, such as SPECT ventilation and perfusion (V/Q) images. The acquisition of SPECT images is very expensive and uses relatively slow machines, and the images have too low spatial resolution. Relying on only the visual appearance (i.e., Hounsfield units [HU]) leads to a late RILI detection that will make the treatment more difficult. As an alternative, detecting early RILI development through monitoring lung functionality and lung texture changes could substantially improve disease management. Four-dimensional computed tomography (4D CT) is acquired as

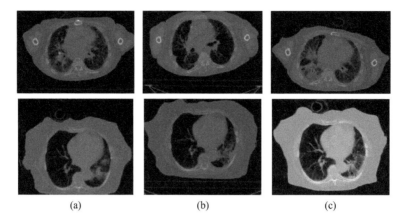

(a)   (b)   (c)

Figure 15.1 Effect of radiation on lung tissues. Two subjects (first and second rows) each with three axial slices from pretreatment (a) and at 3-month (b) and 6-month (c) follow-up scans. Images are cropped from the same position to show the misalignment effects.

part of routine care for lung cancer patients and has gained attention for assessing lung functionality, as the derived ventilation maps provide high spatial resolution and faster acquisition at no cost or with no dose cost to the patient. Moreover, in addition to texture, many other functionality features can be derived from 4D CT scans. Latifi et al. [3] showed that lung ventilation maps based on 4D CT correlate with 3D radiation dose distributions and suggested that these maps can be used in treatment planning to spare functional lung volumes. Reinhardt et al. [4] estimated local lung expansion from multiple respiratory CT images and showed that the Jacobian of the registration displacement field directly relates to a specific volume change. A quantitative study by Cunliffe et al. [5] measured lung reactions to RT and assessed the development of RP by extracting intensity-based information to distinguish between RP and non-RP patients. Vinogradskiy et al. [6] validated the use of 4D CT ventilation maps through the comparison with PFTs. The correlation coefficients for the comparison ranged from 0.63 to 0.72, with the best agreement between forced expiratory volume in 1 second (FEV1) and the coefficient of variation. Sharifi et al. [7] presented a prediction model for radiation-induced lung damage by measuring only the lung tissue density changes per voxel. Hu et al. [8] explored the use of CT perfusion imaging (CTPI) in early diagnosis of acute RILI. They compared the CTPI values at pre- and postradiation time points to measure the mean values of relative regional blood flow, relative regional volume, and relative regional permeability surface.

To overcome the limitations of known methods, such as the lake of PFTs to provide regional functionality, low spatial resolution of nuclear imaging, and sensitivity to noise of conventional voxel-wise descriptors, we propose an efficient computational framework to accurately segment and align lung regions from 4D CT images, extract discriminative features, and perform classification using a deep 3D convolutional neural network (CNN) to detect RILI.

15.2 Methods

The proposed framework (Figure 15.2) was performed sequentially: 4D lung segmentation; deformable image registration (DIR) for the 4D lung data, with a newly developed image model and methodology; extraction of textural and functional features; and detection of RILI by using a trainable deep CNN of lung tissues. Unlike our previous work [9, 10], this framework presents a new 4D CT segmentation and registration technique in addition to the deep 3D CNN for the identification of lung injury. The details of each step are given below.

15.2.1 4D CT Lung Segmentation

The segmentation of the lung fields is a crucial step for any computer-aided diagnostic (CAD) system [11–14] and for all subsequent steps of our framework for many reasons. First, the lung fields are segmented in order to ensure that all potentially injured regions will be examined. Second, determination of the lung fields in CT scans reduces intersubject variations of estimated features, which is achieved by normalizing the features inside the lung fields in each data set by averaging over its chest region. Third, the segmented lung masks at different respiratory phases will be used for the DIR. Finally, lung masks will be used as a volume of interest (VOI) for the analysis of the 3D CNN. Therefore, accurate segmentation is a must for accurate results at each step. We used our 3D lung segmentation framework [15], which is based on combining the segmentations of joint 3D Markov-Gibbs random field (MGRF) models for the original 3D scan and its Gaussian scale spaced-filtered volumes. The joint model integrates voxel-wise visual appearance features, pairwise spatial voxel interactions, and an adaptive shape prior of the lung that accounts for voxel location in addition to its intensity.

In order to segment the lung at different phases of the respiratory cycle, our method [15] is modified to increase its capability to segment 4D CT data as follows.

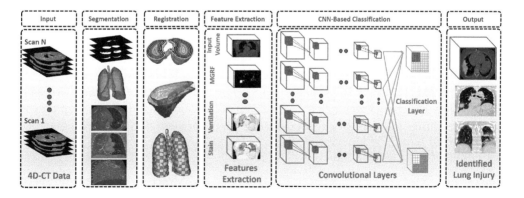

Figure 15.2 Our framework for detecting RILI.

First, the exhale phase of the 4D data is segmented. Then the segmentation labels of the exhale volume are propagated to the subsequent respiratory phases using only the modified adaptive shape prior component, which leads to an accurate and a faster segmentation. Label propagation is based on the visual appearance of the CT images at the different respiratory phases. Namely, each voxel $\mathbf{r}$ of the different phase image $\mathbf{t}$ is mapped to the same location at the exhale lattice. Then an initial search cube $\mathbf{C_r}$ of size $c_{x:i} \times c_{y:i} \times c_{z:i}$ is centered at the mapped location $\mathbf{r}$ for finding in the cube all the exhale voxels with signal deviations within a predefined fixed range, λ, from the mapped input signal, t_r. If such voxels are absent in the exhale, the cube size increases iteratively until the voxels within the predefined signal deviation range are found or the final cube size is reached ($c_{x:i} = c_{y:i} = c_{z:i} = 3$; λ from 50 to 125 with the step of $\Delta_\lambda = 25$, and the final cube size of $c_{x:f} = c_{y:f} = c_{z:f} = 11$ were used in our experiments). Then the voxel-wise probabilities, $P_{sh:r}(k)$; $k \in \mathbf{K}$ for the adaptive shape prior are estimated based on the found voxels of similar appearance and their labels. Let $\mathbb{R}_r = \{\varphi : \varphi \in \mathbf{R}; \varphi \in \mathbf{C_r}; |g_\varphi - t_r| \leq \lambda\}$ be a subset of similar voxels within the cube $\mathbf{C_r}$ in the exhale image. Let $R_r = \mathrm{card}(\mathbb{R}_r)$ denote the cardinality (number of voxels) of this subset; and $\delta(z)$ be the Kronecker's delta function: $\delta(0) = 1$ and 0 otherwise. The final probability for each voxel is calculated as:

$$P_{sh:r}(k) = \frac{1}{R_r} \sum_{\varphi \in \mathbb{R}_r} \delta(k - m_\varphi)$$

15.2.2 Deformable Image Registration

Accurate estimation of regional functional features requires accurate spatial mapping between successive pairs of 3D CT volumes of the respiratory cycle. Traditional 4D CT registration tries to establish direct spatial correspondences between the peak exhale and peak inhale images. However, this may lead to losing some accuracy that can be avoided due to relatively large changes in lung volumes between the two peak phases. To reduce these errors that can affect the estimated features, a sequential DIR has been performed between successive 3D CT volumes of the respiratory cycle. The registration establishes the voxel-wise displacement vector field $\mathbf{U} = \{\mathbf{u}(\mathbf{r}) = \sum_{i=1}^{N-1} \mathbf{u}_i(\mathbf{r}) : \mathbf{r} \in \mathbb{R}\}$, which integrates displacements between successive 3D-CT volumes. The total field, $\mathbf{U}$, and its successive components, $\mathbf{U}_i = \{\mathbf{u}_i(\mathbf{r}) : \mathbf{r} \in \mathbb{R}\}$, defined on the initial 3D-CT volume $\mathbb{R}$, determine gradual changes of image geometry and signals or features along the cycle. We used our developed nonrigid registration technique [16] to get the displacement fields. This is achieved using a two-step registration, which includes a global affine step of the calculated distance map for the segmented lungs followed by a local deformation of each voxel to its correspondence by solving the 3D Laplace equation, $\nabla^2\gamma = \dfrac{\partial^2\gamma}{\partial x^2} + \dfrac{\partial^2\gamma}{\partial y^2} + \dfrac{\partial^2\gamma}{\partial z^2} = 0$; where $\gamma(x,y,z)$ is the estimated electric field between the reference and target surfaces between each two corresponding isosurfaces that generates streamlines from the fixed volume voxels to the moving one. Then the generalized Gaussian Markov random field (GGMRF) smoothing is applied to ensure anatomical consistency and best match using equation 1:

$$\widehat{\mathbf{p}}_s = \arg\min_{\mathbf{p}_s = \left(\widetilde{x}_s^{ref}, \widetilde{y}_s^{ref}, \widetilde{z}_s^{ref}\right)} \left\{ \left(\left| x_s^{ref} - \widetilde{x}_s^{ref} \right|^\alpha \right. \right.$$

$$\left. + \left| y_s^{ref} - \widetilde{y}_s^{ref} \right|^\alpha + \left| z_s^{ref} - \widetilde{z}_s^{ref} \right|^\alpha \right) + \rho^\alpha \lambda^\beta \sum_{r \in N} \eta_{s,r}$$

$$\left(\left| \widetilde{x}_s^{ref} - x_r^{ref} \right|^\beta + \left| \widetilde{y}_s^{ref} - y_r^{ref} \right|^\beta + \left| \widetilde{z}_s^{ref} - z_r^{ref} \right|^\beta \right)$$

$$+ \left| q_{s'}^{tar} - \widetilde{q}_s^{ref} \right|^\alpha + \rho^\alpha \lambda^\beta \sum_{r \in N} \eta_{s,r} \left| \widetilde{q}_{s'}^{tar} - q_r^{ref} \right|^\beta \right\} \qquad (1)$$

where $\mathbf{p}_s = \left(x_s^{ref}, y_s^{ref}, z_s^{ref}\right)$ and $\widehat{\mathbf{p}}_s = \left(\widetilde{x}_s^{ref}, \widetilde{y}_s^{ref}, \widetilde{z}_s^{ref}\right)$ denote the initial 3D locations of the target voxels' correspondences and their expected estimates on the reference; $q_{s'}^{tar}$ and $\widetilde{q}_s^{ref}$ are the target voxel intensity and its estimate correspondences on the reference, respectively; N is the number of the nearest neighbor voxels; $\eta_{s,r}$ is the GGMRF potential, and ρ and λ are scaling factors. The level of smoothing is controlled by the $\beta \in [1.01, 2.0]$ parameter (e.g., $\beta = 1.01$ for relatively abrupt vs. $\beta = 2$ for smooth edges). The prior distribution of the estimator is determined by $\alpha \in \{1, 2\}$ parameter: $\alpha = 2$ for Gaussian, or $\alpha = 1$ for Laplace. The used parameter values are $\rho = 1$, $\lambda = 5$, $\beta = 1.01$, $\alpha = 2$, and $\eta_{s,r} = \sqrt{2}$ for all directions.

15.2.3 Extraction of Texture and Functionality Features

Two categories of discriminative features are extracted using the segmented lung volumes and the calculated deformation fields. These features describe the lung alteration as a result of the RT. The textural feature is modeled in terms of Gibbs energy for the novel seventh-order contrast-offset-invariant MGRF image model, while the functional features are modeled using the Jacobian ventilation, describing the airflow in the lung and functional strain describing the elasticity of the lung tissue. Both of the feature categories are detailed below.

15.2.3.1 The Seventh-Order Textural Feature
To model the changes in visual appearance of the injured parts of the lung, the CT lung voxels are considered samples of a trainable translation- and contrast-offset-invariant seventh-order MGRF [17, 18]. The model relates the Gibbs probability of an image $\mathbf{g} = (g(\mathbf{r}) : \mathbf{r} \in \mathbb{R})$ with the voxel-wise HU $g(\mathbf{r})$ to a general-case seventh-order exponential family distribution is $P_7(\mathbf{g}) = \dfrac{1}{Z} \psi(\mathbf{g}) \exp(-E_7(\mathbf{g}))$, where Z is the normalizing factor and $E_7(\mathbf{g})$ is the Gibbs energy of the image. It describes an image texture in terms of signal dependencies (interactions) between each voxel and its neighbors depending on how the training lungs have been affected. This model accounts for partial ordinal

interactions between voxel-wise signals in each particular voxel and within a radius ρ from it for describing the appearance of the injured parts in the lung CT scans. Given a training image $\mathbf{g}^{\circ}$, Gibbs potentials, $v_{7:\rho}(g(\mathbf{r}'): \mathbf{r}' \in v(\mathbf{r}))$, of translation-invariant subsets of 7 pixels to compute the energy $E_7(\mathbf{g})$ are learned using their approximate maximum likelihood estimates. The latter are obtained by generalizing the analytical approximation of potentials for the general second-order MGRF [19, 20]:

$$v_{7:\rho}(\beta) = \frac{F_{7:\rho:core}(\beta) - F_{7:\rho}\left(\beta \mid \mathbf{g}^{\circ}\right)}{F_{7:\rho:core}(\beta)\left(1 - F_{7:\rho:core}(\beta)\right)}; \beta \in \mathbb{B}_7$$

where β denotes a numerical code of a particular contrast-offset invariant relation between seven signals, $\mathbb{B}_7$ is a set of these codes for all these seven-signal co-occurrences, $F_{7:\rho}\left(\mathbf{g}^{\circ}\right)$ is a marginal probability of the code β; $\beta \in \mathbb{B}_7$, over all the 7-voxel configurations with the radius ρ in the image $\mathbf{g}^{\circ}$, and $F_{7:\rho:core}(\beta)$ is the like probability for the core distribution. The computed energy monitors changes in the tissue signals over time and indicates the RILI development. The computed energy gives an indication of the tissue signals changes over time and the possibility of lung injury development. While a severe radiation effect is suggested by the higher energy, the lower the Gibbs energy, the lower the injury. To quantify the normal and injured regions' appearances, we use the Gibbs energies for the three seventh-order contrast/offset- and translation-invariant MGRFs, each with a single family of central-symmetric, fixed-shape voxel configurations $v(\mathbf{r} = (x, y, z)) = \{(x, y, z); (x \pm \rho, y, z), (x, y \pm \rho, z), (x, y, z \pm \rho)\}$. Their distances, ρ, between the peripheral and central voxels and potentials are learned from $\mathbf{g}^{\circ}$ by modifying the learning process in Liu et al. [17].

15.2.3.2 Functionality Features Extraction

These groups of features are extracted from the calculated voxel-wise deformation fields obtained. After the registration of successive respiratory phases, the obtained voxel-wise deformation fields are used to calculate the following functionality features.

Functional strain can be used for the identification of injured lung regions, as the characteristics of these regions change as a result of the applied RT. The strain describes the elasticity characteristic of the lung tissues. From the gradient of the displacement vector $\mathbf{u}(\mathbf{r})$, which maps the voxel at location $\mathbf{r}$ of the peak exhale to its corresponding peak-inhale image, the Lagrangian strain can be estimated mathematically as follows:

$$S = \begin{bmatrix} \dfrac{\partial u_x}{\partial x} & \dfrac{1}{2}\left(\dfrac{\partial u_x}{\partial y} + \dfrac{\partial u_y}{\partial x}\right) & \dfrac{1}{2}\left(\dfrac{\partial u_x}{\partial z} + \dfrac{\partial u_z}{\partial x}\right) \\[3ex] \dfrac{1}{2}\left(\dfrac{\partial u_y}{\partial x} + \dfrac{\partial u_x}{\partial y}\right) & \dfrac{\partial u_y}{\partial y} & \dfrac{1}{2}\left(\dfrac{\partial u_y}{\partial z} + \dfrac{\partial u_z}{\partial y}\right) \\[3ex] \dfrac{1}{2}\left(\dfrac{\partial u_z}{\partial x} + \dfrac{\partial u_x}{\partial z}\right) & \dfrac{1}{2}\left(\dfrac{\partial u_z}{\partial y} + \dfrac{\partial u_y}{\partial z}\right) & \dfrac{\partial u_z}{\partial z} \end{bmatrix} \qquad (2)$$

where the main diagonal components $\dfrac{\partial u_x}{\partial x}$, $\dfrac{\partial u_y}{\partial y}$, and $\dfrac{\partial u_z}{\partial z}$ define the linear strain along x, y, and z, respectively. The shear strain components are calculated using the off-diagonal components as: $\left(\gamma_{ij} = \dfrac{1}{2}\left(\dfrac{\partial u_i}{\partial j} + \dfrac{\partial u_j}{\partial i} \right) = \gamma_{ji}; \ i,j \in \{x,y,z\}, \ i \neq j \right)$. In terms of $\mathbf{u}(\mathbf{r})$, the strain tensor can be expressed as: $S = \dfrac{1}{2}\left[\nabla \mathbf{u} + (\nabla \mathbf{u})^T \right]$, where:

$$
\nabla \mathbf{u}(\mathbf{r}) =
\begin{bmatrix}
\dfrac{\partial u_x}{\partial x} & \dfrac{\partial u_x}{\partial y} & \dfrac{\partial u_x}{\partial z} \\[2ex]
\dfrac{\partial u_y}{\partial x} & \dfrac{\partial u_y}{\partial y} & \dfrac{\partial u_y}{\partial z} \\[2ex]
\dfrac{\partial u_z}{\partial x} & \dfrac{\partial u_z}{\partial y} & \dfrac{\partial u_z}{\partial z}
\end{bmatrix}
\tag{3}
$$

Jacobian ventilation, as the partial volume changes of the lung voxels, gives a good estimation of regional changes [4]. Incorporating this feature in terms of Jacobian ventilation will help in the detection of injured regions. The voxel-wise volume at the inhale phase is estimated as $V_{in}^{\mathbf{r}} = V_{ex}^{\mathbf{r}} J_{\mathbf{r}}$ and the exhale-to-inhale volume change is $\Delta V_J = V_{in}^{\mathbf{r}} - V_{ex}^{\mathbf{r}} = V_{ex}^{\mathbf{r}}(J_{\mathbf{r}} - 1)$, where $J_{\mathbf{r}}$ is the Jacobian determinant for each voxel, estimated from the gradient of the displacement fields as $J_{\mathbf{r}} = |\nabla \mathbf{u}(\mathbf{r}) + I|$, where I is the identity matrix, and $\nabla \mathbf{u}(\mathbf{r})$ is the gradient of $\mathbf{u}(\mathbf{r})$ for each voxel in equation 3.

15.2.3.3 Tissue Classification and Segmentation Using Deep CNN

To detect and segment the injured tissues, all the estimated features ($E_7(\mathbf{g})$, ΔV_J, and the maximum eigenvalue of the strain matrix of equation 3), in addition to the raw exhale phase (shown in Figure 15.3), are used as 3D input volumes to the deep CNN. The latter learns discriminative characteristics from the different 3D inputs by using the training database containing both injured and normal lungs. A deep 3D CNN is used for the generation of soft segmentation maps followed by fully connected 3D conditional random field to produce the final labeled output of the segmented injuries [21]. The input is sequentially convolved with multiple filters at the cascaded network layers. Each layer consists of a number of channels where each channel is corresponding to the 3D volume of the calculated feature. The 3D input feature volumes at the first layer are considered as the channels of the input. This process can be viewed as convolving 4D volumes (concatenated 3D feature volumes) with 4D kernels. The network architecture is depicted in Figure 15.2. The architecture of the used CNN consists of seven layers with kernels of size 5^3 and the receptive field (input voxel neighborhood influencing the activation of a neuron) of size 17^3. The kernels for the classification layer is 1^3. The advantage of this architecture is its ability to capture 3D contextual information from the provided feature volumes.

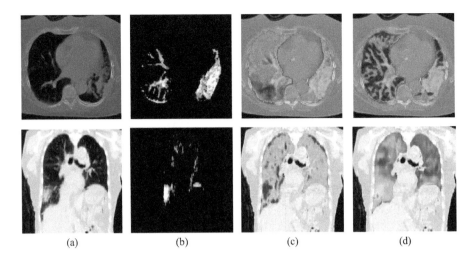

(a)   (b)   (c)   (d)

Figure 15.3 A 2D axial slice for axial (first row) and coronal (second row) (a) with its calculated seventh-order Gibbs energy (b), maximal strain feature (c), and Jacobian ventilation (d).

The configuration parameters have been chosen heuristically similar to those of Kamnitsas et al. [21].

15.3 Experimental Results

4D CT data from 13 lung cancer patients scheduled to receive RT have been used in this study. The 4D CT data were collected using the Philips Brilliance Big Bore CT scanner with the Varian real-time position management system (Varian Medical Systems, Palo Alto, CA, USA) for respiratory traces. The data spacing for the collected data ranges from $1.17 \times 1.17 \times 2.0$ mm to $1.37 \times 1.37 \times 3.0$ mm. To obtain functionality and appearance features for training our CNN network, the CT data were contoured by a radiologist. Then the deep network was applied to the voxels within the VOI determined by the segmented lung mask in a "leave-one-subject-out scenario." The voxels were classified as normal or injured tissue, and morphological operations were used for refinement, removal of scattered voxels, and hole filling. The 3D feature values and the raw exhale volume (its HU values) inside the VOI are normalized to be zero mean and unity standard deviation to accelerate the convergence by reducing the internal covariant shift. Since lung segmentation and DIR are crucial steps in the proposed framework, Figure 15.4 shows a 2D illustration of the 4D CT segmentation that propagates the labels of the exhale phase to the inhale phase along the overlap between the two phase images before and after the DIR registration. The average lung segmentation accuracy in terms of the Dice Similarity Coefficient (DSC) [22], which characterizes spatial overlap, is 99%, with an average speed of 7.3 seconds, while the DIR accuracy in terms of target registration error equals 1.37×1.03 mm. The performance of the deep network tested on our data sets

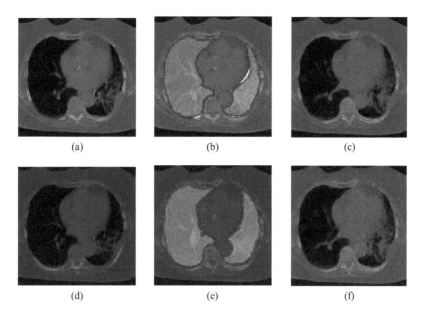

(a) (b) (c)

(d) (e) (f)

Figure 15.4 Two typical axial slices at the same cross section for the exhale phase (a) with its segmentation (b) and the inhale phase (d) with its segmentation (e). Their overlap before the registration (f) and after the registration (c). The color codes are green for true positive, yellow for false positive, pink for false negative, and red for ground truth edges.

has been evaluated in terms of accuracy *Acc*, sensitivity *Sens*, and specificity *Spec*, defined as $Acc = \dfrac{TP + TN}{TP + TN + FP + FN}, Sens = \dfrac{TP}{TP + FN}, pec = \dfrac{TN}{TN + FP}$, where *TP, TN, FP*, and *FN* are the number of true positive, true negative, false positives, and false negatives, respectively. The performance measures are listed in Table 15.1 for different feature groups (FGs), using only the raw exhale phase (FG1), the exhale phase in addition to functionality features (FG2), and FG2 in addition to texture features (FG3). It is clear that combining the features achieves the highest accuracy because these features complement each other in both early and late phases.

TABLE 15.1   Performance of the 3D CNN for Different Feature Groups: FG1 (4D CT Volume), FG2 (4D CT Volume and Functionality Features), and FG3 (4D CT Volume, Functionality, and Appearance Features)

	Performance Metrics						
	Classification Metrics				Segmentation Metrics		
	AUC	Acc	Sens	Spec	Dice	BHD	AVD
FG1	94.1	91.8	79.1	96.3	72.7	19.4	9.5
FG2	96.3	92.6	81.0	96.5	82.9	14.2	6.0
FG3	99.0	95.4	86.8	98.3	88.0	5.2	4.6

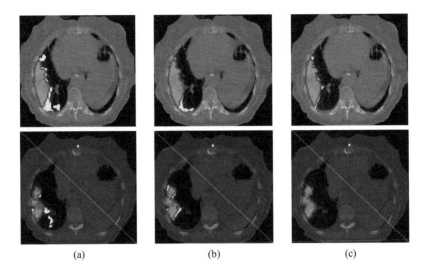

| (a) | (b) | (c) |

Figure 15.5 Typical 2D segmentation results for two axial slices using FG1 (a), FG2 (b), and FG3 (c). The color codes are green for true positive, yellow for false positive, pink for false negative, and red for ground truth edges.

Moreover, the classification accuracy has been evaluated using the area under the curve (AUC) for different FGs. The AUC for using the FG1 equals only 0.94 and for the FG2 equals 0.96. When combining all the features in the classification process, the AUC has increased to 0.99. This enhancement highlights the advantages of integrating both texture and functionality features as discriminatory ones for the detection of RILI.

In addition to the DSC, the segmentation accuracy for the injured tissues has been evaluated for each subject with bidirectional Hausdorff distance (BHD) and percentage volume difference (PVD) [23, 24], which characterize maximum surface-to-surface distances and volume differences, respectively, between the segmented and "ground-truth" injured regions. Table 15.1 summarizes the DSC, BHD, and PVD statistics for all test subjects showing the effect of different FG of our framework. The ground truth borders were outlined manually by a radiologist. The mean ± standard deviation of the DSC, BHD, and PVD for all the test subjects using our proposed framework is 88.0 ± 3.5%, 5.2 ± 1.3 mm, and 4.6 ± 0.7%, respectively. Figure 15.5 shows a sample RILI segmentation using different FGs.

15.4 Conclusion

In conclusion, this chapter introduced a processing pipeline for the detection of RILI using 4D CT lung data. The pipeline consists of 4D CT lung segmentation, DIR, extraction of discriminative feature, and injured tissue segmentation using

3D CNN. The segmentation/detection results in a set of 13 patients who underwent RT confirm that the proposed framework holds the promise for early detection of lung injury. We plan to integrate other clinical biomarkers (e.g., PFTs) to our framework and perform more validation by collecting more data with shorter follow-up scans to evaluate the ability of detecting the RILI before any radiographic evidence.

This work could also be applied to other applications in medical imaging, such as the kidney, the heart, the prostate, and the retina.

One application is renal transplant functional assessment. Chronic kidney disease affects about 26 million people in the United States, with 17,000 transplants being performed each year. In renal transplant patients, acute rejection is the leading cause of renal dysfunction. Given the limited number of donors, routine clinical posttransplantation evaluation is of immense importance to help clinicians initiate timely interventions with appropriate treatment and thus prevent graft loss. In recent years, an increased area of research has been dedicated to developing noninvasive CAD systems for renal transplant function assessment, utilizing different image modalities (e.g., ultrasound, CT, and magnetic resonance imaging [MRI]). Accurate assessment of renal transplant function is critically important for graft survival. Although transplantation can improve a patient's well-being, there is a potential posttransplantation risk of kidney dysfunction that, if not treated in a timely manner, can lead to the loss of the entire graft and even patient death. Thus, accurate assessment of renal transplant function is crucial for the identification of proper treatment. In recent years, an increased area of research has been dedicated to developing noninvasive image-based CAD systems for the assessment of renal transplant function. In particular, dynamic and diffusion MRI-based systems have been clinically used to assess transplanted kidneys with the advantage of providing information on each kidney separately. For more details about renal transplant functional assessment, see references [25–50].

The heart also has an important application to this work. The clinical assessment of myocardial perfusion plays a major role in the diagnosis, management, and prognosis of ischemic heart disease patients. Thus, there have been ongoing efforts to develop automated systems for accurate analysis of myocardial perfusion using first-pass images [51–67].

Another application for this work could be the detection of retinal abnormalities. Most ophthalmologists depend on visual interpretation for the identification of diseases types. However, inaccurate diagnosis will affect the treatment procedure, which may lead to fatal results. Hence, there is a crucial need for CAD systems that yield highly accurate results. Optical coherence tomography has become a powerful modality for the noninvasive diagnosis of various retinal abnormalities, such as glaucoma, diabetic macular edema, and macular degeneration. The problem with diabetic retinopathy is that the patient is not aware of the disease until the changes in the retina have progressed to a level that treatment tends to be less effective. Therefore, automated early detection could limit the severity of the disease and assist ophthalmologists in investigating and treating it more efficiently [68, 69].

Abnormalities of the lung could also be another promising area of research and a related application to this work. RILI is the main side effect of RT for lung cancer patients. Although higher radiation doses increase the effectiveness of RT for tumor control, this can lead to lung injury, as a greater quantity of normal lung tissues is included in the treated area. Almost one-third of patients who undergo RT develop lung injury following radiation treatment. The severity of RILI ranges from ground-glass opacities and consolidation at the early phase to fibrosis and traction bronchiectasis in the late phase. Early detection of lung injury will thus help to improve management of the treatment [9–11, 14, 16, 70–108].

This work can also be applied to other brain abnormalities, such as dyslexia and autism. Dyslexia is one of the most complicated developmental brain disorders that affect children's learning abilities. Dyslexia leads to the failure to develop age-appropriate reading skills in spite of normal intelligence level and adequate reading instructions. Neuropathological studies have revealed an abnormal anatomy of some structures, such as the corpus callosum, in dyslexic brains. There has been a lot of work in the literature that aims at developing CAD systems for diagnosing such a disorder, along with other brain disorders [109–131].

This work could also be applied for the extraction of blood vessels from phase contrast magnetic resonance angiography (MRA). Accurate cerebrovascular segmentation using noninvasive MRA is crucial for the early diagnosis and timely treatment of intracranial vascular diseases [114, 115, 132, 133].

References

1. Larici AR, del Ciello A, Maggi F, et al. Lung abnormalities at multimodality imaging after radiation therapy for non–small cell lung cancer. *Radiographics*. 2011;31(3):771–789.
2. Giridhar P, Mallick S, Rath GK, Julka PK. Radiation induced lung injury: prediction, assessment and management. *Asian Pac J Cancer Prev*. 2015;16(7):2613–2617.
3. Latifi K, Dilling T, Hoffe S, Stevens C, Moros E, Zhang G. SU-E-J-187: evaluation of the effects of dose on 4D CT-calculated lung ventilation. *Med Phys*. 2012;39(6):3695–3696.
4. Reinhardt JM, Ding K, Cao K, Christensen GE, Hoffman EA, Bodas SV. Registration-based estimates of local lung tissue expansion compared to xenon CT measures of specific ventilation. *Med Image Anal*. 2008;12(6):752–763.
5. Cunliffe AR, Armato SG III, Straus C, Malik R, Al-Hallaq HA. Lung texture in serial thoracic CT scans: correlation with radiologist-defined severity of acute changes following radiation therapy. *Phys Med Biol*. 2014;59(18):5387.
6. Vinogradskiy Y, Schubert L, Brennan D, et al. Clinical validation of 4DCT-ventilation with pulmonary function test data. *Int J Radiat Oncol Biol Phys*. 2014;90(1):S61–S62.
7. Sharifi H, Van Elmpt W, Oberije C, et al. Quantification of CT-assessed radiation-induced lung damage in lung cancer patients treated with or without chemotherapy and cetuximab. *Acta Oncol*. 2016;55(2):156–162.
8. Hu X-Y, Fang X-M, Chen H-W, et al. Early detection of acute radiation-induced lung injury with multi-section CT perfusion imaging: an initial experience. *Clin Radiol*. 2014;69(8):853–860.

9. Soliman A, Khalifa F, Shaffie A, et al. Image-based CAD system for accurate identification of lung injury. In: *IEEE International Conference on Image Processing (ICIP)*. 2016:121–125.

10. Soliman A, Khalifa A, Shaffie A, et al. Detection of lung injury using 4D-CT chest images. In: *IEEE 13th International Symposium on Biomedical Imaging (ISBI)*. 2016:1274–1277.

11. El-Baz A, Beache GM, Gimel'farb G, et al. Computer-aided diagnosis systems for lung cancer: challenges and methodologies. *Int J Biomed Imaging*. 2013;2013:1–46.

12. Soliman A, Elnakib A, Khalifa F, El-Ghar MA, El-Baz A. Segmentation of pathological lungs from CT chest images. In: *2015 IEEE International Conference on Image Processing (ICIP)*. 2015:3655–3659.

13. Soliman A, Khalifa F, Alansary A, Gimel'farb G, El-Baz A. Segmentation of lung region based on using parallel implementation of joint MGRF: validation on 3D realistic lung phantoms. In: *2013 IEEE 10th International Symposium on Biomedical Imaging (ISBI)*. 2013:864–867.

14. Abdollahi B, Soliman A, Civelek A, Li X-F, Gimel'farb G, El-Baz A. A novel 3D joint MGRF framework for precise lung segmentation. In: *International Workshop on Machine Learning in Medical Imaging*. 2012:86–93.

15. Soliman A, Khalifa F, Elnakib A, et al. Accurate lung segmentation on CT chest images by adaptive appearance-guided shape modeling. *IEEE Trans Med Imaging*. 2016:36(1):263–276.

16. Soliman A, Khalifa F, Dunlap N, Wang B, El-Ghar MA, El-Baz A. An iso-surfaces based local deformation handling framework of lung tissues. In: *IEEE 13th International Symposium on Biomedical Imaging (ISBI)*. 2016:1253–1259.

17. Liu N, Gimel'farb G, Delmas P. High-order MGRF models for contrast/offset invariant texture retrieval. In: *Proceedings of International Conference on Image Vision Computing New Zealand*. 2014:96–101.

18. Liu N, Soliman A, Gimel'farb G, El-Baz A. Segmenting kidney DCE-MRI using 1st-order shape and 5th-order appearance priors. In: *International Conference on Medical Image Computing and Computer-Assisted Intervention*. 2015:77–84.

19. Gimel'farb G, Farag A. Texture analysis by accurate identification of simple Markovian models. *Cybernet Syst Anal*. 2005;41(1):27–38.

20. El-Baz A, Gimel'farb G, Suri S. *Stochastic Modeling for Medical Image Analysis*. Boca Raton, FL: CRC Press; 2015.

21. Kamnitsas K, Ledig C, Newcombe VF, et al. Efficient multi-scale 3D CNN with fully connected CRF for accurate brain lesion segmentation. arXiv preprint. arXiv:1603.05959, 2016.

22. Zou KH, Warfield SK, Bharatha A, et al. Statistical validation of image segmentation quality based on a spatial overlap index. *Acad Radiol*. 2004;11(2):178–189.

23. Gerig G, Jomier M, Chakos M. Valmet: a new validation tool for assessing and improving 3D object segmentation. In: *International Conference on Medical Image Computing and Computer-Assisted Intervention*. 2001:516–523.

24. Soliman A, Khalifa F, Alansary A, et al. Performance evaluation of an automatic MGRF-based lung segmentation approach. *AIP Conf Proc*. 2013;1559(1):323–332.

25. Ali AM, Farag AA, El-Baz A. Graph cuts framework for kidney segmentation with prior shape constraints. In: *Proceedings of International Conference on Medical Image Computing and Computer-Assisted Intervention (MICCAI'07)*. 2007:384–392.

26. Chowdhury AS, Roy R, Bose S, Elnakib FKA, El-Baz A. Non-rigid biomedical image registration using graph cuts with a novel data term. In: *Proceedings of IEEE International Symposium on Biomedical Imaging: From Nano to Macro (ISBI'12)*. 2012:446–449.

27. El-Baz A, Farag AA, Yuksel SE, El-Ghar MEA, Eldiasty TA, Ghoneim MA. Application of deformable models for the detection of acute renal rejection. In: Farag AA, Suri JS, eds. *Deformable Models*. Vol. 1. New York, NY: Springer; 2007:293–333.

28. El-Baz A, Farag A, Fahmi R, Yuksel S, El-Ghar MA, Eldiasty T. Image analysis of renal DCE MRI for the detection of acute renal rejection. In: *Proceedings of IAPR International Conference on Pattern Recognition (ICPR'06).*2006:822–825.

29. El-Baz A, Farag A, Fahmi R, et al. A new CAD system for the evaluation of kidney diseases using DCE-MRI. In: *Proceedings of International Conference on Medical Image Computing and Computer-Assisted Intervention (MICCAI'08).* 2006:446–453.

30. El-Baz A, Gimel'farb G, El-Ghar MA. A novel image analysis approach for accurate identification of acute renal rejection. In: *Proceedings of IEEE International Conference on Image Processing (ICIP'08).* 2008:1812–1815.

31. El-Baz A, Gimel'farb G, El-Ghar MA. Image analysis approach for identification of renal transplant rejection. In: *Proceedings of IAPR International Conference on Pattern Recognition (ICPR'08).* 2008:1–4.

32. El-Baz A, Gimel'farb G, El-Ghar MA. New motion correction models for automatic identification of renal transplant rejection. In: *Proceedings of International Conference on Medical Image Computing and Computer-Assisted Intervention (MICCAI'07).* 2007:235–243.

33. Farag A, El-Baz A, Yuksel S, El-Ghar MA, Eldiasty T. A framework for the detection of acute rejection with dynamic contrast enhanced magnetic resonance imaging. In: *Proceedings of IEEE International Symposium on Biomedical Imaging: From Nano to Macro (ISBI'06).* 2006:418–421.

34. Khalifa F, Beache GM, El-Ghar MA, et al. Dynamic contrast-enhanced MRI-based early detection of acute renal transplant rejection. *IEEE Trans Med Imaging.* 2013;32(10):1910–1927.

35. Khalifa F, El-Baz A, Gimel'farb G, El-Ghar MA. Non-invasive image-based approach for early detection of acute renal rejection. In: *Proceedings of International Conference Medical Image Computing and Computer-Assisted Intervention (MICCAI'10).* 2010:10–18.

36. Khalifa F, El-Baz A, Gimel'farb G, Ouseph R, El-Ghar MA. Shape-appearance guided level-set deformable model for image segmentation. In: *Proceedings of IAPR International Conference on Pattern Recognition (ICPR'10).* 2010:4581–4584.

37. Khalifa F, El-Ghar MA, Abdollahi B, Frieboes H, El-Diasty T, El-Baz A. A comprehensive non-invasive framework for automated evaluation of acute renal transplant rejection using DCE-MRI. *NMR Biomed.* 2013;26(11):1460–1470.

38. Khalifa F, El-Ghar MA, Abdollahi B, Frieboes HB, El-Diasty T, El-Baz A. Dynamic contrast-enhanced MRI-based early detection of acute renal transplant rejection. In: *2014 Annual Scientific Meeting and Educational Course Brochure of the Society of Abdominal Radiology (SAR'14).* 2014:1855912.

39. Khalifa F, Elnakib A, Beache GM, et al. 3D kidney segmentation from CT images using a level set approach guided by a novel stochastic speed function. In: *Proceedings of International Conference Medical Image Computing and Computer-Assisted Intervention (MICCAI'11).* 2011:587–594.

40. Khalifa F, Gimel'farb G, El-Ghar MA, et al. A new deformable model-based segmentation approach for accurate extraction of the kidney from abdominal CT images. In: *Proceedings of IEEE International Conference on Image Processing (ICIP'11).* 2011:3393–3396.

41. Mostapha M, Khalifa F, Alansary A, Soliman A, Suri J, El-Baz A. Computer-aided diagnosis systems for acute renal transplant rejection: challenges and methodologies. In: El-Baz A, Saba L, Suri J, eds. *Abdomen and Thoracic Imaging*. New York, NY: Springer; 2014:1–35.
42. Shehata M, Khalifa F, Hollis E, et al. A new non-invasive approach for early classification of renal rejection types using diffusion-weighted MRI. In: *IEEE International Conference on Image Processing (ICIP)*. 2016:136–140.
43. Khalifa F, Soliman A, Takieldeen A, et al. Kidney segmentation from CT images using a 3D NMF-guided active contour model. In: *IEEE 13th International Symposium on Biomedical Imaging (ISBI)*. 2016:432–435.
44. Shehata M, Khalifa F, Soliman A, et al. 3D diffusion MRI-based CAD system for early diagnosis of acute renal rejection. In: *IEEE 13th International Symposium on Biomedical Imaging (ISBI)*. 2016:1177–1180.
45. Shehata M, Khalifa F, Soliman A, et al. A level set-based framework for 3D kidney segmentation from diffusion MR images. In: *IEEE International Conference on Image Processing (ICIP)*. 2015:4441–4445.
46. Shehata M, Khalifa F, Soliman A, et al. A promising non-invasive CAD system for kidney function assessment. In: *International Conference on Medical Image Computing and Computer-Assisted Intervention*. 2016:613–621.
47. Khalifa F, Soliman A, Elmaghraby A, Gimel'farb G, El-Baz A. 3D kidney segmentation from abdominal images using spatial-appearance models. *Comput Math Models Med*. 2017;2017:1–10.
48. Hollis E, Shehata M, Khalifa F, El-Ghar MA, El-Diasty T, El-Baz A. Towards non-invasive diagnostic techniques for early detection of acute renal transplant rejection: a review. *Egypt J Radiol Nucl Med*. 2016;48(1):257–269.
49. Shehata M, Khalifa F, Soliman A, El-Ghar MA, Dwyer AC, El-Baz A. Assessment of renal transplant using image and clinical-based biomarkers. In: *Proceedings of 13th Annual Scientific Meeting of American Society for Diagnostics and Interventional Nephrology (ASDIN'17)*. 2017.
50. Shehata M, Khalifa F, Soliman A, El-Ghar MA, Dwyer AC, El-Baz A. Early assessment of acute renal rejection. In: *Proceedings of 12th Annual Scientific Meeting of American Society for Diagnostics and Interventional Nephrology (ASDIN'16)*. 2017.
51. Khalifa F, Beache G, El-Baz A, Gimel'farb G. Deformable model guided by stochastic speed with application in cine images segmentation. In: *Proceedings of IEEE International Conference on Image Processing (ICIP'10)*.2010:1725–1728.
52. Khalifa F, Beache GM, Elnakib A, et al. A new shape-based framework for the left ventricle wall segmentation from cardiac first-pass perfusion MRI. In: *Proceedings of IEEE International Symposium on Biomedical Imaging: From Nano to Macro (ISBI'13)*. 2013:41–44.
53. Khalifa F, Beache GM, Elnakib A, et al. A new nonrigid registration framework for improved visualization of transmural perfusion gradients on cardiac first–pass perfusion MRI. In: *Proceedings of IEEE International Symposium on Biomedical Imaging: From Nano to Macro (ISBI'12)*. 2012:828–831.
54. Khalifa F, Beache GM, Firjani A, Welch KC, Gimel'farb G, El-Baz A. A new non-rigid registration approach for motion correction of cardiac first-pass perfusion MRI. In: *Proceedings of IEEE International Conference on Image Processing (ICIP'12)*. 2012:1665–1668.
55. Khalifa F, Beache GM, Gimel'farb G, El-Baz A. A novel CAD system for analyzing cardiac first-pass MR images. In: *Proceedings of IAPR International Conference on Pattern Recognition (ICPR'12)*. 2012:77–80.

56. Khalifa F, Beache GM, Gimel'farb G, El-Baz A. A novel approach for accurate estimation of left ventricle global indexes from short-axis cine MRI. In: *Proceedings of IEEE International Conference on Image Processing, (ICIP'11)*. 2011:2645–2649.

57. Khalifa F, Beache GM, Gimel'farb G, Giridharan GA, El-Baz A. A new image-based framework for analyzing cine images. In: El-Baz A, Acharya UR, Mirmedhdi M, Suri JS, eds. *Handbook of Multi Modality State-of-the-Art Medical Image Segmentation and Registration Methodologies*. New York, NY: Springer; 2011:69–98.

58. Khalifa F, Beache GM, Gimel'farb G, Giridharan GA, El-Baz A. Accurate automatic analysis of cardiac cine images. *IEEE Trans Biomed Eng*. 2012;59(2):445–455.

59. Khalifa F, Beache GM, Nitzken M, Gimel'farb G, Giridharan GA, El-Baz A. Automatic analysis of left ventricle wall thickness using short-axis cine CMR images. In: *Proceedings of IEEE International Symposium on Biomedical Imaging: From Nano to Macro (ISBI'11)*. 2011:1306–1309.

60. Nitzken M, Beache G, Elnakib A, Khalifa F, Gimel'farb G, El-Baz A. Accurate modeling of tagged CMR 3D image appearance characteristics to improve cardiac cycle strain estimation. In: *19th IEEE International Conference on Image Processing (ICIP)*. 2012:521–524.

61. Nitzken M, Beache G, Elnakib A, Khalifa F, Gimel'farb G, El-Baz A. Improving full-cardiac cycle strain estimation from tagged CMR by accurate modeling of 3D image appearance characteristics. In: *9th IEEE International Symposium on Biomedical Imaging (ISBI)*. 2012:462–465.

62. Nitzken MJ, El-Baz AS, Beache GM. Markov-Gibbs random field model for improved full-cardiac cycle strain estimation from tagged CMR. *J Cardiovasc Magn Reson*. 2012;14(1):1–2.

63. Sliman H, Elnakib A, Beache G, Elmaghraby A, El-Baz A. Assessment of myocardial function from cine cardiac MRI using a novel 4D tracking approach. *J Comput Sci Syst Biol*. 2014;7:169–173.

64. Sliman H, Elnakib A, Beache GM, et al. A novel 4D PDE-based approach for accurate assessment of myocardium function using cine cardiac magnetic resonance images. In: *Proceedings of IEEE International Conference on Image Processing (ICIP'14)*. 2014:3537–3541.

65. Sliman H, Khalifa F, Elnakib A, Beache GM, Elmaghraby A, El-Baz A. A new segmentation-based tracking framework for extracting the left ventricle cavity from cine cardiac MRI. In: *Proceedings of IEEE International Conference on Image Processing, (ICIP'13)*. 2013:685–689.

66. Sliman H, Khalifa F, Elnakib A, et al. Myocardial borders segmentation from cine MR images using bi-directional coupled parametric deformable models. *Med Phys*. 2013;40(9):1–13.

67. Sliman H, Khalifa F, Elnakib A, et al. Accurate segmentation framework for the left ventricle wall from cardiac cine MRI. In: *Proceedings of International Symposium on Computational Models for Life Science (CMLS'13)*. 2013:287–296.

68. Eladawi N, Elmogy MM, Ghazal M, et al. Classification of retinal diseases based on OCT images. *Front Biosci (Landmark Ed)*. 2017;23:247–264.

69. ElTanboly A, Ismail M, Shalaby A, et al. A computer-aided diagnostic system for detecting diabetic retinopathy in optical coherence tomography images. *Med Phys*. 2016;44(3):914–923.

70. Abdollahi B, Civelek AC, Li X-F, Suri J, El-Baz A. PET/CT nodule segmentation and diagnosis: a survey. In: Saba L, Suri JS, eds. *Multi Detector CT Imaging*. New York, NY: Taylor & Francis; 2014:639–651.

71. Abdollahi B, El-Baz A, Amini AA. A multi-scale non-linear vessel enhancement technique. In: *Engineering in Medicine and Biology Society, EMBC, 2011 Annual International Conference of the IEEE.* 2011:3925–3929.

72. Abdollahi B, Soliman A, Civelek A, Li X-F, Gimel'farb G, El-Baz A. A novel 3D joint MGRF framework for precise lung segmentation. In: *International Workshop on Machine Learning in Medical Imaging.* 2012:86–93.

73. Ali AM, El-Baz AS, Farag AA. A novel framework for accurate lung segmentation using graph cuts. In: *Proceedings of IEEE International Symposium on Biomedical Imaging: From Nano to Macro (ISBI'07).* 2007:908–911.

74. El-Baz A, Beache GM, Gimel'farb G, Suzuki K, Okada K. Lung imaging data analysis. *Int J Biomed Imaging.* 2013;2013:1–2.

75. El-Baz A, Elnakib A, Abou El-Ghar M, Gimel'farb G, Falk R, Farag A. Automatic detection of 2D and 3D lung nodules in chest spiral CT scans. *Int J Biomed Imaging.* 2013; 2013:1–11.

76. El-Baz A, Farag AA, Falk R, La Rocca R. A unified approach for detection, visualization, and identification of lung abnormalities in chest spiral CT scans. In: *International Congress Series.* Vol. 1256. New York, NY: Elsevier; 2003:998–1004.

77. El-Baz A, Farag AA, Falk R, La Rocca R. Detection, visualization and identification of lung abnormalities in chest spiral CT scan: phase-I. *Proc Int Conf Biomed Eng (Cairo, Egypt).* 2002;12(1).

78. El-Baz A, Farag A, Gimel'farb G, Falk R, El-Ghar MA, Eldiasty T. A framework for automatic segmentation of lung nodules from low dose chest CT scans. In: *Proceedings of International Conference on Pattern Recognition (ICPR'06).* 2006:611–614.

79. El-Baz A, Farag A, Gimel'farb G, Falk R, El-Ghar MA. A novel level set-based computer-aided detection system for automatic detection of lung nodules in low dose chest computed tomography scans. *Lung Imaging Comput Aided Diagn.* 2011;10:221–238.

80. El-Baz A, Gimel'farb G, Abou El-Ghar M, Falk R. Appearance-based diagnostic system for early assessment of malignant lung nodules. In: *Proceedings of IEEE International Conference on Image Processing, (ICIP'12).* 2012:533–536.

81. El-Baz A, Gimel'farb G, Falk R. A novel 3D framework for automatic lung segmentation from low dose CT images. In: El-Baz A, Suri JS, eds. *Lung Imaging and Computer Aided Diagnosis.* New York, NY: Taylor & Francis; 2011:1–16.

82. El-Baz A, Gimel'farb G, Falk R, El-Ghar M. Appearance analysis for diagnosing malignant lung nodules. In: *Proceedings of IEEE International Symposium on Biomedical Imaging: From Nano to Macro (ISBI'10).* 2010:193–196.

83. El-Baz A, Gimel'farb G, Falk R, El-Ghar MA. A novel level set-based CAD system for automatic detection of lung nodules in low dose chest CT scans. In: El-Baz A, Suri JS, eds. *Lung Imaging and Computer Aided Diagnosis.* New York, NY: Taylor & Francis; 2011:221–238.

84. El-Baz A, Gimel'farb G, Falk R, El-Ghar MA. A new approach for automatic analysis of 3D low dose CT images for accurate monitoring the detected lung nodules. In: *Proceedings of International Conference on Pattern Recognition (ICPR'08).* 2008:1–4.

85. El-Baz A, Gimel'farb G, Falk R, El-Ghar MA. A novel approach for automatic follow-up of detected lung nodules. In: *Proceedings of IEEE International Conference on Image Processing (ICIP'07).* 2007:v–501.

86. El-Baz A, Gimel'farb G, Falk R, El-Ghar MA. A new CAD system for early diagnosis of detected lung nodules. In: *Image Processing, 2007. ICIP 2007. IEEE International Conference on.* Vol. 2. IEEE. 2007:II–461.

87. El-Baz A, Gimel'farb G, Falk R, El-Ghar MA, Refaie H. Promising results for early diagnosis of lung cancer. In: *Proceedings of IEEE International Symposium on Biomedical Imaging: From Nano to Macro (ISBI'08)*. 2008:1151–1154.

88. El-Baz A, Gimel'farb GL, Falk R, Abou El-Ghar M, Holland T, Shaffer T. A new stochastic framework for accurate lung segmentation. In: *Proceedings of Medical Image Computing and Computer-Assisted Intervention (MICCAI'08)*. 2008:322–330.

89. El-Baz A, Gimel'farb GL, Falk R, Heredis D, Abou El-Ghar M. A novel approach for accurate estimation of the growth rate of the detected lung nodules. In: *Proceedings of International Workshop on Pulmonary Image Analysis*. 2008:33–42.

90. El-Baz A, Gimel'farb GL, Falk R, Holland T, Shaffer T. A framework for unsupervised segmentation of lung tissues from low dose computed tomography images. In: *Proceedings of British Machine Vision (BMVC'08)*. 2008:1–10.

91. El-Baz A, Gimel'farb G, Falk R, El-Ghar MA. 3D MGRF-based appearance modeling for robust segmentation of pulmonary nodules in 3D LDCT chest images. In: El-Baz A, Suri JS, eds. *Lung Imaging and Computer Aided Diagnosis*. New York, NY: Taylor & Francis; 2011:51–63.

92. El-Baz A, Gimel'farb G, Falk R, El-Ghar MA. Automatic analysis of 3D low dose CT images for early diagnosis of lung cancer. *Pattern Recognit*. 2009;42(6):1041–1051.

93. El-Baz A, Gimel'farb G, Falk R, et al. Toward early diagnosis of lung cancer. In: *Proceedings of Medical Image Computing and Computer-Assisted Intervention (MICCAI'09)*. 2009:682–689.

94. El-Baz A, Gimel'farb G, Falk R, El-Ghar MA, Suri J. Appearance analysis for the early assessment of detected lung nodules. In: El-Baz A, Suri JS, eds. *Lung Imaging and Computer Aided Diagnosis*. New York, NY: Taylor & Francis; 2011:395–404.

95. El-Baz A, Khalifa F, Elnakib A, et al. A novel approach for global lung registration using 3D Markov Gibbs appearance model. In: *Proceedings of International Conference Medical Image Computing and Computer-Assisted Intervention (MICCAI'12)*. 2012:114–121.

96. El-Baz A, Nitzken M, Elnakib A, et al. 3D shape analysis for early diagnosis of malignant lung nodules. In: *Proceedings of International Conference Medical Image Computing and Computer-Assisted Intervention (MICCAI'11)*. 2011:175–182.

97. El-Baz A, Nitzken M, Gimel'farb G, et al. Three-dimensional shape analysis using spherical harmonics for early assessment of detected lung nodules. El-Baz A, Suri JS, eds. *Lung Imaging and Computer Aided Diagnosis*. New York, NY: Taylor & Francis; 2011:421–438.

98. El-Baz A, Nitzken M, Khalifa F, et al. 3D shape analysis for early diagnosis of malignant lung nodules. In: *Proceedings of International Conference on Information Processing in Medical Imaging (IPMI'11)*. 2011:772–783.

99. El-Baz A, Nitzken M, Vanbogaert E, Gimel'farb G, Falk R, Abo El-Ghar M. A novel shape-based diagnostic approach for early diagnosis of lung nodules. In: *IEEE International Symposium on Biomedical Imaging: From Nano to Macro*. 2011:137–140.

100. El-Baz A, Sethu P, Gimel'farb G, et al. Elastic phantoms generated by microfluidics technology: validation of an image-based approach for accurate measurement of the growth rate of lung nodules. *Biotechnol J*. 2011;6(2):195–203.

101. El-Baz A, Sethu P, Gimel'farb G, et al. A new validation approach for the growth rate measurement using elastic phantoms generated by state-of-the-art microfluidics technology. In: *Proceedings of IEEE International Conference on Image Processing (ICIP'10)*. 2010:4381–4383.

102. El-Baz A, Sethu P, Gimel'farb G, et al. Validation of a new imaged-based approach for the accurate estimating of the growth rate of detected lung nodules using real CT images and elastic phantoms generated by state-of-the-art microfluidics technology. In: El-Baz A, Suri JS, eds. *Lung Imaging and Computer Aided Diagnosis*. New York, NY: Taylor & Francis; 2011:405–420.

103. El-Baz A, Soliman A, McClure P, Gimel'farb G, El-Ghar MA, Falk R. Early assessment of malignant lung nodules based on the spatial analysis of detected lung nodules. In: *Proceedings of IEEE International Symposium on Biomedical Imaging: From Nano to Macro (ISBI'12)*. 2012:1463–1466.

104. El-Baz A, Yuksel SE, Elshazly S, Farag AA. Non-rigid registration techniques for automatic follow-up of lung nodules. In: *Proceedings of Computer Assisted Radiology and Surgery (CARS'05)*. 2005:1115–1120.

105. El-Baz AS, Suri JS. *Lung Imaging and Computer Aided Diagnosis*. Boca Raton, FL: CRC Press; 2011.

106. Soliman A, Khalifa F, Shaffie A, et al. Image-based CAD system for accurate identification of lung injury. In: *Proceedings of IEEE International Conference on Image Processing (ICIP'16)*. 2016:121–125.

107. Soliman A, Khalifa F, Shaffie A, et al. A comprehensive framework for early assessment of lung injury. In: *IEEE International Conference on Image Processing (ICIP)*. 2017:3275–3279.

108. Shaffie A, Soliman A, Ghazal M, et al. A new framework for incorporating appearance and shape features of lung nodules for precise diagnosis of lung cancer. In: *IEEE International Conference on Image Processing (ICIP)*. 2017:1372–1376.

109. Dombroski B, Nitzken M, Elnakib A, Khalifa F, El-Baz A, Casanova MF. Cortical surface complexity in a population-based normative sample. *Transl Neurosci*. 2014;5(1):17–24.

110. El-Baz A, Casanova M, Gimel'farb G, Mott M, Switwala A. An MRI-based diagnostic framework for early diagnosis of dyslexia. *Int J Comput Assist Radiol Surg*. 2008;3(3–4):181–189.

111. El-Baz A, Casanova M, Gimel'farb G, et al. A new CAD system for early diagnosis of dyslexic brains. In: *Proceedings of International Conference on Image Processing (ICIP'2008)*. 2008:1820–1823.

112. El-Baz A, Casanova MF, Gimel'farb G, Mott M, Switwala AE. A new image analysis approach for automatic classification of autistic brains. In: *Proceedings of IEEE International Symposium on Biomedical Imaging: From Nano to Macro (ISBI'2007)*. 2007:352–355.

113. El-Baz A, Elnakib A, Khalifa F, et al. Precise segmentation of 3-D magnetic resonance angiography. *IEEE Trans Biomed Eng*. 2012;59(7):2019–2029.

114. El-Baz A, Farag AA, Gimel'farb GL, El-Ghar MA, Eldiasty T. Probabilistic modeling of blood vessels for segmenting MRA images. In: *Proceedings of IAPR International Conference on Pattern Recognition (ICPR)*. 2006:917–920.

115. El-Baz A, Farag AA, Gimel'farb G, El-Ghar MA, Eldiasty T. A new adaptive probabilistic model of blood vessels for segmenting MRA images. In: *Medical Image Computing and Computer-Assisted Intervention—MICCAI 2006*. Vol. 4191. New York, NY: Springer; 2006:799–806.

116. El-Baz A, Farag AA, Gimel'farb G, Hushek SG. Automatic cerebrovascular segmentation by accurate probabilistic modeling of TOF-MRA images. In: *Medical Image Computing and Computer-Assisted Intervention—MICCAI 2005*. New York, NY: Springer; 2005:34–42.

117. El-Baz A, Farag A, Elnakib A, et al. Accurate automated detection of autism related corpus callosum abnormalities. *J Med Syst*. 2011;35(5):929–939.

118. El-Baz A, Farag A, Gimel'farb G. Cerebrovascular segmentation by accurate proba-bilistic modeling of TOF-MRA images. In: *Image Analysis*. Vol. 3540. New York, NY: Springer; 2005:1128–1137.

119. El-Baz A, Gimel'farb G, Falk R, El-Ghar MA, Kumar V, Heredia D. A novel 3D joint Markov-Gibbs model for extracting blood vessels from PC–MRA images. In: *Medical Image Computing and Computer-Assisted Intervention—MICCAI 2009*. Vol. 5762. New York, NY: Springer; 2009:943–950.

120. Elnakib A, El-Baz A, Casanova MF, Gimel'farb G, Switwala AE. Image-based detec-tion of corpus callosum variability for more accurate discrimination between dyslexic and normal brains. In: *Proceedings of IEEE International Symposium on Biomedical Imaging: From Nano to Macro (ISBI'2010)*. 2010:109–112.

121. Elnakib A, Casanova MF, Gimel'farb G, Switwala AE, El-Baz A. Autism diagnos-tics by centerline-based shape analysis of the corpus callosum. In: *Proceedings IEEE International Symposium on Biomedical Imaging: From Nano to Macro (ISBI'2011)*. 2011:1843–1846.

122. Elnakib A, Nitzken M, Casanova M, Park H, Gimel'farb G, El-Baz A. Quantification of age-related brain cortex change using 3D shape analysis. In: *21st International Conference on Pattern Recognition (ICPR)*. 2012:41–44.

123. Mostapha M, Soliman A, Khalifa F, et al. A statistical framework for the classifica-tion of infant DT images. In: *IEEE International Conference on Image Processing (ICIP)*. 2014:2222–2226.

124. Nitzken M, Casanova M, Gimel'farb G, et al. 3D shape analysis of the brain cortex with application to dyslexia. In: *18th IEEE International Conference on Image Processing (ICIP)*. 2011:2657–2660.

125. El-Gamal FE, Elmogy M, Ghazal M, et al. A novel CAD system for local and global early diagnosis of Alzheimer's disease based on PIB-PET scans. In: *IEEE International Conference on Image Processing (ICIP)*. 2017:3270–3274.

126. Ismail M, Soliman A, Ghazal M, et al. A fast stochastic framework for automatic MR brain images segmentation. *PLoS one*. 12(11): p.e0187391.

127. Ismail MM, Keynton RS, Mostapha MM, et al. Studying autism spectrum disorder with structural and diffusion magnetic resonance imaging: a survey. *Front Hum Neurosci*. 2016;10:211.

128. Alansary A, Ismail M, Soliman A, et al. Infant brain extraction in t1-weighted MR images using BET and refinement using LCDG and MGRF models. *IEEE J Biomed Health Inform*. 2016;20(3):925–935.

129. Ismail M, Barnes G, Nitzken M, et al. 2017, September. A new deep-learning approach for early detection of shape variations in autism using structural MRI. In *2017 IEEE International Conference on Image Processing (ICIP)* (pp. 1057–1061).

130. Ismail M, Soliman A, ElTanboly A, et al. Detection of white matter abnormalities in MR brain images for diagnosis of autism in children. In *2016 IEEE 13th International Symposium on Biomedical Imaging (ISBI)*. 2016:6–9.

131. Ismail M, Mostapha M, Soliman A, et al. Segmentation of infant brain MR images based on adaptive shape prior and higher-order MGRF. In *2015 IEEE International Conference on Image Processing (ICIP)*. 2015:4327–4331.

132. El-Baz A, Shalaby A, Taher F, et al. Probabilistic modeling of blood vessels for segmenting magnetic resonance angiography images. In: *Medical Research Archive—MRA*. KEI; 2017:5(3):34–42, ISSN 2375-1924. Available at: https://www.journals.ke-i.org/index.php/mra/article/view/1031. Date accessed: February 19, 2019.

133. Chowdhury AS, Rudra AK, Sen M, Elnakib A, El-Baz A. Cerebral white matter segmentation from MRI using probabilistic graph cuts and geometric shape priors. In: *IEEE International Conference on Image Processing (ICIP'10)*. 2010:3649–3652.

Index

Note: *Italicized* page numbers refer to figures, **bold** page numbers refer to tables

A